THE GENETICS OF OBESITY

Edited By

Claude Bouchard, Ph.D.

Physical Activity Sciences Laboratory
Laval University
Ste-Foy, Québec, Canada

CRC Press
Boca Raton Ann Arbor London Tokyo

Library of Congress Cataloging-in-Publication Data

The Genetics of obesity / edited by Claude Bouchard.
p. cm.
Includes bibliographical references and index.
ISBN 0-8493-4880-3
1. Obesity—Genetic aspects. I. Bouchard, Claude.
RC628.G46 1994
616.3'98042—dc20 93-21032
CIP

Direct all inquiries to CRC Press, Inc., 2000 Corporate Blvd., N.W., Boca Raton, Florida 33431.

International Standard Book Number 0-8493-4880-3
Library of Congress Card Number 93-21032
Printed in the United States of America 2 3 4 5 6 7 8 9 0
Printed on acid-free paper

PREFACE

This book was developed over a period of about two years with two main objectives in mind: to compile the evidence currently available about the role of genetic differences in the etiology of human obesities and of their metabolic implications; and to identify the most promising research areas, research methods, and strategies that are likely to be of help in the efforts to understand the genetic basis of obesities and of their consequences on human health. It was felt by all those who were consulted over the need for such a volume that it was indeed a timely publication.

To meet these objectives, a team of authors was assembled which included almost all those who have made a significant contribution to our present understanding of the role of biological inheritance in human body mass and body fat content variation. The book includes 16 chapters to which 31 authors and co-authors have contributed. Although several chapters include sections on regional fat distribution, the emphasis is on excess body mass for height and body fat content. Of course, this is a reflection of the small body of knowledge concerning the genetics of fat topography.

The book begins with an introductory chapter (Bouchard), a chapter on the etiology and prevalence of obesities (Bray), and text on the nongenetic determinants of obesity and fat topography (Hill et al.). They are followed by eight chapters that are primarily based on human research and clinical observations addressing the following aspects of the currently available genetic evidence: adoption studies (Sørensen and Stunkard), twin studies (Meyer and Stunkard), family studies (Bouchard and Pérusse), single gene effects (Price), temporal trends and etiologic heterogeneity (Borecki et al.), energy intake and food preference (Pérusse and Bouchard), energy expenditure (Bouchard et al.), and susceptibility to metabolic derangements in the obese state (Williams and collaborators). Four chapters provide an overview of the contributions that have been made or that can be anticipated from animal models and molecular biology technology in the effort to delineate the genetic basis of human obesities. These chapters cover the following areas: animal models of obesity (Gregoire and Johnson), animal models of polygenic obesity and the quantitative trait loci approach (Warden and Fisler), molecular biology of the adipose cell (Ailhaud et al.), and molecular biology in the search of genes involved in animal models of obesity (Chua and Leibel). The last chapter addresses the topic of current status and of future directions of research in the field (Bouchard).

The editor of this collective publication would like to thank Ms. Diane Drolet for her help in putting the material together in a coherent manner and for her assistance in the preparation of several chapters. Thanks are also expressed to CRC Press, Inc. for having expressed to me their interest in the concept of a book on the genetics of obesity, and for their support in its production.

Claude Bouchard

THE EDITOR

Claude Bouchard, Ph.D., is Professor of Exercise Physiology at Laval University, Ste-Foy, Québec, Canada. He is Director of the Biology of Physical Activity Research Unit in the Physical Activity Sciences Laboratory.

Dr. Bouchard graduated in 1962 from Laval University with a B.Ped., and he obtained a M.Sc. from the University of Oregon in 1963, both degrees being in the exercise science area. He then pursued postgraduate work in Cologne, Germany, from 1963 to 1964. He later completed a Ph.D. in anthropology, with a dissertation in anthropological genetics, at the University of Texas at Austin in 1977.

Dr. Bouchard is a member of the American Society of Human Genetics, Human Biology Council, North American Association for the Study of Obesity, American Physiological Society, American Institute of Nutrition, American Society of Clinical Nutrition, a Fellow of the American College of Sports Medicine, Canadian Society of Exercise Physiology, American Association for the Advancement of Science, and Association Canadienne-Française pour l'Avancement des Sciences.

Dr. Bouchard is Vice President for North America of the International Association for the Study of Obesity and a past president of the North American Association for the Study of Obesity and of the Canadian Society of Exercise Physiology. He has received several awards, including a Citation Award from the American College of Sports Medicine, an Honor Award from the Canadian Society of Exercise Physiology, and the Price Benjamin Delessert from France, plus several lecture awards.

Dr. Bouchard has presented over 400 lectures and has published more than 350 research and review papers. He has also authored and edited several books on obesity and exercise science. His current research focuses on the genetics of obesity and of its metabolic complications and on the genetics of the response to regular exercise. His research is funded mainly by the Medical Research Council of Canada and the National Institutes of Health of the United States of America.

CONTRIBUTORS

Gérard Ailhaud, Ph.D.
Centre de Biochimie (UMR 134 CNRS)
Université de Nice-Sophia Antipolis
U.F.R. Sciences
Parc Valrose
Nice, France

Ingrid B. Borecki, Ph.D.
Division of Biostatistics
Washington University School of Medicine
St. Louis, Missouri

Claude Bouchard, Ph.D.
Physical Activity Sciences Laboratory
Laval University
Ste-Foy, Quebec, Canada

George A. Bray, M.D.
President/Executive Director
Pennington Biomedical Research Center
Louisiana State University
Baton Rouge, Louisiana

Streamson C. Chua, Jr., M.D., Ph.D.
Laboratory of Human Behavior and Metabolism
Rockefeller University
New York, New York

Olivier Dériaz, M.D., Ph.D.
Physical Activity Sciences Laboratory
Laval University
Ste-Foy, Quebec, Canada

Janis S. Fisler, Ph.D.
Department of Medicine
Division of Cardiology
University of California
Los Angeles, California

Francine Grégoire, Ph.D.
Department of Nutrition
University of California
Davis, California

Paul A. Grimaldi, Ph.D.
Centre de Biochimie (UMR 134 CNRS)
Université de Nice-Sophia Antipolis
U.F.R. Sciences
Parc Valrose
Nice, France

Sandra J. Hasstedt, Ph.D.
Department of Human Genetics
University of Utah Health Sciences Center
Salt Lake City, Utah

James O. Hill, Ph.D.
Center for Human Nutrition
University of Colorado Health Sciences Center
Denver, Colorado

Paul N. Hopkins, M.D., M.S.P.H.
Department of Medicine
University of Utah Health Sciences Center
Salt Lake City, Utah

Steven C. Hunt, Ph.D.
Department of Medicine
University of Utah Health Sciences Center
Salt Lake City, Utah

Patricia R. Johnson, Ph.D.
Department of Nutrition and
Division of Biological Sciences
University of California
Davis, California

Rudolph L. Leibel, M.D.
Laboratory of Human Behavior and Metabolism
Rockefeller University
New York, New York

Joanne M. Meyer, Ph.D.
Department of Human Genetics
Medical College of Virginia
Virginia Commonwealth University
Richmond, Virginia

Raymond L. Négrel, Ph.D.
Centre de Biochimie (UMR 134 CNRS)
Université de Nice-Sophia Antipolis
U.F.R. Sciences
Parc Valrose
Nice, France

Michael J. Pagliassotti, Ph.D.
Center for Human Nutrition
University of Colorado Health Sciences Center
Denver, Colorado

Louis Pérusse, Ph.D.
Physical Activity Sciences Laboratory
Laval University
Ste-Foy, Quebec, Canada

John C. Peters, Ph.D.
Regulatory and Clinical Development
Food and Beverage Products
The Procter & Gamble Co.
Cincinnati, Ohio

R. Arlen Price, Ph.D.
Department of Psychiatry
University of Pennsylvania
Philadelphia, Pennsylvania

Michael A. Province, Ph.D.
Division of Biostatistics
Washington University School of Medicine
St. Louis, Missouri

D. C. Rao, Ph.D.
Division of Biostatistics
Washington University School of Medicine
St. Louis, Missouri

M. Catherine Schumacher, M.D., M.S.P.H.
Department of Medicine
University of Utah Health Sciences Center
Salt Lake City, Utah

Thorkild I. A. Sørensen, M.D.
Institute of Preventive Medicine
Copenhagen Health Services
Copenhagen Municipal Hospital
Copenhagen, Denmark

Barry M. Stults, M.D.
Department of Medicine
University of Utah Health Sciences Center
Salt Lake City, Utah

Albert J. Stunkard, M.D.
Department of Psychiatry
University of Pennsylvania
Philadelphia, Pennsylvania

Angelo Tremblay, Ph.D.
Physical Activity Sciences Laboratory
Laval University
Ste-Foy, Quebec, Canada

Craig H. Warden, Ph.D.
Department of Medicine
Division of Cardiology
University of California
Los Angeles, California

Roger R. Williams, M.D.
Cardiovascular Genetics Research Clinic
Department of Medicine
University of Utah Health Sciences Center
Salt Lake City, Utah

Lily L. Wu, Ph.D.
Departments of Medicine and Pathology
University of Utah Health Sciences Center
Salt Lake City, Utah

TABLE OF CONTENTS

Chapter 1

GENETICS OF HUMAN OBESITIES: INTRODUCTORY NOTES

Claude Bouchard

TABLE OF CONTENTS

I. OBESITY IS A MAJOR HEALTH CONCERN

The prevalence of overweight and obesity cases in contemporary industrialized nations is strikingly high. This is a fact recognized by all health authorities irrespective of political regime and national wealth. In the U.S., it has been estimated that obesity is responsible for about 5% of total health care costs.[1] Based on 1986 figures, obesity was then responsible for about $40 billion of the total health costs primarily because of the adverse effects of obesity on diabetes, cardiovascular diseases, gall-bladder disease, hypertension, and cancer.

Excess body weight is perceived as a problem by a great number of adults. Thus, as summarized recently by the National Institutes of Health Technology Assessment Conference Panel,[2] based on four U.S. surveys, about 33% of adult women and 20% of adult men are currently trying to lose weight. Moreover, about 25% in each sex are taking measures to maintain their present weight. Among those trying to lose weight, the time spent on a weight loss regimen during the previous year averaged about 6 months. The same surveys also indicated that diet and exercise were the most common methods used when adults attempted to lose weight, each with a frequency ranging from about 60 to 80%. Other methods were cited by about 25% and/or less of the respondents trying to reduce body weight. The Conference Panel also estimated that Americans were spending about $30 billion a year on weight loss efforts.

II. HISTORICAL NOTES

Davenport[3] was among the first investigators to report data pertaining to the problem of heredity in body mass relative to stature. Using a variant of the body mass index (BMI), body weight in kilograms divided by height in centimeters squared, he studied 528 parental matings and their 926 male and 745 female offspring, about 600 of which were adults. He classified subjects into 5 classes of BMI (as specified in Table 1) in an attempt to identify Mendelian segregation from the parental to the filial generations. As suggested by the data summarized in Table 1, Davenport found some evidence for a parental

0-8493-4880-3/94/$0.00+$.50

Table 1. **Body mass index (BMI) of adult offspring from various classes of parental mating[a]**

Parental mating	N offspring	Distribution of BMI of offspring in %				
		VS	S	M	F	VF
VS × S	20	20	60	10	10	
S × S	51	10	69	21		
M × M	332	1	12	60	25	2
F × F	159		9	39	38	14
VF × VF	37			40	27	33

Note: VS = very slender (BMI: 14.0 to 18.0 in kg/m^2); S = slender (BMI: 18.1 to 21.4); M = medium (BMI: 21.5 to 25.4); F = fleshy (BMI: 25.7 to 30.5); VF = very fleshy (BMI: 30.6 and above).

[a] From Davenport, C. B., Body build and its inheritance, 329, 1923, as modified by Bray, G. A., *The Body Weight Regulatory System: Normal and Disturbed Mechanisms,* 1981, 185.

influence on the BMI of adult offspring. However, all matings produced a highly variable progeny in terms of BMI classes.

Several other early studies have considered the genetics of overweight and obesity. Gurney,[4] using a model similar to Davenport's,[3] studied the familial history of 75 women who were classified as being overweight (stout). He observed that 43% had an overweight mother, 15% had an overweight father, and 25% had both an overweight mother and an overweight father; thus 83% had either or both parents overweight. In contrast with the above, percentage figures in a nonstout control group were 30%, 2%, 6%, and 38%, respectively. Gurney also looked for Mendelian segregation among the progeny of different matings. Among 89 offspring of overweight persons, 73% were classified as being overweight and 27% as normal weight. There were 170 children of an overweight and a normal weight parent; of these, 41% were overweight and 59% were normal weight. Finally, of 176 children of matings of normal weight individuals, only 9% could be judged as being overweight. Gurney concluded that the data showed the presence of segregation, which is evidence for Mendelian inheritance of body build. Angel[5] studied 103 adult white females who were classified as obese, with an average of 60% overweight. Familial analysis revealed that one third of the women were already fat in childhood. Studies of parental matings involving these women revealed fat-to-thin ratios of offspring similar to the data reported by Gurney.[4] Angel observed that segregation takes place and that several genes appear to be involved.

In addition to these studies, several authors have also reported on the relationship between parents and children for obesity and overweight phenotypes.[6-9] Bray[10] has reviewed eight of these studies which quite consistently demonstrated that obese children had frequently obese parents. Thus, in about 30% of the cases, both parents of obese children were obese, with a range in frequency of 6 to 43%. Of course, one can readily observe that the fit between the obese state of the children and that of the parents is variable and not very tight. Some of the reasons that can be invoked to account for this state are the small number of subjects in some studies, the various definitions of obesity that were used, the possibility that obesity may not be highly determined by the genotype, differences in lifestyle and energy balance between parents and children, and undoubtedly others.

Along these lines, the earlier data of Reynolds and Schoen[11] on a set of identical triplets had indicated that genes were not sufficient to make these triplets similar in terms of fat diameters measured from roentgenograms of the calf and forearm during growth.

It should be noted that if interindividual differences among the triplets were surprisingly high, especially during puberty, their concordance for fatness tended, however, to increase in the post-pubertal period. This could be interpreted equally well under a genetic hypothesis or under a nutritional and energy balance model with little contribution from the genotype. Reynolds,[12] on the other hand, reported mean differences in standard scores for calf, waist, and forearm fat thickness between children of various degrees of kinship, which seemed to reflect the presence of a certain genetic influence. Thus, the summed standard score differences for fatness at the 3 body sites gave a mean of 15 standard score units for 8 sets of twins and triplets, a mean of 28 units for 27 pairs of full sibs, and a mean of 35 units for 20 pairs of unrelated children.

Garn[13,14] has emphasized the importance of distinguishing between the absolute fat thickness at specific sites, the rate of fat deposition at these sites, and the relative patterning of fat throughout the body. When individual differences in absolute amounts of fat are eliminated, a relative fat pattern emerges. Garn[14] has shown that the relative fat pattern of an individual seems to persist in marked weight loss, suggesting a certain degree of stability in the fat distribution profile of a person. Garn further suggested that the relative fat pattern is probably resistant to nutritional stress and may be genetically determined.

Following these early reports, human biologists, geneticists and obesity scientists became more interested in the topic of heredity and body fat content and obesity. A good number of studies were reported in the 1960s, and even more in the 1970s and 1980s, using a variety of designs (twin studies, adoption studies, family studies, animal models, etc.) and analytical techniques, as evidenced by the content of the various chapters in this volume.

III. OBESITY: THE PHENOTYPES

The interest for the genetics of human obesities has increased considerably during the last decade partly because of the realization that some forms of obesity were associated with high risks for various morbid conditions and mortality rate. Obesity cannot be seen anymore as a homogeneous phenotype. However, a commonly agreed upon classification of the obesity phenotypes does not exist yet. Nonetheless, based on the topography of the adipose tissue and its association with a variety of metabolic characteristics, we have proposed that four different types of human obesity can be recognized.[15-17] We are not referring here to the heterogeneity of the clinical manifestations of obesity or their determinants, but only to the phenotype of body fat itself.

These four types of obesities are outlined in Table 2. Type I is characterized by excess total body fat without any particular concentration of fat in a given area of the body. The other types have to do with excessive accumulation of fat in some areas of the body; that

Table 2. **The types of obesity phenotypes in a health perspective**

Type I Obesity:	Excess body mass or percent fat
Type II Obesity:	Excess subcutaneous truncal-abdominal fat (android)
Type III Obesity:	Excess abdominal visceral fat
Type IV Obesity:	Excess gluteo-femoral fat (gynoid)

is, they are based on the anatomical distribution of body fat. Type II is defined by excess subcutaneous fat on the trunk, particularly in the abdominal area, and is equivalent to the so-called android or male type of fat deposition. Type III is characterized by an excessive amount of fat in the abdominal visceral area and can be labeled abdominal visceral obesity. The last type, Type IV, is defined as gluteo-femoral obesity and is observed primarily in women (gynoid obesity). Thus, excess fat can be stored primarily in the truncal-abdominal area or in the gluteal and femoral area. In other words, for a given excess body fat, one could be either Type II (android), Type IV (gynoid), or Type III (visceral) obese. This implies that a given body fat content, say, 30% or 50 kg, may exhibit different anatomical distribution characteristics. Yet, in almost all genetic studies, individuals with quite different phenotypic characteristics have been lumped together and studied as if they all had the same trait.

Strictly speaking, one should therefore talk about the obesities rather than obesity. However, the situation is even more complex because the phenotypes are not of the simple Mendelian kind. Segregation of the genes is not readily perceived, and whatever the influence of the genotype on the etiology, it is generally attenuated or exacerbated by nongenetic factors. In other words, variation in human body fat is caused by a complex network of genetic, nutritional, metabolic, social, psychological, and energy expenditure variables.

IV. COVARIATION AMONG PHENOTYPES

The evidence accumulated over the last decade indicates that it is useful to distinguish several obesity phenotypes for the evaluation of the relationships between excess body fat and the etiology of cardiovascular diseases and noninsulin dependent diabetes mellitus or the other risk factors for these diseases. However, it is important to recognize that these phenotypes are not fully independent of one another as shown by the data of Figure 1. The level of covariation among the various body fat phenotypes ranges from about 30 to 50%. One implication of the above is that studies designed to investigate the causes of the individual differences in the various body fat phenotypes, including genetic causes, should control for these levels of covariation.

This book focuses largely on the genetics of two commonly used measurements in the field of obesity: the body mass index and percent body fat or fat mass adjusted for stature derived from underwater weighing. In clinical settings, the BMI is commonly used to assess the normality of body weight in patients. The correlation between the BMI and total body fat or percent body fat is reasonable in large and heterogeneous samples. The

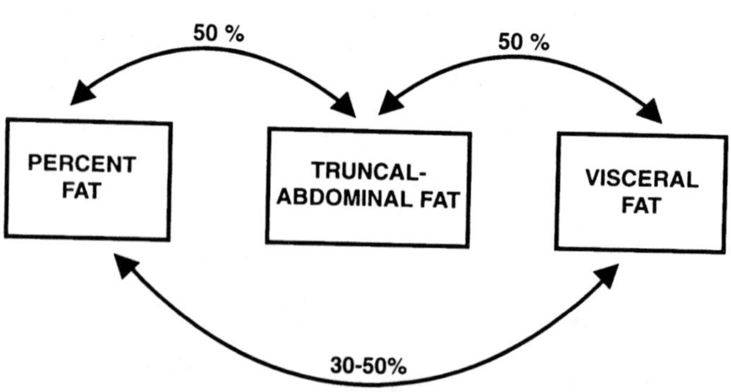

Figure 1. Common variance between three body fat phenotypes. Fat mass estimated from underwater weighing; truncal-abdominal fat assessed from skinfolds or CT scans; abdominal visceral fat estimated by CT scan at the L4/L5 vertebrae.

predictive value of the BMI is, however, much less impressive in a given individual, especially when the BMI is below 30 kg/m^2. Thus, the BMI is an indicator of heaviness and only indirectly an indicator of body fat.[17,18] Any estimate of the genetic effect on BMI is bound to be influenced in unknown proportions by the contribution of the genotype to fat mass, muscle mass, skeletal mass, and other components as well. Nevertheless, the BMI is worth considering because of its clinical use. However, the most appropriate indicator of Type I obesity remains the percentage of body fat.

A properly assessed phenotype is a sine qua non condition for a valid and productive genetic study. The data summarized in Table 3 indicate why the BMI is only a partially acceptable surrogate measure of body fat content. The common variance between BMI and percent body fat derived from underwater weighing in large samples of adult men and women ranging from 35 to 54 years of age attains only about 40%. At the extremes of the body fat content distribution, BMI is more closely associated with percent body fat; that is, the common variance may reach 60% and more. This is not entirely satisfactory as genetic studies deal with individual differences in the phenotype of interest and, for them to be successful, the phenotype of complex multifactorial trait must be measured with a reasonable degree of precision.

The fact that percent body fat remains quite heterogeneous at any level of BMI is further illustrated in Table 4. The table is based on data from young and middle-aged adult males. For instance, in 27 men with a BMI of 28 to 30, the mean percent body fat reached 28, but the range was from 15 to 41%. We have observed the same phenomenon with women.

The same point can be made for regional fat distribution phenotypes. Thus the correlation between the waist-to-hip circumferences ratio (WHR) and abdominal visceral fat is positive and generally significant in various populations, but the association is characterized by a wide scatter of scores. For instance, in a study of 51 adult obese women, the correlation between WHR and CT-assessed abdominal visceral fat reached

Table 3. **Common variance ($r^2 \times 100$) between BMI and body composition in adults, 35 to 54 years of age**

	BMI in 342 males	BMI in 356 females
Percent fat	41	40
Fat-free mass	37	25
Sum 6 skinfolds	58	67
Trunk/limb skinfolds	10	8

Note: Percent fat and fat-free mass were derived from underwater weighing assessment of body density.

Adapted from Bouchard, C., *Obesity in Europe 91, Proceedings of the 3rd European Congress on Obesity,* 1992, 7.

Table 4. **Heterogeneity of body fat content for a given BMI class in adult males**

		% Body Fat[a]		
BMI	**N**	**Mean**	**Minimum**	**Maximum**
20 to 22	27	17	8	32
23 to 25	76	22	11	35
26 to 27	46	26	16	40
28 to 30	27	28	15	41

[a] From underwater weighing.

Table 5. **Variation in amount of abdominal visceral fat measured by CT scan at L4-L5 for given BMI and percent body fat classes in adult males**

N	BMI	% Fat (range)	Visceral Fat in cm^2		
			Mean	Minimum	Maximum
15	21 to 22	14 to 18	58	31	84
19	24 to 25	19 to 24	89	50	140
18	27 to 28	25 to 29	133	63	199
16	30 to 31	30 to 33	153	77	261

Note: % fat derived from underwater weighing.

Adapted from Bouchard, C., Després, J. P., and Mauriège, P., *Endo. Rev.*, 14(1), 72, 1993.

0.55.[19] However, for a WHR of about 0.80, the amount of visceral fat area at the L4-L5 level ranged from a low of about 50 cm^2 to a high of approximately 200 cm^2. Even though the covariation between total body fat and abdominal visceral fat is statistically significant, the relationship is also characterized by a high degree of heterogeneity. As shown in Table 5, when BMI and percent body fat are constrained to narrow ranges, one finds generally a threefold range for the amount of CT-assessed abdominal visceral fat in adult males. Thus in 16 men with BMI values of 30 or 31 and a percentage of body fat ranging from 30 to 33, mean abdominal visceral fat was 153 cm^2 with a range from 77 to 261 cm^2. Again, the same lack of coupling between BMI, percent body fat, and abdominal visceral fat was observed in adult women.

The above data suggest that even though it may be necessary to use the BMI or a prediction of abdominal visceral fat in clinical settings, in field work or large population surveys, the practice should not be recommended in the context of scientific and clinical research designed to understand the causes and metabolic consequences of variation in body fat content or in fat topography.

V. DETERMINANTS OF OBESITY PHENOTYPES

In the context of genetic analysis of the various obesity phenotypes, knowledge about the determinants of these phenotypes can be extremely useful because they can be conceived as intermediate phenotypes that could be involved in the causal chain of factors leading to obesity. There is no common agreement at this time on the list and the hierarchical structure of the determinants for any of the obesity phenotypes. Nonetheless, it is useful to provide at the onset of this book a brief listing of some of these determinants and to draw a tentative picture of the relationships among the most promising intermediate phenotypes. From several lines of evidence,[20] it seems opportune to distinguish between the determinants of excess body fat (Type I obesity) and those associated with fat topography (Types II, III, and IV).

A. EXCESS BODY FAT CONTENT

Some commonly recognized correlates of body fat content are listed in Table 6. It is known that individual differences are determined by variations in energy balance; a positive energy balance over a relatively long period of time resulting in an increase in the phenotype. However, we still do not have a clear understanding of all the complex mechanisms coupling energy intake and energy expenditure. We understand that both are generally not tightly coupled over a short period of time but are reasonably well correlated in the long run in the normal weight individuals. In some cases, apparently high levels

Table 6. **Correlates of body fat content**

Age	Adults and middle-aged individuals are fatter
Gender	Females have more
Positive energy balance	Associated with an increase over time
Negative energy balance	Associated with a decrease over time
Amount of energy intake	Overfeeding leads to a gain
Composition of intake	High-fat intake is associated with an increase
Physical activity level	Low levels associated with high body fat
Resting metabolic rate	A low RMR is associated with gains in body fat
Thermic effect of food	Low effect associated with high body fat in some obesity cases
Lipid oxidation	A high respiratory quotient is associated with gains in body fat
Nutrient partitioning	A high fat mass to fat free mass ratio is associated with gains in body fat
Adipose tissue lipoprotein lipase activity	High in the obese and remains high (perhaps even increases) with loss of body weight
Variety of social and behavioral factors	Associated with socioeconomic status, familial conditions, network of friends, pattern of leisure activities, television time, smoking habits, alcohol intake, etc.
Undetermined genetic components	1. Affecting nutrient partitioning? 2. Affecting energy balance via energy expenditures? 3. Affecting dietary fat intake? 4. Affecting the relative proportion of lipids and carbohydrates oxidized? 5. Affecting other intermediate phenotypes?

of energy intake in sedentary persons do not appear to be accompanied by positive energy balance. In others, low levels of dietary energy while the individuals remain sedentary lead to a state of positive energy balance and weight gain.

The proneness to be in positive energy balance cannot be easily accounted for as shown by factors listed in Table 6: age, gender, and socioeconomic status. Among the correlates identified in the table, composition of the diet, resting metabolic rate, thermic response to food, rate of lipid oxidation, level of activity of adipose tissue lipoprotein lipase, and proneness to store energy in the form of fat or lean tissue are of particular interest.

A high fat diet is becoming increasingly recognized as a factor that enhances the risk of being in positive energy balance.[21,22] The resting metabolic rate is correlated in some studies with weight gain over time.[23] A depressed thermic response to food is observed in a subgroup of obese individuals, but not in all of them.[24] The respiratory exchange ratio, an estimate of the relative proportion of lipid and carbohydrate oxidized, is correlated with weight gain over time in some studies.[25] Finally, the proneness to store excess food energy as fat or lean tissue was correlated with weight gain in an overfeeding experiment.[16] Our own studies of cohorts of large eaters and small eaters indicate that for comparable body weight levels, the small eaters have a higher fat mass to fat free mass ratio.[26,27] These studies seem to suggest that the physically inactive small eaters build progressively over time a larger body fat content and thus retain more of the ingested energy as body energy than the large eaters. As for the adipose tissue lipoprotein lipase activity, it is in fact quite often high in the obese or even the reduced obese.[28,29] However, at this time, one cannot establish whether it is a cause or an effect of the condition.

Type I obesity is therefore a multifactorial phenotype determined by a variety of genetic and nongenetic affectors. Figure 2 describes a simple model designed to integrate the various classes of affectors of Type I obesity as well as their interactions.[30,17] Each affector constitutes a family of components such that the total picture is a very complex one. Energy intake includes not only the total caloric intake, but also the macronutrient composition of the intake, the palatability of the diet, its content of various amino acids and other molecules as they influence the metabolic outcomes of the food ingested, and appetite as well as satiety. Energy expenditures include basal and resting metabolic rates, thermic effect of food, energy cost of exercise and work, level of habitual physical activity, temperature-induced thermogenesis, stress-induced thermogenesis, and other components.

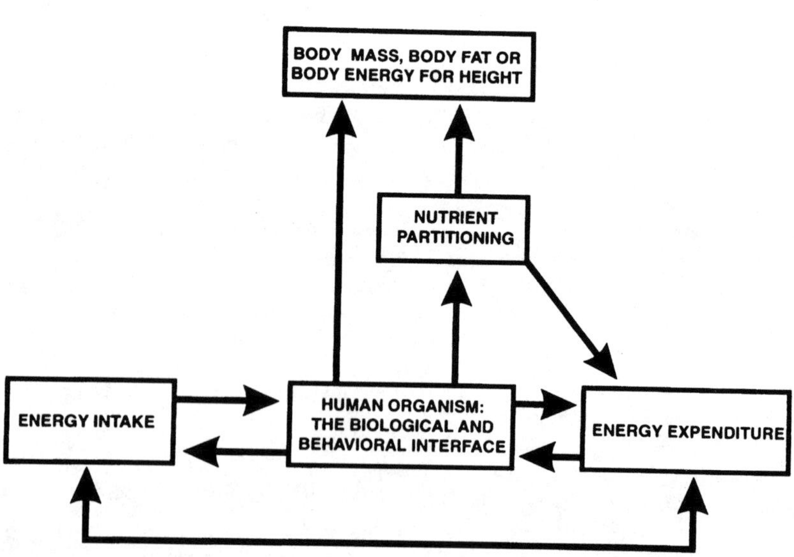

Figure 2. A paradigm of the major affectors of body mass, body fat, or body energy for height.

The next component is probably the most complex. It is defined as the interface between energy (nutrient) intake and expenditure and results from the fact that there are characteristics of the human body that have an impact on the outcome of a given set of energy intake and expenditure conditions. Variations in the biological/behavioral interface can be caused by inherited or acquired conditions. For instance, one could find inherited variants in enzymes of the liver (or other tissues) that may influence the efficiency of lipid metabolism in the carrier individuals and affect substrate utilization under certain dietary conditions. This in turn may impact on energy balance and influence the body fat phenotype. Finally, based on some of our most recent data, it appears that a critical determinant of total body fat is the proneness to store the surplus of ingested energy in the form of triacylglycerides in adipose tissue or as lean tissue.[16]

These considerations have led us to the observation that the epidemiological or population research approach about the role of the genes on body fat content or obesity per se is of limited value. It would be more productive in the future to invest in the study of the primary and secondary affectors of obesity; that is, in the network of intermediate phenotypes. For instance, the genetic analysis of the various components of energy expenditure may yield more conclusive evidence for the presence of inherited susceptibility to be in a positive energy balance than if one was studying only the BMI or body fat per se.

B. REGIONAL FAT DISTRIBUTION PHENOTYPES

The data concerning the true determinants of truncal-abdominal and visceral fat levels in each gender are generally inconclusive at this time. A more coherent picture is perhaps emerging for women than for men although there are many contradictory results and unanswered questions in both genders. Defining specificity from low level relationships is proving to be quite complex. One of the most immediate problems is to identify what is truly causal and specific as opposed to consequence from a network of apparently nonspecific associations. The present state of uncertainty about the true determinants of the phenotypes of regional fat distribution is, of course, a major handicap when trying to define their genetic basis. Moreover, regional fat distribution measurements are complex multifactorial phenotypes that are not easily reduced to single gene systems. We have reviewed this area in detail in two recent publications.[31,20]

Men and women with abdominal subcutaneous or visceral obesity tend to be characterized by large fat cells, increased LPL activity, enhanced lipolysis, and low antilipolytic effect of insulin in these depots. Sex steroid, glucocorticoid, catecholamine, and growth hormone levels are apparently associated with amount of visceral fat, and the relationships may be somewhat different in men and women. It remains to be determined whether blood flow, innervation, and the natural catecholaminergic environment differ between visceral and subcutaneous fat cells from various depots in order to provide a better explanation for regional differences in fat topography.

Björntorp has developed an attractive hypothesis to account for some of the individual differences in regional fat distribution, namely the neuroendocrine dysregulation associated with a state of chronic hypothalamic arousal hypothesis.[32-36] Briefly, the hypothesis states that depressed or unpleasant social conditions, behavioral characteristics such as smoking, alcohol consumption or drug use, and other forms of pressures on the individual are perceived as stressors which engender neuroendocrine responses in preparation for coping reactions. Two types of reactions are commonly observed. One is the well known "fight or flight" response associated with an activation of the sympathetic nervous system. The other is more analogous to the recognition of defeat and the submissiveness attitude with an apparent loss of control. The latter can be considered as a maladaptive response to various environmental, potentially stressfull challenges, and has been associated with increased activity along the CRF-ACTH-cortisol axis and a decrease in sex steroid levels in males but an increase in females.[34,36]

The hypothesis suggests that social, behavioral, and biological stimuli perceived as stressful may initiate chronic neuroendocrine dysregulations resulting over time in a more pronounced android profile of fat deposition with a higher amount of abdominal visceral fat in males and a greater risk of developing the android fat distribution phenotype in females. The main features of the hormonal responses being an increased sympathetic nervous system activity and an augmented glucocorticoid but with altered androgen levels (depressed in men but elevated in women), the growing upper body fat, and visceral fat depots act synergistically with the prevailing hormonal profile leading progressively to metabolic disturbances and eventually to the full blown "metabolic syndrome".[34-36]

Only partial evidence has been found to support the hypothalamic arousal and neuroendocrine dysregulation hypothesis at this time, and cause and effect relationships cannot be established unambiguously. However, a handful of studies have produced consistent findings. Thus, a preponderance of upper body fat (as assessed from WHR) was seen in men and women who smoked or drank alcohol regularly.[37] Others have shown that men and women with upper body fat were more likely to be from a low socioeconomic class, to be less educated with a low income, to be more frequently absent from work, and were more apt to suffer from depression than those with lower body fat.[38,39] It is quite likely that the susceptibility to stress exposure and neuroendocrine dysregulation as well as to their consequences in terms of the modulation of the adipose tissue topography and of the metabolic profile is influenced by DNA sequence variation at a number of loci. This field will undoubtedly become one of active research as our understanding of the mechanisms involved and understanding of the causal chain of events gets better.

Figure 3 provides one view of the various determinants and correlates of abdominal visceral fat that specifies the major relationships in terms of the direction of the effects. Gender differences for the various paths of the model are not delineated on the figure. The potential role of several hormones has not been included, and genotype-environment interaction effects are also not specified in the figure. However, the latter are ubiquitous as shown by the results of our long-term overfeeding and exercise-training studies.[16,40]

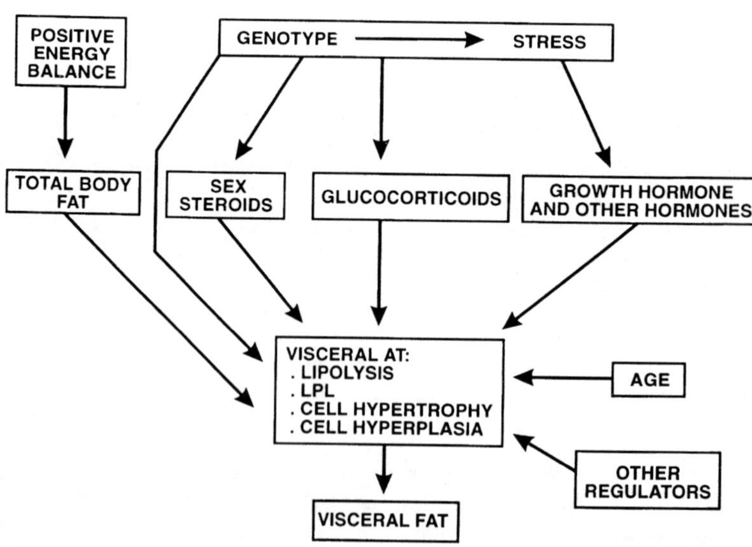

Figure 3. A model of the determinants and correlates of abdominal visceral fat with particular reference to women.

These interaction effects imply that some individuals are more prone to develop truncal-abdominal obesity or to become viscerally obese because of unknown genetic characteristics.

VI. STABILITY WITH AGE

It is commonly recognized that when an excessive amount of body fat has been accumulated, it is very difficult to revert to a normal weight and body composition status. This observation has led to the hypothesis that body fat content during the growing years was a critical determinant of obesity in adulthood. However, it has proven difficult to document the phenomenon and it may not be as strong as originally anticipated. Some studies have reported that body mass index and skinfolds measured during childhood or adolescence were good predictors of adulthood values, but others have found rather low correlations.[41]

An interesting report on this topic was recently published based on samples of males and females from the Harvard Longitudinal Studies of Child Health and Development who were followed for a period of about 50 years.[41] Some of the results of that study are summarized in Table 7. The tracking from childhood to middle age was generally unimpressive, but it was slightly better for males than for females. Thus BMI in childhood accounted for 0% of the variance in female middle age BMI but accounted for about 17% in males. These results are quite compatible with those of an earlier study based on a cohort of children born in one week in March 1946 in England, Wales, and Scotland and then followed over a 36-year period.[42] Only 21% of obese 36-year-olds had been obese at 11 years of age, about 10% of adult obese men and 30% of adult obese women. Another group, i.e., 79% of obese 36-year-olds, first became obese in early adult life. Those men and women were often not the most overweight in childhood.

However, tracking tends to be better when one considers the extremes of the distribution. The relationship between childhood obesity and adult obesity reaches its peak when the probands are teenagers. Being overweight at or around puberty may be indeed an important correlate of adulthood body mass as suggested by a report on a 40-year follow-up of overweight children.[43] In other words, there is some truth to the notion that obese children or adolescents tend to become obese adults while very lean children grow into lean adults, but only when the fattest and leanest children are considered. These trends were also observed by Garn et al.[44] when they analyzed the relationship between obese probands and their parents as a function of age in 1419 such pairs. The tendency toward a greater prevalence of obesity among the parents of obese propositi is related to the age of the propositus in a curvilinear manner. The relationship is least when probands are young, peaks when the sons and daughters are teenagers, and declines thereafter.[44]

Table 7. **Correlations for BMI from childhood to 50 years of age in males and females**

	Males (N from 32 to 55)		Females (N from 35 to 59)	
	5 to 7 years	18 years	5 to 5 years	18 years
30 years	0.41**	0.67***	0.21	0.66***
40 years	0.36*	0.61***	–0.03	0.62***
50 years	0.41*	0.51**	0.05	0.44*

Note: * $p < 0.05$; ** $p < 0.005$; *** $p < 0.0001$.

Adapted from Casey, V. A., Dwyer, J. T., Coleman, K. A., and Valadian, I., *Am. J. Clin. Nutr.*, 56, 14, 1992.

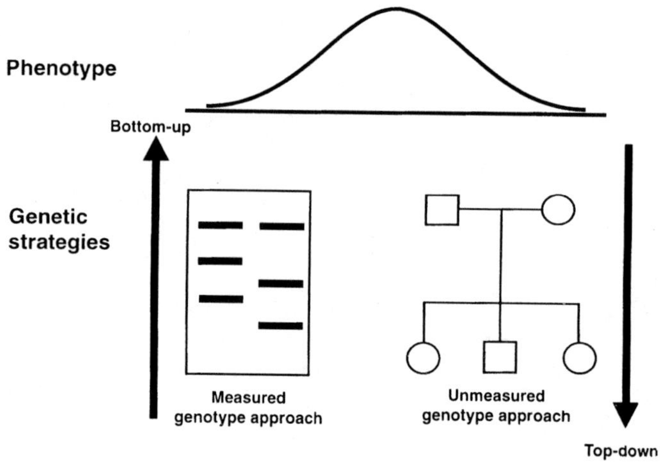

Figure 4. The two main strategies to study the role of genes in continuously distributed phenotypes. (Adapted from Sing, C. F. and Boerwinkle, E. A., *Molecular Approaches to Human Polygenic Disease,* 1987, 99.)

VII. TWO MAIN TYPES OF RESEARCH

Two strategies have been traditionally used by geneticists to study the role of genes in continuously distributed phenotypes in humans. As shown in Figure 4, they are referred to as the unmeasured genotype and the measured genotype approaches.[45,46] The unmeasured genotype approach attempts to estimate the contribution of genetic variation to the phenotypic variance and to find quantitative evidence for single genes with detectable (major) effects on the phenotype. As inference about the contribution of genes is made from the phenotype, this approach is also referred to as the top-down strategy. Here one uses various sampling designs (twins, nuclear families, families with adoptees, extended pedigrees, etc.) in combination with statistical tools such as path analysis, variance component estimation, and complex segregation analysis. On the other hand, the measured genotype approach is based on direct measurement of genetic variation at the protein or DNA levels in an effort to assess the impact of allelic variation on the phenotypic variation. Since inference about the role of genes is made from DNA to the phenotype, this approach is at times referred to as the bottom-up strategy.[46] Direct measures of genetic variation may be obtained by studying gene products or, better still, DNA sequences. Advances in recombinant DNA technology over the last two decades have made possible the measure of genetic variation at the DNA level and have provided the impetus necessary for the extensive use of the measured genotype approach in human genetic studies.

The top-down and bottom-up approaches include a large network of designs and technologies that are used by human geneticists in the effort to understand the genetic basis of complex multifactorial diseases. This topic will also be discussed in the concluding chapter of this book.

REFERENCES

1. **Colditz, G. A.,** Economic costs of obesity, *Am. J. Clin. Nutr.,* 55, 503S, 1992.
2. Technology Assessment Conference Panel, Methods for voluntary weight loss and control: technology assessment conference statement, *Ann. Intern. Med.,* 116, 942, 1992.

3. **Davenport, C. B.,** Body build and its inheritance, *Carnegie Institution of Washington,* Publication No. 329, 1923.
4. **Gurney, R.,** Hereditary factor in obesity, *Arch. Intern. Med.,* 57, 557, 1936.
5. **Angel, J. L.,** Constitution in female obesity, *Am. J. Phys. Anthropol.,* 7, 433, 1949.
6. **Dunlop, D. M. and Lyon, R. M.,** Study of 523 cases of obesity, *Edinburgh Med. J.,* 38, 561, 1931.
7. **Ellis, R. W. B. and Tallerman, K. H.,** Obesity in childhood: study of 50 cases, *Lancet,* 2, 615, 1934.
8. **Rony, H. R.,** *Obesity and Leanness,* Lea & Febiger, Philadelphia, 1940.
9. **Bauer, J.,** *Constitution and Disease,* Grune and Stratton, New York, 1945.
10. **Bray, G. A.,** The inheritance of corpulence, in *The Body Weight Regulatory System: Normal and Disturbed Mechanisms,* Cioffi, L. A., James, W. P. T., and Van Itallie, T. B., Eds., Raven Press, New York, 1981, 185.
11. **Reynolds, E. L. and Schoen, G.,** Growth patterns of identical triplets from 8 through 18 years, *Child Dev.,* 18, 130, 1947.
12. **Reynolds, E. L.,** The distribution of subcutaneous fat in childhood and adolescence, *Monog. Soc. Res. Child Dev.,* 15, Serial 50, No. 2, 1951.
13. **Garn, S. M.,** Fat patterning and fat intercorrelations in the adult male, *Hum. Biol.,* 26, 59, 1954.
14. **Garn, S. M.,** Relative fat patterning and individual characteristics, *Hum. Biol.,* 27, 75, 1955.
15. **Bouchard, C.,** Variation in human body fat: the contribution of the genotype, in *Obesity: Towards a Molecular Approach,* Bray, G., Ricquier, D., and Spiegelman, B., Eds., Alan R. Liss, New York, 1990, 17.
16. **Bouchard, C., Tremblay, A., Després, J. P., Nadeau, A., Lupien, P. J., Thériault, G., Dussault, J., Moorjani, S., Pineault, S., and Fournier, G.,** The response to long-term overfeeding in identical twins, *N. Engl. J. Med.,* 322, 1477, 1990.
17. **Bouchard, C.,** Human obesities: chaos or determinism? in *Obesity in Europe 91, Proceedings of the 3rd European Congress on Obesity,* Ailhaud, G., Guy-Grand, B., Lafontan, M., and Ricquier, C., Eds., John Libbey & Co., Paris, 1992, 7.
18. **Garn, S. M., Leonard, W. R., and Hawthorne, V. M.,** Three limitations of the body mass index, *Am. J. Clin. Nutr.,* 44, 996, 1986.
19. **Ferland, M., Després, J. P., Tremblay, A., Pinault, S., Nadeau, A., Moorjani, S., Lupien, P. J., Thériault, G., and Bouchard, C.,** Assessment of adipose tissue distribution by computed axial tomography in obese women: association with body density and anthropometric measurements, *Br. J. Nutr.,* 61, 139, 1989.
20. **Bouchard, C., Després, J. P., and Mauriège, P.,** Genetic and nongenetic determinants of regional fat distribution, *Endo. Rev.,* 14(1), 72, 1993.
21. **Romieu, I., Willett, W. C., Stampfer, M. J., Colditz, G. A., Samson, L., Rosner, B., Hennekens, C. H., and Speizer, F. E.,** Energy intake and other determinants of relative weight, *Am. J. Clin. Nutr.,* 47, 406, 1988.
22. **Dreon, D. M., Frey-Hewitt, B., Ellsworth, N., Williams, P. T., Terry, R. B., and Wood, P. D.,** Dietary fat: carbohydrate ratio and obesity in middle-aged men, *Am. J. Clin. Nutr.,* 47, 995, 1988.
23. **Ravussin, E., Lillioja, S., Knowler, W. C., Christin, L., Freymond, D., Abbott, W. G. H., Boyce, V., and Howard, B.,** Reduced rate of energy expenditure as a risk factor for body weight gain, *N. Engl. J. Med.,* 318, 467, 1988.
24. **Jéquier, E. and Schutz, Y.,** New evidence for a thermogenic defect in human obesity, in *Regulation of Energy Expenditure,* Horton, E. S. and Danforth, E., Jr., Eds., John Libbey, London, 1985, 1.
25. **Zurlo, F., Lilioja, S., Esposito-Del Puente, A., Nyomba, B., Ray, I, Saad, M., Swinburn, B., Kmowler, W., Bogardus, C., and Ravussin, E.,** Low ratio of fat to

carbohydrate oxidation as predictor of weight gain, *Am. J. Physiol.*, 259, E650, 1990.

26. **George, V., Tremblay, A., Després, J. P., Leblanc, C., Pérusse, L., and Bouchard, C.,** Evidence for the existence of small eaters and large eaters of similar fat-free mass and activity level, *Int. J. Obes.*, 13, 43, 1989.
27. **George, V., Tremblay, A., Després, J. P., Landry, M., Allard, L., Leblanc, C., and Bouchard C.,** Further evidence for the presence of small and large eaters among women, *Am. J. Clin. Nutr.*, 53, 425, 1991.
28. **Kern, P. A., Ong, J. M., Saffari, B., and Carty, J.,** The effects of weight loss on the activity and expression of adipose tissue lipoprotein lipase in very obese humans, *N. Engl. J. Med.*, 322, 1053, 1990.
29. **Eckel, R. H. and Yost, T. J.,** Weight reduction increases adipose tissue lipoprotein lipase responsiveness in obese women, *J. Clin. Invest.*, 80, 992, 1987.
30. **Bouchard, C.,** Current understanding of the etiology of obesity: genetic and nongenetic factors, *Am. J. Clin. Nutr.*, 53, 1561S, 1991.
31. **Bouchard, C., Després, J. P., Mauriège, P., Marcotte, M., Chagnon, M., Dionne, F.T., and Bélanger, A.,** The genes in the constellation of determinants of regional fat distribution, *Int. J. Obes.*, 15, 9, 1991.
32. **Björntorp, P.,** Possible mechanisms relating to fat distribution and metabolism, in *Fat Distribution During Growth and Later Health Outcomes*, Bouchard, C. and Johnston, F. E., Eds., Alan Liss, New York, 1988, 176.
33. **Björntorp, P.,** The association between obesity, adipose tissue distribution and disease, *Acta Med. Scand., Suppl.*, 723, 121, 1988.
34. **Björntorp, P.,** Visceral fat accumulation: the missing link between psychosocial factors and cardiovascular disease? *J. Intern. Med.*, 230, 195, 1991.
35. **Björntorp, P.,** Metabolic implications of body fat distribution, *Diabetes Care*, 14, 1132, 1991.
36. **Björntorp, P.,** Visceral obesity: a "civilization syndrome", *Obes. Res.*, 1, 206, 1993.
37. **Seidell, J. C.,** Environmental influences on regional fat distribution, *Int. J. Obes.*, 15, 31, 1991.
38. **Larsson, B., Seidell, J., Svärdsudd, K., Welin, L., Tibblin, G., and Björntorp, P.,** Obesity, adipose tissue distribution, and health in men: the study of men born in 1913, *Appetite*, 13, 37, 1989.
39. **Lapidus, L., Bengtsson, C., Hällström, T., and Björntorp, P.,** Obesity, adipose tissue distribution, and health in women: results from a population study in Gothenburg, Sweden, *Appetite*, 12, 25, 1989.
40. **Bouchard, C., Dionne, F. T., Simoneau, J. A., and Boulay, M. R.,** Genetics of aerobic and anaerobic performances, in *Exercise and Sport Sciences Reviews*, Holloszy, J. O., Ed., Williams and Wilkins, 1992, 20, 27.
41. **Casey, V. A., Dwyer, J. T., Coleman, K. A., and Valadian, I.,** Body mass index from childhood to middle age: a 50-year follow-up., *Am. J. Clin. Nutr.*, 56, 14, 1992.
42. **Braddon, F. E. M., Rodgers, B., Wadsworth, M. E. J., and Davies, J. M. C.,** Onset of obesity in a 36-year birth cohort study, *Br. Med. J.*, 293, 299, 1986.
43. **Mossberg, H. O.,** 40-Year follow-up of overweight children, *Lancet*, 491, 1989.
44. **Garn, S. M., Sullivan, T. V., and Hawthorne, V. M.,** Fatness and obesity of the parents of obese individuals, *Am. J. Clin. Nutr.*, 50, 1308, 1989.
45. **Sing, C. F. and Boerwinkle, E. A.,** Genetic architecture of inter-individual variability in apolipoprotein, lipoprotein and lipid phenotypes, in *Molecular Approaches to Human Polygenic Disease*, Weatherall, D., Ed., Ciba Foundation Symposium 130, John Wiley & Sons, Chichester, 1987, 99.

46. **Sing, C. F., Boerwinkle, E., Moll, P. P., and Templeton, A. R.,** Characterization of genes affecting quantitative traits in humans, in *Proceedings of the Second International Conference on Quantitative Genetics,* Weir, B. S., Eisen, E. J., Goodman, M. M., and Namkoong, G., Eds., Sinauer Associates, Sunderland, MA, 1988, 250.

Chapter 2

Etiology and Prevalence of Obesity

George A. Bray

TABLE OF CONTENTS

I. INTRODUCTION AND DEFINITION

During this century several approaches have been proposed to classify obesity.[1] The terms exogenous and endogenous were originally introduced at the beginning of the 20th century by Von Noorden[2] and have been widely used to separate those cases of obesity which result from external causes from those due to internal causes. As our understanding of obesity has increased, the need for more persuasive classifications has become apparent. The classification which will form the basis for the discussion in this chapter is presented in Table 1. This classification includes three parts — an anatomic classification, an etiologic classification, and a functional classification.

0-8493-4880-3/94/$0.00+$.50

Table 1. **Classification of Obesity**

I. Anatomic classification
    A. Microscopic
        1. Fat cell size
        2. Fat cell number
    B. Macroscopic
        1. Total body fat
        2. Subcutaneous fat distribution
        3. Visceral fat
        4. Abnormal or unusual fat deposits
II. Etiologic classification
    A. Hypothalamic
    B. Endocrine
    C. Dietary
    D. Physical inactivity
    E. Genetic
    F. Drug-induced
III. Functional classification
    A. Degree of risk estimated from BMI
        1. Very low (class 1 or grade 0) — BMI 20 < 25 kg/m^2
        2. Low (class 2 or grade 1) — BMI 25 to < 30 kg/m^2
        3. Moderate (class 3 or grade 2) — BMI 30 to < 35 kg/m^2
        4. High (class 4 or grade 2) — BMI 35 to < 40 kg/m^2
        5. Very high (class 5 or grade 3) — BMI > 40 kg/m^2
    B. Associated risks
        1. High blood pressure
        2. Insulin resistance or diabetes
        3. Low HDL-C/LDL-C ratio
        4. LVH by ECG
        5. Sleep apnea or high P_{ACO_2}
        6. Hirsutism or high LH/FSH ratio
        7. Smoking
        8. Restrained eaters
        9. Low physical activity

Note: BMI, body mass index; HDL-C, high-density lipoprotein cholesterol; LDL-C, low-density lipoprotein cholesterol; LVH, left ventricular hypertrophy; ECG, electrocardiogram; P_{ACO_2}, arterial CO_2 pressure; LH, luteinizing hormone; FSH, follicle-stimulating hormone.

Overweight can be expressed in several ways, and the prevalence of obesity depends on which one is selected. Relative weight is the ratio or percentage of actual weight to some standard weight which is most often obtained from the life insurance industry tables. Of these tables, the Metropolitan Life Insurance Company table of 1959 and its 1983 revision are the most commonly used. A second relative weight standard is the 85th percentile of weight for height for a given age group. Using the 85th percentile of 20 to 29 year olds as the standard for comparison, the National Center for Health Statistics in the U.S.[3] has published data on the percentage of people within other age groups who are overweight. One problem with this approach is that it automatically defines no less than 15% of Americans as being overweight.

Weight and height also can be related by various other ratios such as weight divided by height, weight divided by the cube root of height (ponderal index), or weight divided by height to some power. The most widely used of these is the body mass index (BMI) or Quetelet index (QI), defined as body weight divided by the square of the height. Using the body mass index, overweight can be conveniently classified or graded by intervals of 5 BMI units above a BMI of 25 kg/m^2, as shown in Table 1.

Obesity or fatness can be measured by a number of techniques.[4] A summary of these methods is shown in Table 2, which lists the various methods and provides an estimate of cost and difficulty as well as noting whether the method can measure body fat distribution. For epidemiologic studies, fat is usually estimated using skinfold measurements. When the body mass index is above 30 kg/m,[2] skinfold measurements for the top 5% of the population and BMI are almost superimposable. The sum of the triceps plus subscapular skinfold measurements totaling greater than 45 mm in males and 65 mm in females also can be used to define obesity. Where measurements of body fat are available, a body fat above 25% for males and above 35% for females also can define obesity.

In addition to measurements of body fatness, regional fat distribution also plays an important role in health risks. Regional fat distribution can be estimated by several techniques. Either a computed tomographic (CT) scan or a magnetic resonance imaging (MRI) scan at the level of the L-4/L-5 vertebral space is the most accurate, but is also the most expensive (Table 2). The ratio of the circumference of the waist to the circumference of the hips has been used widely in epidemiologic studies. Ratios above 0.80 in women and above 0.95 in men put them in the high risk category. The ratio of skinfolds on the trunk to that on the limbs and the sagittal diameter are two other techniques used to estimate central and visceral fat. Widely accepted standards for fat distribution do not exist.

Table 2. **Methods of estimating body fat and its distribution**

Method	Cost[a]	Ease of use	Accuracy	Measures regional fat
Height and weight	$	Easy	High	No
Skin folds	$	Easy	Low	Yes
Circumferences	$	Easy	Moderate	Yes
Ultrasound	$$	Moderate	Moderate	Yes
Density				
Immersion	$	Moderate	High	No
Plethysmography	$$$	Difficult	High	No
Heavy water				
Tritiated	$$	Moderate	High	No
Deuterium oxide, or heavy oxygen	$$$	Moderate	High	No
Potassium isotope (^{40}K)	$$$$	Difficult	High	No
Total body electrical conductivity (TOBEC)	$$$	Moderate	High	No
Bioelectric impedance (BIA)	$$	Easy	High	No
Fat-soluble gas	$$	Difficult	High	No
Absorptiometry (dual-energy X-ray absorptiometry = DEXA; dual-photon absorptiometry = DPA)	$$$	Easy	High	No
Computed tomography (CT)	$$$$	Difficult	High	Yes
Magnetic resonance imaging (MRI)	$$$$	Difficult	High	Yes
Neutron activation	$$$$	Difficult	High	No

[a] $ = low cost, $$ = moderate cost, $$$ = high cost, $$$$ = very high cost.

II. ETIOLOGIC CLASSIFICATION

There are a number of etiologic causes of obesity which are summarized in Table 1.

A. HYPOTHALAMIC OBESITY

Hypothalamic obesity has been reported in human beings after a variety of injuries.[5,6] The major hypothalamic injuries are trauma, malignancy, and inflammatory diseases. Three groups of findings accompany the syndrome of hypothalamic obesity. The first is related to the increased intracranial pressure and includes headaches and diminished vision due to papilledema or swelling of the optic nerve. The second group of symptoms are manifestations of endocrine alterations following disturbance of the hypothalamic pituitary axis and include amenorrhea, impotence, diabetes insipidus, thyroid insufficiency, and adrenal insufficiency. The third group of symptoms are a variety of neurological and physiological derangements including convulsions, coma, somnolence, temperature disturbances, and abnormalities of thirst. Treatment of the syndrome requires treating the underlying disease and giving appropriate endocrine and neurologic support.

B. ENDOCRINE OBESITY

1. Cushing's Disease

Cushing's disease results from adrenocorticotropic hormone (ACTH)-secreting pituitary adenomas, from ectopic production of ACTH or corticotropin-releasing hormone (CRH), or from adrenal tumors which hypersecrete cortisol. In clinical series of patients with Cushing's syndrome due to a pituitary adenoma, obesity is a common finding, and in some cases it can be the presenting symptom.[7] One 4-year-old boy was brought to our endocrine clinic by his mother because of weight gain. He had an elevated plasma and urinary free cortisol and exhibited loss of the diurnal rhythm for cortisol. The most common cause of hypercortisolemia in children is an adrenal tumor, but this boy proved to be suffering from a pituitary tumor for which appropriate treatment was given, leading to the disappearance of his obesity.

2. Polycystic Ovary Syndrome

The syndrome of polycystic ovaries was originally described in 1844 as sclerocsystic ovaries. It is characterized clinically by oligomenorrhea or amenorrhea, hirsutism, hyperandrogenism, an elevated luteinizing hormone follicle-stimulating hormone (LH)/(FSH) ratio, and polycystic ovaries.[8] Obesity is present in 16 to 49% of the cases in various series. When a group of very obese women with polycystic ovaries was compared to a group of women with a similar degree of obesity but without polycystic ovaries, the SHBG (Sex Hormone Binding Globulin) concentration was found to be reduced in both groups compared to control women. However, testosterone and albumin-bound testosterone levels were higher than normal, as were Δ^4-androstenedione levels in the women with polycystic ovaries. The level of dehydroepiandrosterone-sulfate (DHEA-S) was not increased. Estradiol and estrone were significantly higher in the women with polycystic ovaries than in the control women. An increased and pulsatile pattern of LH secretion was seen in both groups, but the value was higher in the less obese women.

Insulin resistance is a characteristic of the polycystic ovary syndrome. These changes are not due to alterations in the insulin receptors. Insulin secretion over 24 h is higher in women with polycystic ovaries than in control-matched obese women. The levels of insulin-like growth factor binding proteins (IGFBP) are altered in women with polycystic ovaries. The level of one of these binding proteins, IGFBP-1, is low and may be associated with the high degree of insulin resistance observed in some of these patients. Obese women with polycystic ovaries show a blunted secretion of growth hormone and a low growth hormone response to the injection of growth hormone releasing hormone

(GHRH). This contrasts with the normal levels of growth hormone and normal response to GHRH in normal-weight women with polycystic ovaries, suggesting an important role of obesity. One sequence relating these events may be the following: the increased insulin resistance associated with this syndrome leads to a decrease in IGFBP-1, which in turn leads to increased bioavailability of insulin-like growth factor (IGF-1) to its receptors. Since IGF-1 can stimulate the ovary to increase androgen production, this would lead to the syndrome of polycystic ovaries.

3. Hypogonadism

Hypogonadism is associated with reduced gonadal steroid hormone production and with increased body fat in both males and females. Appropriate replacement therapy will restore the lean-to-fat ratios to normal.

4. Growth Hormone Deficiency

Growth hormone deficiency is likewise associated with increased subcutaneous adipose tissue deposition. Treatment with growth hormone has been shown to reduce the level of subcutaneous adipose tissue.

5. Insulinoma

Insulin treatment has been noted to increase body fat. In patients with insulinomas, however, the degree of increase of body fat is very modest, suggesting that an elevation in insulin levels alone is not sufficient to be a major cause of obesity.

C. HIGH FAT INTAKE

In experimental animals, one of the most robust techniques for producing obesity is to give animals a high-fat diet. The association of obesity with the high-fat Western-type of diet is also suspected to be important in humans, but documenting this has been difficult. The most clearcut example is an epidemiologic study from Brazil which showed a definite relationship between obesity and the intake of dietary fat.[9] Support for this concept also comes from the increasing prevalence of obesity in Japan as the fat content of the Japanese diet has increased from below 15% in the early years after World War II to values above 25% at the present time. Several other reports also suggest this relationship.[10]

D. DRUG TREATMENT

There are a number of drugs which can produce weight gain or weight loss. These are summarized in Table 3. The two largest and most important groups are the psychotropic drugs and the steroids. The involvement of norepinephrine, serotonin, histamine, and a variety of peptides in regulating food intake provides a basis for understanding the receptor systems through which drugs can modulate food intake and body weight when these drugs are used as treatment for depression and psychotic disturbances. The

Table 3. **Drugs that increase body weight**

- Phenothiazines (chlorpromazine > thioridazine ≥≥ trifluoperazine mesoridazine > promazine ≥ mepazine ≥ perphenazine ≥ prochlorperazine > haloperidol ≥ loxapine)
- Antidepressants (amitriptyline > imipramine = doxepin = phenelzine > amoxapine = desipramine = trazodone = tranylcypromine)
- Antiepileptics (valproate; carbamazepine)
- Steroids (glucocorticoids; megestrol acetate; estrogens)
- Antihypertensives (terazosin)

phenothiazine drugs characteristically cause some weight gain, but the tricyclic antidepressant amitriptyline leads to the most weight gain. Amitriptyline not only results in increased weight, it also increases the preference for carbohydrate.

E. PHYSICAL INACTIVITY

Surgery or other events which impede physical activity are frequently noted as times where individual patients say their obesity began. Since physical activity is an important element in the energy balance equation, such an observation would not be surprising. The epidemiologic data of Kromhout[11] support a role for decreased activity in weight gain during middle adult life. In a 10-year interval between the ages of 50 and 60 the energy intake of a cohort of Dutch men declined on average 500 kcal/day. Over this same interval of time body weight increased 3.5 kg, suggesting that energy expenditure must have declined by slightly more than 500 kcal/day.

F. GENETIC FACTORS IN OBESITY

1. Dysmorphic Obesities

There are a group of rare diseases, with associated obesity and dysmorphic features, for which there is evidence suggesting that genetic factors are of major importance.[12]

a. The Bardet-Biedl Syndrome

The Lawrence-Moon and Bardet-Biedl syndromes are often considered together, but probably represent distinct entities. In 1866, Laurence and Moon described four patients with retinal degeneration of the pigment cells, mental retardation, hypogenitalism, and a neurologic defect characterized as spastic paraplegia, but without obesity or digital anomalies. Obesity was present in two, spastic paraplegia in one, and ataxia in two patients. Nearly 60 years later Bardet described a syndrome consisting of retinitis pigmentosa, obesity, and polydactyly, and 2 years later Biedl independently described two cases with additional findings of genital hypoplasia, mental retardation, and anal atresia. There have subsequently been more than 500 cases which fit into this group of syndromes.[13] Although often lumped together, the Bardet-Biedl and Lawrence-Moon syndromes differ in a number of important ways and should be considered as separate entities. Both are inherited as autosomal recessive traits. Pigmentary retinopathy is present in the Lawrence-Moon syndrome, but tapetoretinal degeneration occurs in the Bardet-Biedl syndrome. Spastic paraplegia is present in the Lawrence-Moon syndrome, but does not occur in the Bardet-Biedl syndrome. Obesity, which is an almost uniform feature of the Bardet-Biedl syndrome, is uncommon in the Lawrence-Moon syndrome. In addition, the Bardet-Biedl syndrome may be associated with congenital heart disease and nephropathy, which has been reported to be as high as 71% in one autopsy series.[14]

The Ahlstrom-Hallgren syndrome is different from the Bardet-Biedl syndrome, although both are associated with obesity.[15] Blindness in childhood, sensory nerve deafness, and diabetes mellitus characterize the Ahlstrom-Hallgren syndrome. The absence of polydactyly and mental retardation and the presence of nerve deafness and diabetes mellitus also help separate these conditions. Obesity in the Ahlstrom-Hallgren syndrome usually begins between the ages of 2 and 10 years, and body weight ranges between 116 and 230% of "ideal". The obesity subsided in three of the ten patients when they reached adulthood. Acanthosis nigricans, baldness, and hypogonadism also may be present.

b. Cohen Syndrome

The cardinal features of Cohen syndrome are hypotonia, truncal obesity, mental retardation, and a characteristic craniofacial appearance, characterized by a high nasal bridge, high arched palate, short philtrum, small jaw, and a characteristic open mouth.[16] The obesity is truncal and begins at approximately 5 years of age. Delayed puberty occurs, but there is normal gonadal function or, in some cases, hypogonadotropic hypogonadism.

Mental retardation is only mild. This syndrome is probably inherited as an autosomal recessive trait. Friedman and Sack have raised the possibility that it may have a higher prevalence among Ashkenazi Jews.[17]

c. Carpenter Syndrome

Carpenter syndrome belongs to the wider entity known as acrocephalopolysyndactyly. It is rare and transmitted as an autosomal recessive trait. The characteristics of this syndrome include craniosynostosis with a peculiar facies and apparent exophthalmus. Dysmorphic features include a flat nasal ridge, low-set ears, retrognathism, a high arched palate, and partial syndactyly with brachymesophalangy.[18]

d. Prader-Willi Syndrome

Prader-Willi syndrome (PWS) is among the most common of the dysmorphic forms of human obesity. It is characterized by obesity, hypotonic musculature, mental retardation, hypogonadism, short stature, and small hands and feet.[19,20] On the basis of infants with hypotonia referred for evaluation in the state of Iowa, Zellweger has put the prevalence at between 1:25,000 and 1:30,000 births.[21]

Reduced intrauterine fetal movements, hypotonia at birth, and typical facies raised the possibility that this syndrome might be genetic. Deletions or translocations involving the short arm of chromosome 15 (q-11 to q-13) have been reported by several groups in nearly 50% of these individuals. Two quite different syndromes, PWS and Angers syndrome, both appear to involve a chromosomal defect in the same region of chromosome 15. Patients with PWS are obese and appear to reflect paternal transmission. Patients with the Angers syndrome, on the other hand, are not obese, but have much more severe mental retardation which appears to result from maternal transmission of a defective chromosome. The imprinting which occurs after fertilization produces the different syndromes.[22]

Most patients with PWS are short and have an adult height which averages 59 inches in girls and 61 inches in boys. Body weight is increased to a mean of 80 kg in girls and 98 kg in boys.[20] Affected individuals are mentally retarded, but the degree of this retardation is highly variable. Hyperphagia is characteristic of these individuals, and emotional problems — including temper tantrums — are well known, particularly related to food. Levels of pancreatic polypeptide are low, and Zipf and his colleagues have provided suggestive evidence that pancreatic polypeptide can lower food intake, particularly in girls with PWS.[23] Scoliosis has been observed in many patients, but bone age is usually the same as the chronological age or only slightly retarded. Advanced dental caries and hypoplastic enamel have been observed, as has dysplasia of the hip.[20] The profound hypotonia present at birth usually improves somewhat during the first 2 or 3 years of life.

Diabetes mellitus has been described in a number of patients with PWS. A total of 5 of the first 46 patients in one study manifested diabetes. A subsequent series showed only one mild case among 14 individuals tested. The earliest onset of diabetes was at 2½ years of age, and two deaths from diabetes were reported in patients with PWS. The diabetes is type II, non-insulin-dependent-type diabetes; however, in spite of this, one individual has developed ketoacidosis, and the development of microaneurysms has been noted. It thus seems clear that there is an increased incidence of diabetes mellitus in individuals with PWS, but that a major part of this results from their obesity.

Hypogonadism and cryptorchidism are characteristic features.[20] The penis is usually small, and other components of the male reproductive system are present, but small. Histologic examination of the testis showed immaturity without germinal cells. The Sertoli cells are present, and there are diminutive tubules. Menarche and menstruation have both been reported, and precocious puberty has been noted in several clinics.[24] These reports of precocious pubertal development may represent a variant of PWS in which the hypothalamic-pituitary-gonadal axis functions normally with premature onset of menarche; however, there is an alternative explanation for this phenomenon. The initial phases of sexual development are produced by adrenal steroids and are called the "adrenarche". Among these changes are development of pubic hair and the beginnings of axillary hair. This is normally followed by production of ovarian estrogen with completion of the pubertal sequence. In patients with PWS, adrenal function will certainly be adequate to permit the adrenarche to appear. Formation of estrogen also may occur to some extent by conversion of adrenal steroids in peripheral tissues. Adipose tissue stromal cells can convert Δ^4-androstenedione to estrone by aromatization. As the quantity of adipose tissue increases, the amounts of estrogenic compounds produced will also increase. It is conceivable that breakthrough bleeding occurring in a partially estrogenized uterus might be interpreted as menstruation. It would be more likely to occur in the more obese girls with PWS.

Several reports of autopsy findings provide a little insight into the nature of the problem in PWS. The hyperphagia, hypogonadism, and short stature have suggested a hypothalamic problem, but careful histologic examination of the brain by routine methods has failed to show any neuropathologic lesions. However, use of immunologic techniques showed a decrease in the vasopressin content in the VMN (ventromedical nucleus).[22]

e. X-Linked Obesity

Four reports have documented cases of X-linked obesity, usually in association with severe mental retardation. Borjeson et al.[25] reported an individual with X-linked recessively inherited obesity, severe mental retardation, hypogonadism with low or normal levels of gonadotropin, and short stature. Most of these cases have coarse facial features with large ears and microcephaly. In 1979 Vasquez et al.[26] reported an X-linked type of obesity with profound mental retardation, true gynecomastia, and short stature with many other features similar to PWS, except for the mode of inheritance and the normal hands and feet. More recently, Young and Hughes[27] reported four cases of X-linked mental retardation with short stature, obesity, and hypogonadism.[27] Seizures were present in three of the four individuals, and mental tests revealed an IQ of approximately 25. Gonadotropins were high in these individuals, and testosterone, measured in one case, was low. In a recent publication, Wilson et al.[28] have reported 14 males in three generations who have X-linked mental retardation, obesity, gynecomastia, speech difficulties, emotional lability, tapering fingers, and small feet. In contrast with the other reports, the mental retardation in these men was only mild to moderate. The gene is located near the centromere of the X chromosome. These cases are thus different from the three earlier ones.

2. Genetic Predisposition

There is clearly an underlying genetic basis for the development of most cases of obesity. Since the major thrust of this volume is the genetics of obesity, the reader should consult appropriate chapters for additional details on this subject.

III. PREVALENCE

Data on means for BMI have been compiled from a number of countries around the world and are presented in Table 4. Prevalence data using a BMI of 25 to 30 kg/m^2 to define overweight and a BMI > 30 kg/m^2 to define obesity are presented in Table 4.

A. FACTORS AFFECTING WEIGHT WITHIN COUNTRIES

Within any country there are a number of clearcut differences in frequency of obesity. These differences are related to age, sex, ethnic factors, and socioeconomic status.

Table 4. **Mean body mass index in several countries**

Country/region	Age	Male	Female	Ref.
North America				
U.S.	16–50	24.9 ± 3.6	24.1 ± 6.5	30
U.S. Cardio Study				
White	18–30	24.1	23.0	31
Black	18–30	24.7	25.9	31
Europe				
France	16–50	23.5 ± 2.6	22.1 ± 4.0	30
United Kingdom	16–50	23.8 ± 2.9	23.2 ± 4.6	30
Sweden	16–24	22.3 ± 1.80	21.5 ± 1.75	32
	25–34	23.7 ± 1.89	22.2 ± 1.90	32
	35–44	24.8 ± 2.05	23.3 ± 2.12	32
	45–54	25.6 ± 2.63	25.0 ± 2.97	32
	55–64	25.8 ± 2.62	26.2 ± 3.05	32
	65–74	25.6 ± 2.78	26.1 ± 3.23	32
	75–84	25.1 ± 1.67	25.4 ± 1.82	32
Czechslovakia				
1985	25–64	26.9	26.9	33
1988		27.5	27.4	33
Asia				
Fiji				
Urban	>40	30.1 ± 5.2	30.9 ± 5.9	34
Rural	>40	25.4 ± 3.3	25.8 ± 5.1	34
India (Bombay)	15–76	23.9 ± 3.8	24.8 ± 4.3	35
Hawaii	20–29	30.6	28.7	36
	30–39	30.4	30.3	36
	40–49	31.6	31.6	36
	50–59	31.1	30.2	36
	>60	33.2	—	36
	20–24	30.4 ± 4.6	29.9 ± 5.8	37
	25–34	31.3 ± 6.0	34.3 ± 7.8	37
	35–44	32.6 ± 5.4	35.8 ± 7.7	37
	45–54	31.3 ± 5.7	34.7 ± 6.5	37
	55–64	32.1 ± 5.0	34.1 ± 5.5	37
	65–74	31.6 ± 8.9	33.4 ± 6.9	37
Samoa	20–24	24.6 ± 2.8	25.3 ± 3.9	37
	25–34	25.1 ± 3.2	26.7 ± 4.1	37
	35–44	26.5 ± 4.3	29.0 ± 4.7	37
	45–54	27.1 ± 4.9	29.6 ± 4.8	37
	55–64	28.8 ± 5.4	31.0 ± 8.4	37
	65–74	26.5 ± 3.9	28.6 ± 4.1	37
Manu	20–24	26.4 ± 2.6	29.5 ± 7.9	37
	25–34	30.7 ± 4.4	32.3 ± 6.0	37
	35–44	29.2 ± 4.7	35.1 ± 5.8	37
	45–54	27.2 ± 4.7	33.8 ± 7.4	37
	55–64	28.0 ± 5.9	30.7 ± 6.1	37
	65–74	28.7 ± 4.5	29.5 ± 5.8	37
Tutuila	20–24	26.5 ± 3.6	27.9 ± 4.9	37
	25–34	30.2 ± 5.0	32.4 ± 6.6	37
	35–44	30.4 ± 5.5	34.4 ± 6.6	37

Table 4 (continued). **Mean body mass index in several countries**

Country/region	Age	Male	Female	Ref.
	45–54	32.0 ± 6.4	35.3 ± 6.7	37
	55–64	28.8 ± 5.5	33.3 ± 7.5	37
	65–74	28.6 ± 6.2	32.3 ± 5.9	37
Africa				
South Africa				
CORIS Study	15–24	22.9 ± 3.3	22.8 ± 3.6	38
	25–34	25.9 ± 3.7	23.2 ± 4.6	38
	35–44	26.4 ± 3.6	25.7 ± 5.1	38
	45–54	27.2 ± 4.1	27.4 ± 5.6	38
	55–64	27.0 ± 4.0	28.1 ± 5.1	38
Japan	30–39	23.1	21.9	39
	40–49	23.2	22.9	39
	50–59	23.1	23.5	39
	60–69	22.6	23.5	39
Nauru	20–29	32.3 ± 0.7	34.3 ± 1.0	40
	30–39	33.1 ± 0.9	35.6 ± 1.0	40
	40–49	31.6 ± 1.1	35.7 ± 1.0	40
	50–59	30.2 ± 1.3	33.8 ±1.3	40
	60+	31.3 ± 1.4	29.7 ± 2.3	40

1. Age

BMI increases with age in both males and females. Using data from Sweden or the Pacific Islands it is clear that the increase in mean BMI with age is greater in females than in males. This also applies to most other countries as well. Black women have a higher prevalence of obesity at most ages compared to white women in the U.S. (Table 5).

2. Sex

In almost all populations the mean BMI of women is higher than men, particularly at older ages (Table 4). Among Caucasians there is higher prevalence of overweight men than women, but a higher prevalence of obesity in women than men, reflecting the difference in the BMI distribution curves for men and women. Among black Americans, a higher percentage of men are overweight than women between age 20 and 50. More older black women are overweight than black men, and more African-American women are obese at all ages.

3. Ethnic Factors

Obesity is a more common problem in blacks and Hispanics than in whites. It is also more common in native Americans, particularly the Indians living in the southwestern U.S. and in Polynesians and Micronesians (Table 5).

4. Socioeconomic Status

Socioeconomic status plays an important role in the prevalence of obesity. Studies in North America and Europe have almost uniformly demonstrated the importance of socioeconomic status in the development of obesity in females and, to a lesser extent, in males. This is clearly illustrated in data from the U.S. (Table 5). Women living below the poverty line assigned by the U.S. government have a higher prevalence of obesity (BMI > 30 kg/m^2) at almost all ages, whether they are black American, Hispanic American, or

Caucasian American, than those living above the poverty line. The differences among males were small and not statistically significant.

5. Time Trends in Obesity

Several studies suggest that there has been a progressive increase in weight for height throughout the past 100 years.[1] For example, the weight of men 5 feet 8 inches tall inducted into the U.S. military service rose from 147 pounds in 1863 to 168 pounds in 1962. A similar increase has been observed in the Framingham cohort, with males showing a steady increase throughout the early part of this century and females showing a slight downward average weight. Life insurance data and the data from the National Center for Health Statistics (NCHS) also report a small increase in average body weight for height.

Table 5. **Prevalence of obesity**

Country/region	Age	Overweight (BMI 25 to <30 kg/m^2)		Obese (BMI > 30 kg/m^2)		Ref.
		Male	Female	Male	Female	
North America						55
U.S.						
1976–1980						
White	20–74					
	20–29	29.83	15.14	7.85	7.63	
	30–39	41.69	19.06	12.03	14.89	
	40–49	45.33	24.13	14.82	16.39	
	50–59	46.53	29.66	13.63	20.22	
	60–69	45.16	33.72	13.37	20.66	
	70–74	39.45	37.34	13.82	18.62	
Black	20–74					
	20–29	22.99	19.23	8.36	19.25	
	30–39	32.91	25.86	13.09	29.33	
	40–49	45.47	38.56	23.09	33.04	
	50–59	43.53	37.61	19.76	41.75	
	60–69	33.77	36.21	16.81	41.00	
	70–74	37.83	56.71	11.56	18.35	
Below Poverty						
White	20–74					
	20–29	18.8	16.3	5.2	5.9	
	30–39	41.7	29.8	19.3	28.0	
	40–49	42.2	18.4	4.3	34.6	
	50–59	35.3	29.0	13.9	29.5	
	60–69	37.2	30.2	14.1	25.1	
	70–74	27.7	35.6	11.3	29.4	
Black	20–74					
	20–29	17.6	9.5	3.7	22.0	
	30–39	26.9	22.8	15.2	31.6	
	40–49	45.9	41.0	12.2	40.7	
	50–59	24.4	34.7	11.5	43.7	
	60–69	33.0	28.8	19.9	42.3	
	70–74	42.8	54.0	12.9	29.5	

Table 5 (continued). **Prevalence of obesity**

Country/region	Age	Overweight (BMI 25 to <30 kg/m²) Male	Female	Obese (BMI > 30 kg/m²) Male	Female	Ref.
Hispanic	20–74					
	20–29	21.0	26.1	13.17	16.2	
	30–39	44.1	37.0	20.67	27.0	
	40–49	47.2	34.0	18.55	38.7	
	50–59	36.8	36.1	19.50	42.8	
	60–69	47.0	43.3	14.88	37.0	
Above Poverty						
White	20–74					
	20–29	30.9	14.9	8.1	7.9	
	30–39	41.5	17.7	11.8	13.6	
	40–49	45.7	24.7	15.8	15.1	
	50–59	46.8	29.6	13.7	19.0	
	60–69	45.8	33.7	13.5	20.3	
	70–74	42.0	37.3	13.1	16.4	
Black	20–74					
	20–29	3.0	25.8	8.9	18.0	
	30–39	26.7	34.2	9.4	28.2	
	40–49	37.3	45.9	26.7	29.1	
	50–59	34.6	48.1	24.1	46.8	
	60–69	38.2	33.3	16.2	41.2	
	70–74	55.8	37.6	7.4	12.8	
Hispanic	20–74					
	20–29	34.6	26.4	9.8	11.9	
	30–39	46.4	35.6	15.0	20.5	
	40–49	61.2	36.4	14.7	30.4	
	50–59	48.3	36.7	21.9	31.1	
	60–69	49.6	43.5	18.3	33.0	
	70–74	34.0	14.9	21.3	44.2	
Canada				12.0	15.0	41
	35–44	46	21	12.0	16.0	42
				8.5	9.3	41
	35–44	43	21	11.0	8.0	42
Europe						
France						30
Sweden	16–84	35	26	7.0	8.0	32
Italy	15–44			4.8	3.9	41
	45–64			9.9	11.1	41
Northwest	15–80	27	15	4.1	5.1	43
East		31	17	4.4	5.0	43
Central		31	19	5.0	6.4	43
South		31	20	7.8	8.7	43
Netherlands	20–34			1.9	2.0	41
	35–49			4.2	5.0	41
	50–64			5.4	10.3	41
	19–31	22	12	2.0	2.0	44
1974–1988	37–43	40–45	25–30	5–6	7–8	45

Table 5 (continued). **Prevalence of obesity**

Country/region	Age	Overweight (BMI 25 to <30 kg/m²) Male	Female	Obese (BMI > 30 kg/m²) Male	Female	Ref.
1981–1986	33–37	35–40	—	5–6	—	45
1981–1988	35–49	38	21	5.0	6.0	46
	19–35	34	24	4.0	6.0	47
U.K.	20–34			4.0	4.7	41
	35–49			7.9	8.6	41
	50–64			7.4	14.3	41
	35–44	38	24	8.0	8.0	42
Germany	25–69	49	45	16	16	48
South America						
Costa Rica	20–25			0.0	2.8	41
	40–45			5.7	14.4	41
El Salvador	20–25			0.0	1.3	41
	40–45			0.0	1.5	41
Guatemala	20–45			0.0	0.0	41
	40–45			0.0	5.6	41
Honduras	20–45			0.0	1.0	41
	40–45			2.8	6.0	41
Nicaragua	20–45			2.3	3.0	41
	40–45			3.1	16.4	41
Panama	20–25			0.0	0.0	41
	40–45			2.3	1.7	41
Trinidad	40			—	32.0	41
	74			—	27.0	41
Australia	25			4.0	5.7	41
	25–64	42.8	23.0	8.6	13.3	49
Africa						
Seychelles	25–34			3.8	8.9	50
	35–44			4.7	29.4	50
	45–54			2.8	26.9	50
	55–64			6.6	33.1	50
	Age standard			4.2	20.9	50
South Africa						
Black	25–45				19.0	51
Cape Peninsula	15–24	5.3	24.3	2.1	6.8	52
	25–34	19.8	41.5	1.0	17.0	52
	35–44	29.2	46.5	5.8	20.5	52
	45–54	35.8	40.4	6.3	42.6	52
	55–64	26.6	34.7	15.6	45.3	52
	15–64	23.8	37.8	6.1	25.9	52
	15–24	17.0	23.1	3.6	4.6	38
	25–34	42.1	29.9	13.2	10.5	38
	35–44	49.5	40.0	14.3	15.6	38
	45–54	50.0	48.2	20.9	23.8	38
	55–64	49.0	48.0	19.8	31.7	38
	15–64	41.9	38.8	14.7	18.0	38

Table 5 (continued). **Prevalence of obesity**

Country/region	Age	Overweight (BMI 25 to <30 kg/m²) Male	Female	Obese (BMI > 30 kg/m²) Male	Female	Ref.
Asia						
Solomon Islands						
Munda	18–34			7.0	34.0	53
Melanesia urban	35–54			19.0	43.0	53
	>55			10.0	33.0	53
Paradise	18–34			5.0	43	53
Melanesia traditional	35–54			12.0	53.0	53
	>55			19.0	31.0	53
Solstar	18–34			33.0	63.0	53
Micronesia	35–54			51.0	80.0	53
	>55			38.0	48.0	53
India (Bombay)	15–76	28.5	31.8	6.2	10.7	35
Thailand	>30	30.5	30.5	11.1	11.1	54

B. PREVALENCE BETWEEN COUNTRIES

Kluthe and Schubert[29] showed that in Europe the prevalence of obesity in females ranged from 2% to more than 50%, while the data for males ranged from 2% to over 40%. These differences were in part related to the criteria used to define obesity. Data on the prevalence between countries can be best evaluated using the same index derived from population-based studies. In Table 5, overweight is defined as a BMI of 25 to 30 kg/m^2 and obesity as a BMI > 30 kg/m.^{2}

There are some striking regional differences. Among women in the Micronesian and Melanesian populations the prevalence of obesity is between 30 and 80%. This is substantially higher than in any other region. The prevalence of obesity is also very high in South Africa, the Seychelles, and Trinidad. In contrast, the lowest figures are seen in several Central American countries. Males in the U.S. have a higher prevalence of obesity than in any European country except Germany. American women are also more obese than European women with the exception of German women, where the prevalence is almost identical.

ACKNOWLEDGMENTS

The author thanks Dr. Robert Kuczmarski for providing the data on prevalence of obesity by BMI groupings using NCHS data. Ms. Millie Cutrer and Ms. Terry Hodges were essential in preparing the manuscript.

REFERENCES

1. **Bray, G. A.,** Major problems in internal medicine, in *The Obesity Patient,* Vol. 9, W. B. Saunders, Philadelphia, 1976, 1.
2. **Von Noorden, C.,** Obesity, in *Metabolism and Practical Medicine,* Von Noorden, C., Ed., W. T. Keener, Chicago, 1907, 693.
3. **Abraham, S., Johnson, C. L., and Najjar, M. F.,** Weight and height of adults 18–74 years of age: United States, 1971–74, in Vital and Health Statistics, Ser. 11, No.

21, DHEW Publ. No. PHS-79-1659, National Center for Health Statistics, U.S. Public Health Service, U.S. Department of Health, Education, and Welfare, Hyattsville, MD, 1979, 49.

4. **Bray, G. A. and Gray, D. S.,** Obesity: part I — pathogenesis, *West. J. Med.,* 149, 429, 1988.
5. **Bray, G. A. and Gallagher, T. F., Jr.,** Manifestations of hypothalamic obesity in man: a comprehensive investigation of eight patients and a review of the literature, *Medicine,* 54, 301, 1975.
6. **Bray, G. A.,** Syndromes of hypothalamic obesity in man, *Pediatr. Ann.,* 13(7), 525, 1984.
7. **Franks, S., Kiddy, D., Sharp, P., Singh, A., Reed, M., Seppala, M., Koistinen, R., and Hamilton-Fairley, D.,** Obesity and polycystic ovary syndrome, *Ann. N.Y. Acad. Sci.,* 626, 201, 1991.
8. **Yen, S. C. C.,** The polycystic ovary syndrome, *Clin. Endocrinol.,* 12, 177, 1980.
9. **World Health Organization,** Diet, Nutrition, and Prevention of Chronic Diseases, Tech. Rep. Ser. 797, World Health Organization, Geneva, 1990.
10. **Lissner, L., Levitsky, D. A., Strupp, B. J., Kalkwark, H. J., and Roe, D. A.,** Dietary fat and the regulation of energy intake in human subjects, *Am. J. Clin. Nutr.,* 46(6), 886, 1987.
11. **Kromhout, D.,** Changes in energy and macronutrients in 871 middle-aged men during 10 years of follow-up (the Zutphen Study), *Am. J. Clin. Nutr.,* 37, 287, 1983.
12. **Bray, G. A.,** Obesity, in *The Genetic Basis of Common Diseases,* King, R. A., Rotter, J. I., and Motulsky, A. G., Eds., Oxford University Press, New York, 1992, 507.
13. **Stiggelbout, W.,** The Bardet-Biedl syndrome, including Hutchinson-Laurence-Moon syndrome, in *Handbook of Clinical Neurology,* Vinkin, P. K. and Bruyn, G .W., Eds., Elsevier/North-Holland, New York, 1972, 380.
14. **Nadjimi, B., Flanagan, M. J., and Christian, J. R.,** Laurence-Moon-Biedl syndrome associated with multiple genitourinary tract abnormalities, *Am. J. Dis. Child.,* 117, 352, 1968.
15. **Goldstein, J. L. and Fialkow, P. J.,** The Alstrom syndrome. Report of three cases with further delineation of the clinical, pathophysiological, and genetic aspects of the disorder, *Medicine,* 52, 53, 1973.
16. **Cohen, M. M., Hall, B. D., Smith, D. W., Graham, C. B., and Lampert, K. L.,** A new syndrome with hypotonia, obesity, mental deficiency, and facial, oral, ocular, and limb anomalies, *J. Pediatr.,* 83, 280, 1973.
17. **Friedman, E. and Sack, J.,** The cohen syndrome: report of five new cases and a review of the literature, *J. Craniofac. Genet. Dev. Biol.,* 2, 193, 1982.
18. **Temtamy, S. A.,** Carpenters syndrome: acrocephalopolysyndactyly. An autosomal recessive syndrome, *J. Pediatr.,* 69, 111, 1966.
19. **Prader, A., Labhart, A., and Willi, H.,** Ein Syndrom von Adipositas, Kleinwuchs, Kryptorchismus und Oligophrenie nach myatonieartigem zustandin Neugeborenenalter, *Schweiz. Med. Wochenschr.,* 44, 1260, 1956.
20. **Bray, G. A., Dahms, W. T., Swerdloff, R. S., Fiser, R. H., Atkinson, R. L., and Carrel, R. E.,** The Prader-Willi Syndrome: A study of 40 patients and a review of the literature, *Medicine,* 62(2), 59, 1983.
21. **Zellweger, H.,** Diagnosis and therapy in the first phase of Prader-Willi syndrome, in *Prader-Willi Syndrome,* Holm, V. A., Sulzbacher, S., Pipes, P., and Steffes, M. J., Eds., University Park Press, Baltimore, 1981, 55.
22. **Bray, G. A.,** Genetic, hypothalamic and endocrine features of clinical and experimental obesity, in *Progress in Brain Research,* Swaab, D. F., Hofman, M. A., Mirmiran, M., Ravid, R., van Leeuwen, F. W., Eds., Elsevier, Amsterdam, 1992, 93.

23. **Zipf, W. B., O'Dorisio, T. M., and Berntson, G. G.,** Short-term infusion of pancreatic polypeptide: effect on children with Prader-Willi syndrome, *Am. J. Clin. Nutr.,* 51(2), 162, 1990.
24. **Wannarachue, N., Ruvalcaba, R. H. A., and Kelley, V. C.,** Hypogonadism in Prader-Willi syndrome, *Am. J. Ment. Defic.,* 79, 592, 1975.
25. **Borjeson, M., Forssman, H., and Lehman, O.,** An X-linked, recessively inherited syndrome characterized by grave mental deficiency, epilepsy, and endocrine disorder, *Acta Med. Scand.,* 171, 13, 1962.
26. **Vasquez, S. B., Hurst, D. J., and Sotos, J. R.,** X-Linked hypogonadism, gynecomastia, mental retardation, short stature and obesity — a new syndrome, *J. Pediatr.,* 94, 52, 1979.
27. **Young, I. D. and Hughes, H. E.,** Sex-linked mental retardation, short stature, obesity and hypogonadism: report of a family, *J. Ment. Defic. Res.,* 25, 153, 1982.
28. **Wilson, M., Mulley, J., Gedeon, A., Robinson, H., and Turner, G.,** New X-linked syndrome of mental retardation, gynecomastia, and obesity is linked to DXS255, *Am. J. Med. Genet.,* 40, 406, 1991.
29. **Kluthe, R. and Schubert, A.,** Obesity in Europe, *Ann. Intern. Med.,* 103, 1037, 1985.
30. **Laurier, D., Guiguet, M., Chau, N. P., Wells, J. A., and Valleron, A.,** Prevalence of obesity: a comparative survey in France, the United Kingdom and the United States, *Int. J. Obes.,* 16, 565, 1992.
31. **Burke, G. L., Jacobs, D. R., Sprafka, J. M., Savage, P. J., Sidney, S., and Wagenke, L. E.,** Obesity and overweight in young-adults — the cardia study (Technical Note), *Prev. Med.,* 19, 476, 1990.
32. **Kuskowska-Wolk, A. and Rossner, S.,** Prevalence of obesity in Sweden — cross sectional study of a representative adult population, *J. Intern. Med.,* 227(4), 241, 1990.
33. **Skodova, Z., Pisa, Z., Berka, L., Cicha, Z., Emrova, R., Pikhartova, J., Vorlicek, J., Wiesn'er, E., Vojtisek, P., Petrilkova, Z., Cerovska, J., and Valenta, Z.,** Trends in body weight in the population of the Czech Republic, *Cas. Lek. Cesk.,* 129(33), 1033, 1990.
34. **Russell-Jones, D. L., Hoskins, P., Kearney, E., Morris, R., Katoaga, S., Slavin, B., and Turtle, J. R.,** Rural/urban differences of diabetes — impaired glucose tolerance, hypertension, obesity, glycosolated haemoglobin, nutritional proteins, fasting cholesterol and apolipoproteins in Fijian Melanesians over 40, *Q. J. Med.,* 74(273), 75, 1990.
35. **Dhurandhar, N. V. and Kulkarni, P. R.,** Prevalence of obesity in Bombay, *Int. J. Obes.,* 16, 367, 1992.
36. **Aluli, N. E.,** Prevalence of obesity in a native Hawaiian population, *Am. J. Clin. Nutr.,* 53(6), 1556, 1991.
37. **McGarvey, S. T.,** Obesity in Samoans and a perspective on its etiology in Polynesians, *Am. J. Clin Nutr,* 53, 15865, 1991.
38. **Jooste, P. L., Steenkamp, H. J., Benade, A. J. S., and Rossouw, J. E.,** Prevalence of overweight and obesity and its relation to coronary heart disease in the CORIS study, *S. Afr. Med. J.,* 74, 101, 1988.
39. **Horibe, H.,** Trend of average height, weight and skinfolds in the Japanese, *Diabetes Res. Clin. Pract.,* 10, S113, 1990.
40. **Sircree, R. A., Zimmet, P. Z., King, H., and Coventry, J. S.,** Weight change amongst Nauruans over 6.5 years: extent, and association with glucose intolerance, *Diabetes Res. Clin. Prac.,* 3, 327, 1987.
41. **Gurney, M. and Gorstein, J.,** The global prevalence of obesity — an initial overview of available data, *World Health Stat. Q.,* 41, 251, 1988.
42. **Millar, W. J. and Stephens, T.,** The prevalence of overweight and obesity in Britain, Canada, and United States, *Am. J. Public Health,* 77(7), 38, 1987.

43. **Pagano, R., Godi, L., and Cairella, M.,** Obesity in Italy, *Public Health,* 102, 555, 1988.
44. **Kluthe, R. and Schubert, A.,** Obesity in Europe, *Ann. Intern. Med.,* 103, 1037, 1985.
45. **Blokstra, A. and Kromhout, D.,** Trends in obesity in young-adults in The Netherlands from 1974 to 1986, *Int. J. Obes.,* 15(8), 513, 1991.
46. **Verweij, G. C. G.,** Gezondheidsinquetes. Ontwikkelingen in onderen overgewicht, 1981–1988, *Maandbericht Gezondheidsstat,* 11, 5, 1989.
47. **Deurenberg, P. and Hautvast, J. G.,** Prevalence of overweight and obesity in The Netherlands in relation to sociodemographic variables, lifestyle and eating behavior: starting points for the prevention and treatment of obesity, *Bibl. Nutr. Dieta,* 44, 8, 1989.
48. **Greiser, E., Joeckel, K. H., Giersiepen, K., Maschewsky-Schneider, U., and Zachcial, M.,** Cardiovascular disease risk factors, CHD morbitity and mortality in the Federal Republic Germany, *Int. J. Epidemiol.,* 18(Suppl. 1), S118, 1989.
49. **Schwarz, B., Bischof, H. P., and Kunze, M.,** Overweight and coronary risk-factors results from a Western Austrian survey, *Soz. Praeventivmed.,* 36(6), 322, 1991.
50. **Tappy, L., Bovet, P., and Shamlaye, C.,** Prevalence of diabetes and obesity in the adult-population of the Seychelles, *Diabetes Med.,* 8(5), 448, 1991.
51. **Walker, A. R., Walker, B. F., Walker, A. J., and Vorster, H. H.,** Low frequency of adverse sequelae of obesity in South African rural black women, *Int. J. Vitam. Nutr. Res.,* 59(2), 224, 1989.
52. **Steyn, K., Fourie, J., Rossouw, J. E., Langenhoven, M. L., Joubert, G., and Chalton, D. O.,** Anthropometric profile of the coloured population of the Cape Peninsula, *S. Afr. Med. J.,* 78, 68, 1990.
53. **Eason, R. J., Pada, J., Wallace, R., Henry, A., and Thornton, R.,** Changing patterns of hypertension, diabetes, obesity and diet among Melanesians and Micronesians in the Solomon Islands, *Med. J. Aust.,* 146, 465, 1987.
54. **Bunnag, S. C., Sitthi-Amorn, C., and Chandraprasert, S.,** The prevalence of obesity, risk factors and associated diseases in Klong-Toey government apartment houses, *Diabet. Res. Clin. Pract.,* 10(S1), S81, 1990.
55. **Kuczmarski, R.,** personal communucation.

Chapter 3

Nongenetic Determinants of Obesity and Body Fat Topography

James O. Hill, Michael J. Pagliassotti, and John C. Peters

TABLE OF CONTENTS

I. INTRODUCTION

Obesity results from the combined effects of genetic and nongenetic factors, with the relative contribution of each being unclear. Adoption studies[1] and studies of monozygotic human twins[2,3] have convincingly demonstrated that genotype has an important influence on body fat and on almost every aspect of energy balance. Bouchard[2] estimates the variability in percent body fat among humans to be 25% genetic, 30% due to cultural transmission, and 45% due to nontransmissible factors. Thus, as much as 75% of the

0-8493-4880-3/94/$0.00+$.50

variation in body fatness may be influenced by nongenetic factors. Nongenetic influences on the development of obesity can be seen in studies of populations that either have migrated to different cultural and geographical locations[4] or have undergone social and cultural evolution, e.g., Westernization.[5] In these populations, increased total energy intake, increased dietary fat intake, and decreased physical activity are potential nongenetic contributors to the increased incidence of obesity.[4,5]

II. INTERACTION OF GENETIC AND NONGENETIC INFLUENCES IN OBESITY DEVELOPMENT

An understanding of obesity requires an understanding of how the genotype and the environment interact to affect body weight and body composition. Our view is that the genotype defines the boundary conditions or capacity of the system that determines body weight and body composition to respond to the environment. Nongenetic factors determine at what point within these boundaries the system operates. In other words, the genotype determines what can happen and the environment determines what does happen. This chapter will focus on nongenetic factors involved in determining body weight and body composition.

In the most rudimentary sense, obesity can be viewed as the result of a cumulative positive energy balance (i.e., energy ingested in excess of energy expended). In order to understand nongenetic influences on the degree of positive energy balance, i.e., energy stored (E_{stored}), it is necessary to study nongenetic influences on energy intake (E_{in}) and energy expenditure (E_{out}). E_{in} refers to the amount, composition, and pattern of food eaten, and the nongenetic component of E_{in} is largely dependent on behavior. E_{out} refers to the amount and composition of fuel oxidized and is influenced both by metabolic processes and behavior (physical activity).

Viewed in this way, obesity is not solely a metabolic or a behavioral problem, and it cannot be understood without studying both metabolism and behavior. Whether or not a person becomes obese under a given set of environmental and nutritional circumstances is determined by an interaction between the behavioral response to those circumstances and the metabolic response to the behavior. These processes determine how much and what type of energy enters the system and the disposition of that energy within the body. Whether or not body weight and body composition remain the same, increase or decrease over time depends on how closely metabolism matches behavior so that $E_{in} = E_{out}$.

In understanding obesity it is important to account for individual differences in how body weight and body composition respond under different conditions. This involves understanding how different people exposed to similar environmental and nutritional conditions achieve and maintain different levels of body weight and body composition.

III. THE NATURE OF THE SYSTEM WHICH DETERMINES BODY WEIGHT AND BODY COMPOSITION

The model shown in Figure 1 depicts how genetic and nongenetic influences on behavior and metabolism interact to influence energy intake, energy expenditure, and ultimately, body weight and composition. As shown at the top of the figure, the characteristics of the organism, which can be partitioned into behavioral and metabolic components, are determined by both genetic and nongenetic factors.

The behavioral phenotype reflects characteristics of the organism which influence the amount and composition of food consumed and the amount of physical activity. The specific eating and exercise behavior exhibited by a person is determined by an interaction between the physiological state (hunger drive), the immediate environmental and nutritional conditions, and the behavioral phenotype.

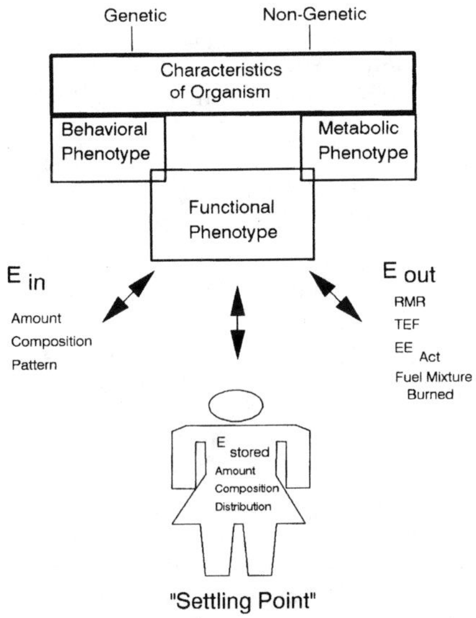

Figure 1. This model depicts the way in which genetic and nongenetic factors combine to influence body weight and body composition. The characteristics of the organism can be separated into behavioral and metabolic aspects, each influenced by genetic and nongenetic factors. The combination of behavioral and metabolic characteristics comprises the functional phenotype. The interaction between the immediate environment and the functional phenotype determines the level at which body weight and body composition will be maintained. E_{in}, energy input; E_{out}, energy output; RMR, resting metabolic rate; TEF, thermic effect of food; EE_{ACT}, energy expenditure associated with physical activity; E_{stored}, energy stored.

The metabolic phenotype reflects characteristics of the organism which determine the fate of ingested energy, including amount and composition of fuel burned and the fate of excess energy. Thus, it represents the current state of a variety of metabolic processes involved in digestion, absorption, oxidation, storage, and interconversion of nutrients.

On the whole-organism level, the behavioral and metabolic components are not expressed separately, but simultaneously. The integrated expression of these components can be termed the functional phenotype, and it represents the current behavioral and metabolic state of an individual. These system characteristics determine how the organism responds to a given set of environmental and nutritional conditions.

A. BODY WEIGHT AND BODY COMPOSITION AS A "SETTLING POINT"

Figure 1 depicts a system in which behavior and metabolism interact to determine body weight and body composition. In this model there is no need to hypothesize that body weight and body composition are regulated directly; rather, body weight and body composition are the product of many other regulated processes. The body weight and body composition achieved under a particular set of environmental and nutritional conditions can be viewed as a "settling point", a concept introduced by Wirtshafter and Davis.[6] The settling point represents the body weight and body composition associated with the condition in which the average energy intake and energy expenditure are equivalent and the average intakes of protein, carbohydrate, and fat are matched by an equivalent oxidation of each. The model depicted in Figure 1 is a complex one in which a change in any single component must either (1) produce compensation which allows the settling point to be maintained or (2) alter the settling point.

IV. NONGENETIC INFLUENCES ON THE SYSTEM

In most people the settling point remains constant over time. This suggests either that these people resist wide variations in behavior despite being exposed to wide variations in environmental and nutritional conditions or that the system has some ability to compensate for effects of the environment without necessitating a change in E_{stored}. An example of such compensation would be an increase in food intake in response to an increase in physical activity. Alternatively, the incidence of adult-onset obesity is sufficiently high[5] to suggest that many people respond to nutritional and environmental conditions with behaviors for which the system cannot compensate completely and which necessitate changes in E_{stored}.

A. NONGENETIC INFLUENCES ON AMOUNT AND COMPOSITION OF ENERGY INTAKE

1. Acute Influences of Environment on Eating Behavior

Human eating is a learned habitual behavior[7] thought to stem from conditioning of responses based on previous experience in which the postingestive consequences of a particular food act as unconditioned stimuli.[8] Properties of the food itself (e.g., orosensory properties), as well as social and cultural factors associated with food, can be associated with the metabolic effects of that food to form the basis of a learned conditioned response that can guide eating behavior. This associative learning is essential for controlling food intake and maintaining energy balance in a sociocultural environment in which meals are taken only at particular times. This is because there is a temporal separation between the orosensory properties and context in which food is eaten (which occur immediately) and the metabolic consequences of the food (which may take many hours to complete).

There is no doubt that the immediate context in which food consumption occurs (i.e., the environmental and nutritional conditions that exist) can influence the amount and composition of what is eaten.[9] The appearance and aroma of food, time of day, and the number of people present are examples of environmental factors that can affect the amount of food eaten at a given meal.[9] The variety and nutrient composition of available food are examples of nutritional variables which can influence food intake. For example, a number of studies have found that diets high in fat increase total energy intake above levels seen when lower fat foods are available.[10-12] For a given physiological state (e.g., hunger drive), the exact response of the system to the immediate context is determined by the interaction between this context and the behavioral phenotype of the individual (i.e., genotype × previous life experience).

Beyond these immediate environmental and nutritional conditions, there are other factors that contribute to the behavioral phenotype of the individual that can affect food intake and selection. For example, cognitive factors such as body awareness, self-image, and beliefs about particular foods can influence both short- and long-term food intake.[7,14,15] The prevalence of eating disorders among teenage girls is an example of how cognitive factors can affect eating behavior.[10]

Finally, cultural and social factors, such as ethnic and religious group and social class, can exert important effects on food intake and selection.[9,16] For example, in Western societies, overeating and obesity are more prevalent among lower social classes, in which negative attitudes about being overweight are not as prominent as in upper classes.[16] The opposite relationship is observed in developing countries, so that the incidence of obesity increases with increasing social status.[17] An individual's cultural history and social status are also part of the complex set of variables which determine the behavioral phenotype.

It should not be surprising, given the myriad of factors that contribute to an individual's behavioral phenotype, that there is no single "obese" eating style or behavioral phenotype. Numerous studies have been unsuccessful in identifying a single lean or obese eating style.[7] It may be possible, however, to distinguish groups of individuals who share common characteristics in eating behavior. For example, Schlundt et al.[18] used cluster analysis to identify five distinct types of eating behavior in obese females. These kinds of classifications may be useful in classifying individuals as to their behavioral susceptibility to obesity and in designing treatment and prevention strategies to help them avoid obesity development.

2. Plasticity of Eating Behavior

A permanent alteration in eating behavior would create a new behavioral phenotype and functional phenotype and might disrupt the steady state between intake and expenditure. The new steady state achieved following the behavioral shift would be a consequence of many factors, including the degree of behavior change, the resulting effect on the metabolic phenotype, and the resulting change in E_{stored}.

Obesity treatment programs illustrate how acute vs. permanent changes in eating behavior can affect the functional phenotype and the settling point. It is not difficult to produce acute changes in amount and composition of food eaten by overweight human subjects (i.e., dieting). Substantial changes in body weight and body composition can occur as a consequence of such changes.[19] However, the majority of overweight persons who lose weight regain it,[19] suggesting that the changes in food intake were not permanent and did not produce a permanent change in the steady state of the system. Not everyone, however, fails in weight reduction attempts, and those who succeed may be the ones who are able to permanently change the eating behavior and force a change in the steady state of the system at a lower level of body weight and body fat content than preweight reduction.

B. NONGENETIC INFLUENCES ON METABOLISM

There are a number of factors involved in determining the amount and composition of fuel burned by an individual. These include metabolic processes related to fuel absorption, digestion, storage, and interconversion as well as an individual's body composition and level of physical activity.

1. Environmental Influences on Amount of Fuel Burned

The amount of fuel burned (total energy expenditure) is an integrated sum of fuel oxidation occurring in all of the body's tissues and organ systems. These metabolic processes, which have been reviewed previously,[20] involve a variety of enzyme systems. The expression of these various metabolic processes under a given set of environmental and nutritional conditions represents the metabolic phenotype of the individual.

Total daily energy expenditure can be subdivided into resting metabolic rate (RMR), the thermic effect of food (TEF), and the energy expenditure associated with physical activity (EE_{ACT}).[21] Fat-free mass (FFM) can explain approximately 60 to 90% of the between-subject variation in RMR,[22,23] and RMR does not appear to be directly affected by the amount or composition of food eaten[24,25] or the amount or type of physical activity.[26-28]

The TEF may comprise 6 to 10% of total energy intake[29] and includes costs of digestion, absorption, and metabolism of ingested food.[20] Both the amount[24] and composition[30] of the diet can influence the TEF, but the effect is likely to be small.[31]

EE_{ACT} (amount of physical activity × energy cost of each unit of activity) is the most variable component of energy expenditure.[22,32] Differences in amount of voluntary physical activity are likely to be the major source of variability in EE_{ACT}, accounting for individual differences in daily energy expenditure as great as 1000 kcal/day.[22,28] Future research must focus on potential environmental and nutritional influences on this component of energy expenditure.

2. Determinants of the Composition of Fuel Burned

The amount of body fat mass[33] and the amount and composition of lean body tissue (e.g., skeletal muscle fiber type distribution[34,35]) are among the known chronic determinants of the composition of fuel burned. Among the acute determinants of the fuel composition burned are the amount and composition of food eaten,[11,25] the amount and type of physical activity,[36] and the state of energy balance of the organism.[11,25]

Maintenance of a consistent body composition requires that, on average over time, the fuel mixture ingested equals the fuel mixture burned.[36] This is important for understanding obesity development because acute changes in protein and carbohydrate intake produce rapid changes in the oxidation of each,[11,37,38] while fat oxidation is not acutely affected by changes in fat intake.[29,38,39] Substantial changes in fat oxidation in response to alterations in fat intake are seen only after the body fat mass is altered.[33] Because fat and carbohydrate differ in the effects on their own oxidation, the composition of the diet chosen can affect the composition of fuel burned and can alter the steady state of the entire system. Thus, the composition of food eaten can play an important role in regulation of body weight.

3. Modification of the Amount and Composition of Fuel Burned

Changes in diet composition can influence the composition of fuel burned, but some investigators believe that such changes (specifically, an increase in the fat/carbohydrate ratio) require an increase in the body fat mass before the composition of fuel burned is equal to the composition of energy ingested.[33] In this sense, a change from a low- to a high-fat diet may require an increase in body fat mass before the system can equilibrate such that $E_{in} = E_{out}$ and intake and oxidation of each macronutrient are equal. Several research groups are currently using whole-room indirect calorimeters to evaluate how changes in the composition of food eaten influence the composition of the fuel burned and the consequences for body weight and body composition.[11,33,40] Hill et al.[25] demonstrated that if total energy intake remains fixed at maintenance levels, a change in the fat/carbohydrate ratio of the diet can rapidly (within 3 days) produce a compensatory change in the fat/carbohydrate ratio of fuel burned. However, if energy intake is not fixed, changes in diet composition may produce both changes in energy intake[11-13] and in fuel oxidation,[11] and the specific changes may depend on the overall state of energy balance. For example, Hill and colleagues studied subjects eating a high-carbohydrate diet ad libitum for 7 days and the same subjects eating a high-fat diet ad libitum for 7 days. Total energy intake was higher on the high-fat diet than on the high-carbohydrate diet. Additionally, after 7 days of high-carbohydrate feeding, carbohydrate oxidation was increased to nearly match carbohydrate intake. Conversely, after 7 days of high-fat feeding, fat oxidation was only slightly increased, leaving subjects in substantial positive fat balance. Thus, when eaten ad libitum, high-fat diets tend to promote body fat accumulation as compared to high-carbohydrate diets because they produce greater positive energy and fat balances.

The composition of energy ingested in excess of usual energy expenditure also may be a factor in development of obesity. Horton et al. demonstrated[41] that 14 days of feeding excess energy as fat produced a greater amount of positive energy and fat balance than feeding a similar excess as carbohydrate in lean and obese men. This is because (1) fat oxidation is not rapidly stimulated by fat overfeeding, whereas carbohydrate oxidation is rapidly increased by carbohydrate overfeeding; and (2) excess fat is stored as body fat very efficiently, whereas excess carbohydrate is stored as body fat far less efficiently.

4. Changes in the Metabolic Phenotype

Theoretically, the metabolic phenotype can be modified at any time and such modification can affect the fate of ingested energy. However, the extent to which modifications in the metabolic phenotype can occur is probably related to the age of the individual. During childhood, it is likely that the metabolic phenotype develops as a consequence of the feeding behavior acquired by the child. In adulthood, the well-established metabolic phenotype will defend itself and will likely be less responsive to nongenetic influences. A clear demonstration of this can be seen with undernutrition, where early in life it can produce stunted growth[42] and permanent reductions in fat cell number.[43] Alternatively, undernutrition later in life results only in temporary reductions in fat cell size.[44]

There are several examples of the profound mutability of many metabolic processes of the fetus during pregnancy and of the infant in the neonatal period. The type of fat consumed during pregnancy and lactation can determine the carcass composition and fatty acid profile of the developing progeny.[45] Several studies have demonstrated the impact of overfeeding during the suckling period on adipose cellularity.[43] The characteristic insulin resistance of the suckling period can be removed by switching rats to a high-carbohydrate diet, but is maintained by continued intake of a high-fat diet.[46] Finally, several studies have demonstrated the ability to express enzymes prematurely by dietary manipulation during the suckling period.[47] In the developing rat (i.e., during growth), dietary manipulation (e.g., high-fat, high-protein, high-sucrose diets) can induce insulin resistance.[48,49] In addition, high-fat diets can increase adipose tissue lipoprotein lipase activity[50] and some oxidative enzymes in skeletal muscle.[51] All of these modifications have the ability to alter the metabolic fate of ingested energy.

A nonobese adult who has maintained a stable weight for a period of time has, by definition, adjusted the mixture of fuel burned to match the mixture of fuel ingested. Any changes in behavior that occur over time (such as declining physical activity or a change in self-selected diet composition) require further system adjustments in order to prevent changes in body composition. In this sense, an important aspect of the amount and composition of fuel burned is that this determines whether, and in what form, excess energy is available for storage in the body.

V. FUNCTIONAL PHENOTYPE

A. THE NATURE OF THE FUNCTIONAL PHENOTYPE

The functional phenotype represents the interaction between the behavioral and metabolic phenotypes. The behavioral phenotype determines the energy and nutrient input to the system under a given set of environmental conditions, and the metabolic phenotype determines what happens to the ingested fuel. The functional phenotype can be considered as the characteristics of the system which determine the body weight and body composition that result from a given set of environmental and nutritional conditions.

B. MODIFICATIONS TO THE FUNCTIONAL PHENOTYPE

As an individual interacts with and responds to a given environment, the functional phenotype constantly changes within the limits defined by the genotype. These changes may or may not alter the settling point. An important aspect of the functional phenotype is that it is responsible for maintaining the steady state within the system. Since the environmental and nutritional conditions that an individual encounters are not constant, the functional phenotype must continuously compensate for perturbations in the system due to changing environmental and nutritional conditions. The maintenance of a constant settling point depends on the functional phenotype being able to do this successfully.

The functional phenotype is modified when the individual engages in cumulative or chronic behaviors that alter E_{in} or E_{out} in such a way that the existing functional phenotype cannot compensate without changing E_{stored}. In adults, modification of the functional phenotype appears to be driven by behavior. For example, chronic changes in diet composition or chronic alterations in physical activity can influence the metabolic phenotype directly via alterations in insulin sensitivity,[52,53] the oxidative vs. storage capacity of individual tissues,[35,48,51] and the chronic hormonal environment.[54,50] For example, increases in chronic exercise improve the capacity of muscle to oxidize fats,[55] and increase muscle lipoprotein lipase activity and triglyceride deposition.[56] Thus, increases in exercise not only increase energy expenditure, but provide a means to reorganize the fuel partitioning system via shunting lipid fuel to muscle for storage and oxidation. Conversely, a sedentary lifestyle might establish a metabolic phenotype which favors the diversion of lipid fuel to adipose tissue rather than to muscle. These chronic changes in behavior alter both the behavioral and metabolic phenotypes and may cause the settling point to change as the system reaches a different steady state.

C. COMPENSATION FOR CHANGES IN ENVIRONMENTAL AND NUTRITIONAL CONDITIONS

In order to maintain a constant settling point over some specified interval, the individual must be able to adjust, either behaviorally or metabolically, for perturbations to the system over this interval. If the system cannot compensate for perturbations, then the system and the settling point must change. The new settling point would represent a new steady state with different system characteristics, the nature of which would depend on the amount of change necessary. The fact that most people maintain a constant body weight and body composition suggests that the functional phenotype has a good capacity to compensate for day-to-day fluctuations in environmental and nutritional conditions.

1. Compensations for Perturbations to Energy Input

When environmental and nutritional perturbations affect the amount and composition of food eaten, the system can compensate through alterations in either behavior or metabolism. For example, changing the meal patterning (the size and number of meals eaten) without changing the total amount of energy consumed can alter many metabolic processes, such as lipogenic enzyme activity and sensitivity of adipose tissue to insulin.[57,58] Changes in meal patterning may or may not produce changes in body weight and body composition, depending on whether the changes exceed the adaptive capacity of the metabolic phenotype.

Another example of metabolic compensation is seen when people alter the fat/carbohydrate ratio of their diet. For example, if an individual switches from a low- to a high-fat diet, E_{stored} may or may not change, depending on the behavioral and metabolic compensation of the system. If compensation is sufficient to maintain energy and nutrient balance, a change in E_{stored} may be avoided. The ability of human subjects to compensate for alterations in diet composition has been examined by Hill et al. When energy intake is fixed at maintenance, the type of compensation required is that the fuel mixture burned equals the fuel mixture ingested. Under these conditions, humans can indeed rapidly alter the fuel mixture burned in the direction of the fuel mixture ingested.[25] The more rapidly and completely such metabolic changes can occur the greater the likelihood of maintaining a constant settling point.

However, when energy intake is not fixed, a switch from a low- to a high-fat diet requires both behavioral and metabolic compensation. For example, high-fat diets generally are associated with greater ad libitum energy intake than low-fat diets.[11-13] When an individual changes from a low- to a high-fat diet, behaviorally the individual can compensate by maintaining constant energy intake (i.e., not increasing E_{in}). Metabolic adjustment can occur via altering the composition of fuel burned to match the composition of the diet. Both compensatory responses are necessary in order to avoid changing body fat stores.

2. Compensations for Perturbations To Energy Output

The major perturbations to E_{out} occur through variations in physical activity. The example most relevant to obesity development is a decline in physical activity; this appears to occur in many adults with advancing age.[59] Any decline in voluntary physical activity will reduce total energy expenditure and potentially alter the composition of fuel burned. The specific effect on the fuel mixture burned will depend on the type of physical activity eliminated and the degree of positive energy balance. Complete compensation for a reduction in physical activity would require an individual to reduce total E_{in} and alter the composition of the diet to match the composition of the fuel burned. Compensation also may be necessary when the type, but not the amount, of physical activity changes. This is because different types of physical activity have different effects on the fuel mixture burned.[55]

D. CONSEQUENCES OF INCOMPLETE COMPENSATION

When perturbations to the system exceed the capacity of the functional phenotype to compensate via behavioral and metabolic responses, an excess or surfeit of energy exists; this is a situation that must produce changes in body energy stores. The extent and nature of such changes depend on the functional phenotype and, in particular, on the metabolic phenotype, since the latter determines the immediate fate of excess energy and the source of E_{stored} to be used for oxidation. Moreover, the specific changes that occur in E_{stored} will in part determine the new characteristics of the functional phenotype.

Individual differences in the capacity of the functional phenotype for behavioral and metabolic compensation may be important in determining whether obesity develops. Again, a distinction is made between compensatory responses developed in early life vs. those developed in later life. In many instances in early life, little or no behavioral compensation is allowed because of parental influences on the amount and composition of food available. Alternatively, substantial metabolic compensation is likely to occur as the system attempts to achieve a steady state under the conditions of the imposed behavior. It is possible that in many adults behavioral compensation is inadequate because they failed to learn appropriate behavioral compensation early in life. Such an individual may be particularly susceptible to obesity since behavior is the driving force determining energy and nutrient input.

1. Determining the Fate of Excess Energy — Nutrient Partitioning

The metabolic phenotype can be described as the machinery which determines the partitioning of nutrients between oxidation and storage. Nutrients which are not oxidized can be stored in the body in different forms (protein, carbohydrate, fat) and in many different locations. It is the metabolic phenotype that determines, given a specific amount of excess nutrient, how and where it is stored in the body. Similarly, the way in which excess energy is stored can have a chronic influence on the functional phenotype. For example, Bouchard et al.[2,3] found wide variation in the fat/FFM ratio of body weight gained during 100 days of overfeeding in identical twins. The subjects whose weight gain consisted of a greater proportion of FFM would develop a more obesity-resistant functional phenotype than subjects whose weight gain was largely fat. This is because the added FFM would stimulate total energy expenditure to a greater extent than added fat mass.

Similarly, the site of storage of additional body fat can influence the functional phenotype. Central fat deposition, by virtue of providing a greater supply of free fatty acids to the liver, may decrease hepatic insulin clearance, a determinant of insulinemia and insulin sensitivity.[60] Individuals metabolically prone to obesity not only may store more fat centrally, but may have a reduced capacity for fat mobilization.[61]

VI. INTERACTION OF BEHAVIOR AND METABOLISM IN THE DEVELOPMENT OF OBESITY

A. HOW DO THE COMPONENTS OF THE SYSTEM INTERACT AT DIFFERENT STAGES OF LIFE TO AFFECT THE SETTLING POINT?

An important aspect of the model presented in Figure 1 is that the functional phenotype, and therefore the settling point, is modifiable at any time in life. However, we believe the greatest potential for modification of the functional phenotype occurs early in life. Most frequently, the eating behavior learned by the child is the behavior taught by the parents, who determine when, where, what, and how much the child eats throughout much of childhood.[62,63] This complex conditioned learning process is difficult to change later in life.[64] Similarly, the most significant factor determining the early metabolic phenotype is the early eating behavior imposed on the child. It is likely that the "metabolic slate" of the neonate is cleaner than it will be at any other time in life. The transition from the fetal to the neonatal environment involves beginning to consume food, which is probably the greatest stimulus for determining aspects of the many metabolic processes involved in fuel metabolism (e.g., establishing capacity for enzyme systems, etc.). Thus, the early years of life are a time when the behavioral and metabolic phenotypes can be moved easily within the genetically defined limits. The functional phenotype acquired in early life is difficult to modify later in life since it requires altering existing behavioral and metabolic systems.

In adulthood, changes in behavior appear to be the early events leading to obesity. In Western societies, the most likely culprits are a decline in amount of physical activity and an increase in the fat/carbohydrate ratio in the diet. However, the effects of such changes in behavior on body weight and body composition also depend on the individual's metabolic phenotype, and two individuals may respond quite differently to the same change in behavior.

B. THE INTERACTION OF BEHAVIOR AND METABOLISM IN DETERMINING SUSCEPTIBILITY TO OBESITY

In summary, whether or not an individual will develop obesity depends in large part on that individual's functional phenotype. This represents the combination of an individual's tendency to engage in behaviors that produce positive energy balance and his or her tendency to store excess energy as body fat. This is illustrated in Figure 2, where behavioral phenotype is represented on one axis and metabolic phenotype on the other. The probability of developing obesity increases as either phenotype favors accumulation of body fat. However, the greatest probability of becoming obese occurs when the behavioral phenotype favors being in positive energy balance and the metabolic phenotype favors storage of excess energy as body fat.

Although the functional phenotype has strong genetic determinants, the nongenetic determinants are sufficiently strong to encourage efforts to modify it in such a way as to

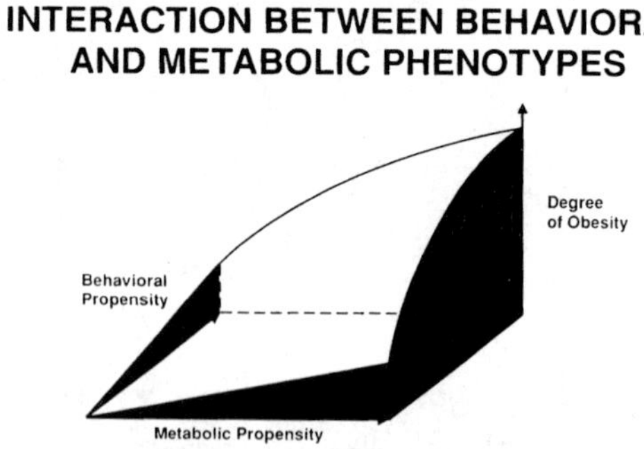

Figure 2. This model illustrates that susceptibility to obesity is a function of both propensity to engage in behaviors leading to positive energy balance (behavioral propensity) and propensity to metabolically store excess energy as body fat (metabolic propensity). The greatest likelihood of developing obesity occurs in an individual with a high propensity to engage in behaviors leading to positive energy balance and with a high propensity to store excess energy as body fat.

decrease the likelihood of obesity development. One major effort should be to identify specific markers of the behavioral and metabolic phenotypes that predispose different individuals to develop obesity. Once obesity-susceptible individuals are identified, specific interventions can be developed. Such modifications will likely involve efforts to insure that "appropriate" eating and exercise behaviors are learned early in life.

We may be more successful in preventing than in treating obesity. According to the system described in this chapter, a permanent reduction in body fat stores requires a permanent change in the steady-state nature of the system involved in body weight regulation. This can occur with a permanent change in behavior (eating or exercise behavior) or a permanent change in metabolism (e.g., pharmacological agents which increase energy expenditure). It is difficult to produce permanent changes in behavior (especially in adults), and no pharmacological agents are currently available to increase energy expenditure in human subjects.

Finally, the system described in this chapter can explain why two individuals could encounter similar environmental and nutritional conditions and differ either in the level of body fat stores maintained over time or in how body fat stores change in response to positive or negative energy balance.

REFERENCES

1. **Stunkard, A. J.,** Genetic contributions to human obesity, in *Genes, Brain, and Behavior,* McHugh, P. R. and McKusick, V. A., Eds., Raven Press, New York, 1991, 205.
2. **Bouchard, C.,** Genetic factors in obesity, *Med. Clin. North Am.,* 73, 67, 1989.
3. **Bouchard, C., Tremblay, A., Després, J.-P., Nadeau, A., Lupien, P. J., Thériault, G., Dussault, J., Moorjani, S., Pinault, S., and Fournier, G.,** The response to long-term overfeeding in identical twins, *N. Engl. J. Med.,* 322, 1477, 1990.
4. **Curb, J. D. and Marcus, E. B.,** Body fat and obesity in Japanese Americans, *Am. J. Clin. Nutr.,* 53(Suppl.), 1552S, 1991.
5. **Kuczmarski, R. J.,** Prevalence of overweight and weight gain in the United States, *Am. J. Clin. Nutr.,* 55(Suppl.), 495S, 1992.
6. **Wirtshafter, D. and Davis, J. D.,** Set points, settling points and the control of body weight, *Physiol. Behav.,* 19, 75, 1977.
7. **Rodin, J. and Marcus, J.,** Psychological factors in human feeding, *Pharmacol. Ther.,* 16, 447, 1982.
8. **Booth, D. A.,** Satiety and appetite are conditioned reactions, *Psychosom. Med.,* 39, 76, 1977.
9. **Rodin, J.,** Determinants of food intake regulation in obesity, in *Obesity,* Björntorp, P. and Brodoff, B. N., Eds., Lippencott, Philadelphia, 1992, 220.
10. **Rolls, B. J. and Hetherington, M.,** The role of variety in eating and body weight regulation, in *Handbook of Psychophysiology of Human Eating,* Shepherd, R., Ed., John Wiley & Sons, Sussex, 1989, 57.
11. **Thomas, C. D., Peters, J. C., Reed, G. W., Abumrad, N. N., Sun, M., and Hill, J. O.,** Nutrient balance and energy expenditure during ad libitum feeding of high-fat and high-carbohydrate diets in humans, *Am. J. Clin. Nutr.,* 55, 934, 1992.
12. **Lissner, L., Levitsky, D. A., Strupp, B. J., Kalkwarf, H. J., and Roe, D. A.,** Dietary fat and the regulation of energy intake in human subjects, *Am. J. Clin. Nutr.,* 46, 886, 1987.
13. **Tremblay, A., Plourde, G., Despres, J. P., and Bouchard, C.,** Impact of dietary fat content and fat oxidation on energy intake in humans, *Am. J. Clin. Nutr.,* 49, 799, 1989.
14. **Ogden, J. and Wardle, J.,** Cognitive restraint and sensitivity to cues for hunger and satiety, *Physiol. Behav.,* 47, 477, 1990.

15. **Polivy, J.,** Perception of calories, *Addict. Behav.,* 1, 237, 1976.
16. **Garn, S. M.,** Family-line and socioeconomic factors in fatness and obesity, *Nutr. Rev.,* 44, 381, 1986.
17. **Stunkard, A. J.,** Obesity and social environment, in *Recent Advances in Obesity Research,* Vol. 1, Howard, A., Ed., John Libbey, London, 1974.
18. **Schlundt, D. G., Taylor, D., Hill, J. O., Sbrocco, T., Pope-Cordle, J., Kasser, T., and Arnold, D.,** A behavioral taxonomy of obese female participants in a weight-loss program, *Am. J. Clin. Nutr.,* 53, 1151, 1991.
19. **Wadden, T. A., Foster, G. D., Wang, J., Pierson, R. N., Yang, M. U., Moreland, K., Stunkard, A. J., and Van Itallie, T. B.,** Clinical correlates of short- and long-term weight loss, *Am. J. Clin. Nutr.,* 56(Suppl.), 271S, 1992.
20. **Flatt, J. P.,** The biochemistry of energy expenditure, in *Recent Advances in Obesity,* Vol. 2, Gray, G. S., Ed., Newmann, London, 1978, 211.
21. **Hill, J. O.,** Exercise, energy expenditure and fat oxidation, in *The Science of Food Regulation,* Bray, G. A. and Ryan, D. H., Eds., Louisiana State University Press, Baton Rouge, 1992, 67.
22. **Ravussin, E., Lillioja, S., Anderson, T. E., Christin, L., and Bogardus, C.,** Determinants of 24-hour energy expenditure in man. Methods and results using a respiratory chamber, *J. Clin. Invest.,* 78, 1568, 1986.
23. **Cunningham, J. J.,** Body composition as a determinant of energy expenditure: a synthetic review and a proposed general prediction equation, *Am. J. Clin. Nutr.,* 54, 963, 1991.
24. **Hill, J. O., Heymsfield, S. B., McManus, C. B., III, and DiGirolamo, M.,** Meal size and thermic response to food in male subjects as a function of maximum aerobic capacity, *Metabolism,* 33, 743, 1984.
25. **Hill, J. O., Peters, J. C., Reed, G. W., Schlundt, D. G., Sharp, T., and Greene, H. L.,** Nutrient balance in humans: effects of diet composition, *Am. J. Clin. Nutr.,* 54, 10, 1991.
26. **Broeder, C. E., Burrhus, K. A., Svanevik, L. S., and Wilmore, J. H.,** The effects of either high-intensity resistance or endurance training on resting metabolic rate, *Am. J. Clin. Nutr.,* 55, 802, 1992.
27. **Schulz, L. O., Nyomba, B. L., Alger, S., Anderson, T. E., and Ravussin, E.,** Effect of endurance training on sedentary energy expenditure measured in a respiratory chamber, *Am. J. Physiol.,* 260, E257, 1991.
28. **Sharp, T., Reed, G. W., Abumrad, N. N., Sun, M., and Hill, J. O.,** Relationship between aerobic fitness level and daily energy expenditure in weight-stable humans, *Am. J. Physiol.,* 263, E121, 1992.
29. **Bennett, C., Reed, G. W., Peters, J. C., Abumrad, N. N., Sun, M., and Hill, J. O.,** Short-term effects of dietary-fat ingestion on energy expenditure and nutrient balance, *Am. J. Clin. Nutr.,* 55, 1071, 1992.
30. **Welle, S., Lilavivat, U., Hana, R., and Campbell, R. G.,** Thermic effect of feeding in man. Increasing plasma norepinephrine levels following glucose but not protein or fat consumption, *Metabolism,* 30, 953, 1981.
31. **Hill, J. O., Drougas, H., and Peters, J. C.,** Obesity treatment: can diet composition play a role?, *Ann. Intern. Med.,* 119, 694, 1993.
32. **Sun, M. and Hill, J. O.,** Measurement of mechanical work and work efficiency in humans, *J. Biomech.,* 26, 229, 1993.
33. **Schutz, Y., Tremblay, A., Weinsier, R. L., and Nelson, K. M.,** Role of fat oxidation in the long-term stabilization of body weight in obese women, *Am. J. Clin. Nutr.,* 55, 670, 1992.
34. **Wade, A. J., Marbut, M. M., and Round, J. M.,** Muscle fibre type and aetiology of obesity, *Lancet,* 335, 805, 1990.

35. **Abou Mrad, J., Yakubu, F., Lin, D., Peters, J. C., Atkinson, J. B., and Hill, J. O.,** Skeletal muscle composition in dietary obese-susceptible and dietary obesity-resistant rats, *Am. J. Physiol.,* 262, R684, 1992.
36. **Flatt, J. P.,** The difference in the storage capacities for carbohydrate and for fat, and its implications in the regulation of body weight, in *Human Obesity,* Wurtmen, R. J. and Wurtmen, J. J., Eds., *Ann. N.Y. Acad. Sci.,* 499, 1987, 104.
37. **Acheson, K. J., Schutz, Y., Bessard, T., Anantharaman, K., Flatt, J. P., and Jequier, E.,** Glycogen storage capacity and de novo lipogenesis during massive carbohydrate overfeeding in man, *Am. J. Clin. Nutr.,* 48, 240, 1988.
38. **Schutz, Y., Flatt, J. P., and Jequier, E.,** Failure of dietary fat intake to promote fat oxidation: a factor favoring the development of obesity, *Am. J. Clin. Nutr.,* 50, 307, 1989.
39. **Flatt, J. P., Ravussin, E., Acheson, K. J., and Jequier, E.,** Effects of dietary fat on postprandial substrate oxidation and on carbohydrate and fat balances, *J. Clin. Invest.,* 76, 1019, 1985.
40. **Zurlo, F., Lillioja, S., Esposito-Del Puente, A., Nyomba, B. L., Raz, I., Saad, M. F., Swinburn, B. A., Knowler, W. C., Bogardus, C., and Ravussin, E.,** Low ratio of fat to carbohydrate oxidation as predictor of weight gain: study of 24-h RQ, *Am. J. Physiol.,* 259, E650, 1990.
41. **Horton, T. J., Reed, G. W, Drougas, H., Brachey, A., Sun, M., Carlson, M., Peters, J. C., and Hill, J. O.,** Nutrient balance during fat and carbohydrate overfeeding in lean and obese males, *Obes. Res.,* 1(Suppl. 1), 11S, 1993.
42. **Widdowson, E. M. and McCance, R. A.,** Some effects of accelerating growth. I. General somatic development, *Proc. R. Soc. London Ser. B,* 152, 188, 1960.
43. **Knittle, J. L. and Hirsch, J.,** Effect of early nutrition on the development of rat epididymal fat pads: cellularity and metabolism, *J. Clin. Invest.* 47, 2091, 1968.
44. **Hirsch, J. and Han, P. W.,** Cellularity of rat adipose tissue: effects of growth, starvation, and obesity, *J. Lipid Res.,* 10, 77, 1969.
45. **Hausman, D. B., McCloskey, H. M., and Martin, R. J.,** Maternal dietary fat type influences the growth and fatty acid compensation of newborn and weanling rats, *J. Nutr.,* 121, 1917, 1991.
46. **Issad, T., Coupe, C., Ferre, P., and Girard, J.,** Insulin resistance during suckling period in rats, *Am. J. Physiol.,* 253, E142, 1987.
47. **Iynedjian, P. B., Ucla, C., and Mach, B.,** Molecular cloning of glucokinase cDNA: developmental and dietary regulation of glucokinase mRNA in rat liver, *J. Biol. Chem.,* 262, 6032, 1987.
48. **Rossetti, L., Rothman, D. L., DeFonzo, R. A., and Shulman, G. I.,** Effect of dietary protein on in vivo insulin action and liver glycogen repletion, *Am. J. Physiol.,* 257, E212, 1989.
49. **Wright, D. W., Hansen, R. I., Mondon, C. P., and Reaven, G. M.,** Sucrose-induced insulin resistance in the rat: modulation by exercise and diet, *Am. J. Clin. Nutr.,* 38, 879, 1983.
50. **Bray, G. A., Stern, J. S., and Castonguay, T. W.,** Effect of adrenalectomy and high-fat diet on the fatty Zucker rat, *Am. J. Physiol.,* 262, E32, 1992.
51. **Nemeth, P. M., Rosser, B. W. C., Choksi, R. M., Norris, B. J., and Baker, K. M.,** Metabolic response to a high-fat diet in neonatal and adult rat muscle, *Am. J. Physiol.,* 262, C282, 1992.
52. **Storlien, L. H., James, D. E., Burleigh, K. M., Chisholm, D. J., and Kraegen, E. W.,** Fat feeding causes widespread *in vivo* insulin resistance, decreased energy expenditure, and obesity in rats, *Am. J. Physiol.,* 251, E576, 1986.
53. **Chang, S., Graham, B., Yakubu, F., Lin, D., Peters, J. C., and Hill, J. O.,** Metabolic differences between obesity-prone and obesity-resistant rats, *Am. J. Physiol.,* 259, R1103, 1990.

54. **Bhathena, S. J., Berlin, E., Judd, J., Nair, P. P., Kennedy, B. W., Jones, J., Smith, P. M., Jones, Y., Taylor, P. R., and Campbell, W. S.,** Hormones regulating lipid and carbohydrate metabolism in premenopausal women: modulation by dietary lipids, *Am. J. Clin. Nutr.,* 49, 752, 1989.
55. **Holloszy, J. O. and Coyle, E. F.,** Adaptations of skeletal muscle to endurance exercise and their metabolic consequences, *J. Appl. Physiol.,* 56, 831, 1984.
56. **Parizkova, J. and Kovtewk, Y.,** The effect of age and different motor activity on fat content, lipoprotein lipase activity and relative weight of internal organs, heart and skeletal muscle, *Physiol. Bohemoslov.,* 17, 179, 1968.
57. **Wilhelmine, P. H. G.,** Influence of the feeding frequency on nutrient utilization in man: consequences for energy metabolism, *Eur. J. Clin. Nutr.,* 45, 161, 1991.
58. **Leville, G. A.,** Adipose tissue metabolism: influence of periodicity of eating and diet composition, *Fed. Proc.,* 29, 1294, 1970.
59. **de Vries, H. A.,** *Physiology of Exercise,* William C. Brown, Dubuque, IA, 1974.
60. **Björntorp, P.,** Metabolic abnormalities in visceral obesity, *Ann. Med.,* 24, 3, 1992.
61. **Hirsch, J., Fried, S. K., Edens, N. K., and Leibel, R. L.,** The fat cell, *Med. Clin. North Am.,* 73, 83, 1989.
62. **Birch, L. L.,** Obesity and eating disorders: a developmental perspective, *Bull. Psychosom. Soc.,* 29, 265, 1991.
63. **Klesges, R. C., Stein, R. J., Eck, L. H., Isbell, T. R., and Klesges, L. M.,** Parental influence on food selection in young children and its relationships to childhood obesity, *Am. J. Clin. Nutr.,* 53, 859, 1991.
64. **Stasch, A. R., Johnson, M. M., and Spangler, G. J.,** Food practices and preferences of some college students, *J. Am. Diet. Assoc.,* 57, 523, 1970.

Chapter 4

Overview of the Adoption Studies

Thorkild I. A. Sørensen and Albert J. Stunkard

TABLE OF CONTENTS

I. INTRODUCTION

The possible contribution of genetic factors to individual differences in human fatness or its extreme variant, obesity, must be seen on the background of the evident strong environmental influences, even under conditions of unrestricted food supply (see Chapter 2). The suspicion that genetic factors are important stems from observations in animals (see Chapter 12) and numerous studies demonstrating familial resemblance in fatness, assessed by various weight-for-height measures, skinfold thicknesses, and determination of body composition (see Chapter 6).[1-5] Parents and offspring usually show correlations between 0.20 and 0.25 and siblings correlations between 0.25 and 0.35. This resemblance could be due to the genes they have in common or to shared environmental influences. The study of individuals separated from their biological parents at birth and adopted by an unrelated family provides an opportunity to disentangle these influences.

II. THE PRINCIPLE AND STRENGTH OF THE ADOPTION METHOD

The idea of the adoption method is that resemblance in the trait between the adoptee and the members of the biological family presumably is due to shared genes, whereas resemblance between the adoptee and the members of the adoptive family presumably is due to shared family environment. The resemblance may be expressed by the correlations between the adoptees and their biological and adoptive relatives, respectively. The

0-8493-4880-3/94/$0.00+$.50

pertinent statistical analysis for testing of the presence of genetic or family environmental effects is to examine whether the correlations are significantly different from zero.

However, until recently the adoption studies of fatness have had access only to the adoptive relatives of the adoptee. This kind of study is called a partial adoption study, in contrast to the above-mentioned complete adoption study which is based on access to both adoptive and biological relatives. The partial adoption study utilizes the fact that a genetic effect may lead to greater resemblance of the biological relatives in natural families (who share both genes and family environment) than between the adoptee and members of the adoptive family (who only share the family environment). The natural families used for comparison have been either the adoptive parents and their own biological offspring or members of different natural families (not involving the adoptees and their adoptive family). The genetic effects here are only expressed indirectly by the difference between the correlations of the adoptee and adoptive relatives on the one hand and the correlations among the members of the natural families on the other hand. The pertinent statistical analysis would be a test of whether this difference is significantly greater than zero. Influence of the shared environment is, as in the complete adoption study, expressed in correlations between the adoptee and the adoptive relatives that are statistically different from zero.

In addition to simply testing the hypotheses about presence or absence of genetic or shared environmental effects, it is of interest to assess the extent to which the correlations found in the large population studies of natural families can be attributed to either of these effects. The degree to which genetic differences account for the individual differences in fatness in the total population is measured by the heritability of the trait, which, however, relies on several assumptions.[6]

Two other approaches have been used to address the question of genetic and shared environmental influences on human fatness — the twin method (see Chapter 5) and the model analysis of extended natural families,[7] which may include twins.[8] A weakness of these methods is their assumption that shared environmental effects and genetic effects are not confounded. The strength of the adoption method is the possibility of avoiding this problem. The advantages of the twin and adoption methods are combined in the study of twins reared apart; however, such twins are very rare, and there may be doubt about how effective the separation of the twins has been.[9]

III. ADOPTION STUDIES

Since 1964 nine studies have used adoptees or foster children in the study of fatness.[10-31] The study by Shenker et al.[11] suggested that the degree of overweight of foster mothers influences the development of obesity during infancy, but the study did not allow assessment of genetic influences and is therefore not discussed further. In the following, each of the other eight studies will be described and a conclusion regarding their evidence for the relative contributions of genetic and family environment influences to the familial resemblance will be drawn (Table 1).

A. PARTIAL ADOPTION STUDIES

1. The London Study[10]

In this study all 300 parents, listed in one British adoption society, who had adoptees aged 8 to 13 years received a mailed questionnaire about their weight and height and those of their children. The results were compared with those obtained from two samples of natural families. One sample consisted of 250 women volunteers working at factories in a London suburb whose relatives were also contacted. The other sample consisted of children aged 10 to 18 from schools in a London borough, who reported their own age, height, and weight and those of their first-degree relatives. Percentage overweight relative

Table 1. **List of adoption studies of obesity and their main conclusion regarding the relative contribution of genetic and environmental factors to familial resemblance as judged from the size of the correlations, irrespective of statistical significance**

Study	Genetic effects	Family environment effects	Ref.
Partial adoption studies			
London Study			10
Parent-offspring in childhood	+	+++	
Tecumseh Study			12–14,17
Parent-offspring in childhood	++	++	
TOPS Study			15
Parent-offspring in childhood	++	++	
Siblings in childhood	+	+++	
Montreal Study			16,18
Parent-offspring in childhood	+++	+	
Siblings in childhood	++++	0	
Quebec City Study			19,22
Parent-offspring in adolescence	+	+++	
Siblings in adolescence	++++	0	
Colorado Study			30
Siblings in childhood	++++	0	
Complete adoption studies			
Danish Study			20,23–29
Parent-adult offspring	++++	0	
Adult siblings	++++	0	
Parent-offspring in childhood	+++	+	
Siblings in childhood	+++	+	
Iowa Study			21
Parent-adult offspring	+++	+	
Colorado Study			30
Parent-offspring in childhood	++++	0	

Note: Expressed on a semiquantitative scale, from ++++ to 0 that add up to ++++ for the combined genetic and family environment effects.

to British tables of average weight for given sex, age, and height were used in the analysis. The correlations with the adoptee were 0.11 for adoptive fathers and 0.16 for adoptive mothers, and for the natural families the median parent-offspring correlations were 0.19 (range 0.14 to 0.42), but the significance of the differences was not tested.

2. The Tecumseh Study[12-14,17]

The Tecumseh Study is an ongoing health screening of the total population of the town of Tecumseh, MI. In the first round in 1959 to 1960 there were 13,659 participants, who reported the nature of their familial relationship, which, in addition to natural families, included stepchildren and adoptees. Garn et al. conducted analyses of skinfold thickness on parents and on children aged 0 through 18 years. The correlations between 160 adoptive parents and adoptees were 0.11 for triceps and 0.09 for subscapular skinfolds. The corresponding natural parent-offspring correlations were 0.21 and 0.19, respectively. The correlations for 155 stepparent-stepchildren pairs were 0.23 and 0.21, respectively.[17]

The significance of the differences between the adoptive and natural pair correlations was not tested. Further analyses presented in this and other papers by Garn et al.[12-14] did not distinguish between adoptees and stepchildren.

3. The Take-Off-Pounds-Sensibly (TOPS) Study[15]

From the data base of the TOPS Study in 1969 and 1970, which included 73,532 women and their children, the authors selected families in which there were at least two children aged 4 to 11 years, 10,337 with natural children and 254 with unrelated children. A telephone survey of 23 mothers with 45 unrelated children indicated that 87% were adoptees, of whom 73% had been placed before the age of 6 months. Percentage overweight was calculated from reported height and weight using published tables of sex-, age-, and height-specific average weights. The correlations between parents and unrelated children were 0.03 for fathers and 0.11 for mothers, and those between the parents and their natural children were 0.11 and 0.10, respectively. Once again the significance of the differences between the correlations was not tested. The correlation between the unrelated children was 0.16 and between the natural children 0.20 (derived from the estimated family index), and this difference was not statistically significant. The correlations were possibly underestimated because of the truncation of the distributions caused by restriction of the sample to mothers with weight problems.

4. The Montreal Study[16,18]

In 1972 to 1974, adopted children at least 1 year old and their biologically unrelated adoptive families of the same French-Canadian background were located through an adoption agency in Montreal. Median age at adoption was 3 months, and 75% had been adopted before 1 year of age. For comparison, natural families were randomly sampled from the same community. Height and weight were measured at home visits, and body mass indices and weight adjusted for height, age, and sex were calculated. The first analysis included only adoptive families and accepted children aged 1 to 21 years.[16] The final analysis was restricted to families with children aged 1 to 10 years, and data from 53 out of 606 families in which the body mass index (BMI = weight/height^2) of one or more member exceeded 4 SD were excluded from the analysis.[18]

In the first analysis, the correlations for weight/height as well as for standardized weight between the adoptees and the adoptive parents and adoptive siblings were essentially 0, whereas the natural parent-offspring correlations were 0.26 and 0.31, respectively, and the natural sibling correlations were 0.37 and 0.39, respectively.

In the final analysis, the correlations in BMI between adoptees on one hand and adoptive fathers, mothers, and their offspring on the other hand were –0.03, 0.10, and 0.26, respectively. The corresponding correlations for natural parents and siblings were 0.02, 0.18, and 0.40. The results of the analysis of standardized weight showed the same pattern, although with somewhat different correlations. Thus, the correlations involving the adoptees were 0.01, 0.06, and 0.07, respectively, and those for the natural family members were 0.11, 0.24, and 0.13. In 119 pairs of adoptees the correlations between them were 0.01 for BMI and –0.03 for standardized weight. The statistical significance of the departure from zero correlation was tested, but none of the differences relevant for testing genetic influences was tested.

A comprehensive genetic variance component model that distinguished additive genetic effects from various components of the environmental effects was analyzed.[18] Resemblance in standardized weight could be entirely ascribed to additive genetic effects (29% of the variance), whereas in the model for BMI the genetic effect could be removed. On the other hand, in the complete BMI model, comprising both genetic and various environmental components, the genetic contribution was the greatest (17% of the variance).

5. The Quebec City Study[19,22]

In this study, public media advertisement recruited 409 families containing 727 parents and 971 offspring (including twins) or adopted children. No distinction was made between adoption of children biologically unrelated to both parents and a stepparent's adoption of stepchildren. A total of 94% of the adoptees were adopted before 1 year of age. Age range of children was 8 to 26 years, with an average age of 15 years. Measurements included height and weight, from which BMI was computed, thickness of six different skinfolds, and body composition by underwater weighing.

The first analysis estimated correlations for three types of sibling pairs — adopted pairs, unrelated pairs (including the adopted pairs), and natural siblings.[19] The correlations in sum of the six skinfolds for the three types of sibships were 0.01, 0.11, and 0.27, respectively, and for body density they were 0.14, –0.04, and 0.20, respectively.

The second analysis allowed two kinds of comparisons.[22] One comparison was between the correlations for foster parent-adopted child pairs and the correlation between natural parents and offspring. The second comparison was between the correlation for siblings by adoption (corresponding to the unrelated siblings in the previous analysis) and the correlation for natural siblings. The adopted pairs were not kept separate in this analysis. For the BMI, the correlations for parents and offspring were 0.22 vs. 0.23 and for siblings 0.08 vs. 0.26, respectively. For the sum of six skinfolds they were 0.26 vs. 0.22 and 0.12 vs. 0.26, respectively, and for fat mass 0.16 vs. 0.22 and 0.01 vs. 0.16, respectively. Percentage body fat showed almost the same correlations as the total fat mass. The significance of the difference between correlations was not tested.

A comprehensive path model, which also included data on second-degree relatives and twins and took into account various environmental effects, was developed.[22] It is described in the chapter on twin studies (see Chapter 5).

6. The Colorado Study[31]

This is both a partial adoption study (as regards the sibling analysis, since no biological siblings of the adoptees were included) and also a complete adoption study of the parent-offspring relationships. It will be discussed as a complete adoption study.

B. COMPLETE ADOPTION STUDIES

1. The Danish Study[20,23-30]

This study is based on the Danish Adoption Register, which contains official records of every nonfamilial adoption granted in Denmark between 1924 and 1947 and includes information on the adoptee, adoptive parents, and biological parents.[32] A total of 90% of the adoptees had been transferred to the adoptive home within the first year of life. Questionnaires on height, current weight, and maximum weight were mailed to 4643 adoptees from Copenhagen, and 3651 responded. On the basis of current BMI, 540 adoptees were selected within sex-age strata; they belonged to four groups, each comprising 4% of the population: thin, medium, overweight, and obese.[20] Similarly, 532 adoptees were selected on the basis of their maximum BMI; thereby 240 adoptees were selected according to both current and maximum BMI.[26] Mailed questionnaires obtained information on height and weight and a silhouette score of the adoptive parents, the biological parents, full siblings, and half siblings. The parents were asked for the weight of the adoptee when he or she started school. In addition, annual measurements of height and weight in school from ages 7 through 13 years were obtained for the adoptees and their biological and adoptive siblings.[27]

The mean BMI of the biological parents, full siblings, and half siblings increased significantly as the weight class of the adoptee increased. By contrast, there was no increase in BMI of the adoptive parents as the weight class increased.[20,23] The mean silhouette scores showed the same pattern.[29]

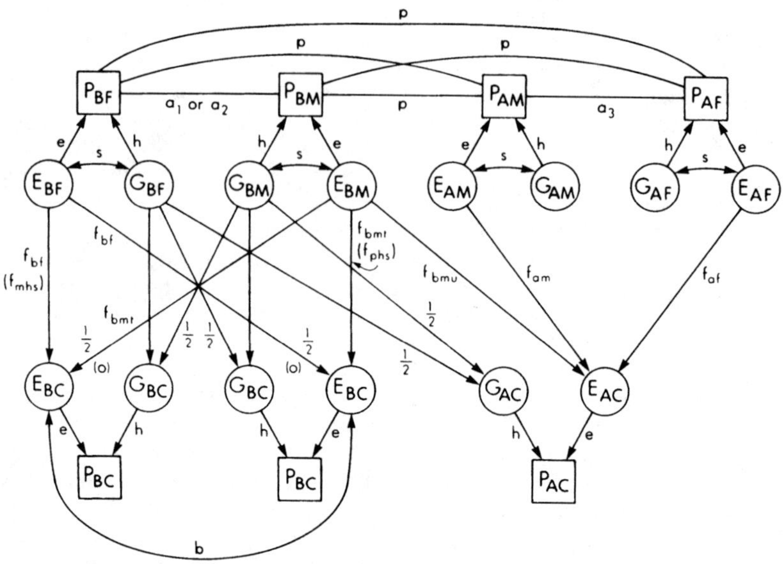

Figure 1. Path diagram of a model of familial resemblance in an adoption design with biological mother (BM), biological father (BF), adoptive mother (AM), adoptive father (AF), adoptive child (AC), and biological children (BC) of the biological parents, either full siblings or paternal or maternal half siblings of the adoptee. The observed phenotype (P, in square) is assumed to be a function of linear additive effects of the genotype G (encircled) and the familial and nonfamilial environment E (encircled), and the parameters for these effects are h and e, respectively, as indicated with the arrows. Genetic heritability is estimated as h^2 and the environmental influences by $e^2 = 1 - h^2$. The model further includes parameters for effects of selective placement of the adoptee (p), phenotypic assortative mating (a_1 for married and a_2 for unmarried parents), genotype-environment correlation (s) that is induced by direct assortative mating, transmission of environmental influences from parent to child (f), each of which are specified according to the parent it concerns (parameters in parentheses refer to effects related to maternal and paternal half siblings), and correlation between sibling shared environment (b). In the Danish Adoption Study this model could be reduced to include only the effect of the genotype on the phenotype,[24,30] with an estimated genetic heritability of $h^2 = 0.34$.

The current adult BMI showed significant positive correlations between the adoptee and the biological relatives (0.15 for mothers, 0.11 for fathers, 0.23 for full siblings, and 0.07 for maternal half siblings). The correlation of 0.06 for paternal half siblings did not reach statistical significance. By contrast, correlations of adoptees with their adoptive relatives were small and statistically insignificant (0.00 for mothers and –0.05 for fathers). The analysis based on maximum BMI gave almost the same correlations.[26]

In childhood, the correlations between the adoptee and the biological relatives were somewhat higher and significant for the first-degree relatives (mean across ages 7 to 13 years: 0.17 for mothers, 0.16 for fathers, 0.59 for full siblings, 0.16 for maternal and 0.08 for paternal half siblings).[27] Correlations between adoptees and their adoptive relatives were positive (mean across ages 7 to 13 years: 0.10 for mothers, 0.03 for fathers, and 0.14 for adoptive siblings), and a few of the adoptive mother and adoptive sib correlations with the adoptee in late childhood were significant.

Both in adulthood and childhood the correlations between adoptees and their various biological relatives were approximately the same as the correlations between these biological relatives themselves.[26,27]

The data on adults were analyzed by a comprehensive path model incorporating linear additive effects of genes and various environmental components (see Figure 1).[24,30] The model could be reduced to one in which genetic effects alone accounted for the familial resemblance. The heritability was estimated at 0.34, corresponding to a correlation of 0.17 between the adoptees and their first-degree biological relatives.

2. The Iowa Study[21]

Two Iowa adoption agencies identified 357 adoptees aged 18 to 38 years who had been separated from their biological parents at birth. One half were selected because of a record of psychopathology in the biological family; one half (sex and age matched) had no such records. Adoptees and usually one adoptive parent reported their own height and weight in an interview at the time of the study. Data on biological parents had been reported to the agency, usually by the mother, at the time of adoption. There were no difference in BMI between the adoptees selected for the two groups.

The correlations between adoptees and biological parents were positive: for mother-daughter, 0.40, for mother-son, 0.15, for father-daughter, 0.18, and for father-son, 0.08. Only the mother-daughter correlation reached statistical significance. The correlations between adoptee and adoptive parents were around zero (0.06, 0.04, 0.09, and –0.09, respectively). There was a significant relationship between BMI of adoptees and biological mothers also in regression analysis, which controlled for BMI of adoptive parents and other environmental factors of some influence on BMI of the adoptee (e.g., rural vs. urban upbringing, occurrence of psychosocial disturbances in the adoptive home).

3. The Colorado Study[31]

The Colorado Adoption Project included 245 adoptive and 245 nonadoptive families matched to the adoptive families by age, education, occupational status of the father, gender of the adopted child, and number of older children in the family. The adoptees were separated from their biological parents a few days after birth and placed in the adoptive homes within 1 month. The sibling categories included 239 adoptees, 221 nonadopted children, 92 unrelated siblings, and 82 natural siblings. Data on height and weight were available annually from birth through age 7 and then at 9 years. Height and weight were measured except at ages 5, 6, and 9, when the parents reported the data. Data on parents were measured. BMI was used for analysis (multivariate analysis of weight and height together gave similar results). The analysis addressed the question whether the continuity of BMI over time is determined by common genetic or environmental factors operating throughout the age period investigated or by genetic and/or environmental effects operative at specific times and transmitted at older ages. Two separate models were developed: one for siblings and one for parents and offspring.

In the sibling model, the data were explained by genetic transmission and genetic occasion-specific factors (but not common or constant genetic factors) together with unique occasion-specific environmental factors. There were great genetic influences at birth; however, their effect did not persist. From age 1 through 9 there were genetic influences that dissipated over time and were continuously replenished by the occasion-specific effects.

In the parent-offspring model the genetic influences were weak during infancy, but increased to stable "sibling" level at age 4 and afterwards. There was no difference between maternal and paternal cultural transmission, which was weak and sometimes even negative.

IV. ASSUMPTIONS OF THE ADOPTION METHOD

Early and continued separation of the adoptee from the biological parents — Adoption usually occurred within the first year of life for most adoptees.[15,16,19,20,31] Adoptees were often separated from their biological parents at birth and may have stayed with foster parents or in foster homes until adoption.[20,21,31] Continued separation of the adoptee and the biological family later in life has been addressed only in a subsample from the Danish adoption register, which showed that the contact between them was negligible or nonexistent.[33]

No selective placement of the adoptee — This implies that selection of the adoptive family does not depend on the phenotype at issue, common environmental factors or genetic relationships. No evidence of selective placement was found in the three complete adoption studies,[20,21,26,31] but it seems likely that it did occur in some of the partial adoption studies.[12,15,19]

No sustained effects of preadoptive, pre- or postnatal environmental factors shared with the biological family — Such effects, usually considered specific maternal effects, would simulate a genetic effect. Perinatal conditions may influence body weight at later ages,[11,34,35] but several large population studies found no greater correlations between mothers and their offspring than between fathers and their offspring.[2-5,7,8] In two studies the correlations between biological mothers and the adoptees were higher than between biological fathers and adoptees.[21,26] Although these findings suggest a maternal effect, it also could be due to reporting bias and particularly to uncertain paternity. Analysis based on comprehensive genetic models of the Danish Study and the Colorado Project did not support the existence of specific maternal effects.[24,30,31]

Representativeness of the study population — It is assumed that the biological-adoptee-adoptive family set is representative of the background population of natural families in terms of the role of genetic and environmental factors affecting the trait. A number of studies have shown that the members of these family sets are similar to the population of members of natural families with regard to measures of obesity.[18,22,26,27] Support for representativeness is provided by the finding in the Danish adoption study of correlations between the adult adoptee and the biological relatives compatible with the correlations found among these relatives and among natural families in the larger population studies.

No assortative mating of biological parents — Resemblances between the adoptee and the biological relatives would be exaggerated by assortative mating of biological parents. In the partial adoption studies, assortative mating of the parents whose parent-offspring correlations are compared with parent-adoptee correlations will also inflate the estimated genetic effects. Most studies have found some evidence of assortment with regard to measures of fatness, both on the biological and the adoptive side, as occurs also in natural families. However, when taken into account in multivariate analysis, the assortative mating had only minimal effects on the estimates of genetic effects.[18,21,22,24,30,31]

Correct paternity assignment — Incorrect paternity will reduce the resemblance between the adoptees and the biological fathers and their offspring (biological full siblings and paternal half siblings of the adoptee). This may have played a role in the Danish and Iowa adoption studies.[21,26]

Special assumptions of the partial adoption study — The partial adoption method requires additional assumptions regarding the shared environmental effects: they must be equal for the adoptee and for the members of the natural families with whom they are compared, and they must act additively on the genetic effects. There is reason to believe that these assumptions often have not been met. Thus, the finding of genetic effects in the complete adoption studies is incompatible with the results of some of the partial adoption studies (see Table 1). Moreover, correlations between stepchildren and natural children are higher than correlations between adoptees and natural children,[17] and the latter correlations are higher than correlations between children who are both adoptees.[18,19] These differences could be due to special rearing of adoptees and stepchildren and, for the correlations involving stepchildren, also assortative mating of the natural parent and the stepparent.[7]

V. GENDER- AND AGE-RELATED GENETIC EFFECTS

Large population studies show minor gender-related differences[2-5,7,8] which the available adoption studies probably do not have the power to detect. In two of the complete adoption studies[21,26] there was a tendency towards greater correlations between biological mothers and biological offspring than between biological fathers and biological offspring and for greater correlations for daughters than for sons. However, as noted above, this pattern may be due as well to greater accuracy of the measurements for the female relationships and the uncertainty regarding paternity. In the Colorado Study there were no such differences.[30] There was no consistent gender-related pattern in the results of the partial adoption studies.

The cross-sectional adoption studies do not suggest a clear age-related pattern of genetic effects. The Danish Adoption Study included longitudinal data both from ages 7 through 13 years and for adulthood, analyzed as repeated cross-sectional data. Neither indicated age-related effects.[27] The only study using longitudinal analysis was the Colorado Study,[30] which showed genetic effects throughout the age period from birth to 9 years, although of different nature in the earlier years. The issue of temporal trends in genetic effects will be addressed further in a later chapter (Chapter 8).

VI. NONADDITIVE GENETIC EFFECTS

Genetic influences on fatness are believed to be due to many genes, each with rather small effects (polygenic effect), which may be additive or nonadditive. Most of the large family population studies of fatness show greater full sibling correlations than parent-offspring correlations. This pattern may reflect either separate environmental effects shared by siblings, and not by parent and offspring, or nonadditive genetic effects.

Adoption studies that include both biological parents and biological siblings of the adoptee allow a distinction between the two effects. If the only genetic effects on obesity were additive ones, the correlation between adoptees and their biological parents should be similar to the correlation between adoptees and their biological full siblings and double the correlation between the adoptees and their biological half siblings. The Danish study is the only one that includes these biological relationships.[23,26,27] It showed the pattern found in natural families, suggesting the presence of nonadditivity and major gene effects.[25] The comprehensive model analysis, however, does not support such effects,[24,30] although there is some evidence to support the existence of major single gene effects (see Chapter 7).

VII. COHABITATION AND GENE-ENVIRONMENT INTERACTION

Some of the partial adoption studies suggested an effect of the shared rearing environment, which seems reasonable since they primarily contained children and adolescents who were living in the family at the time of study.[7,17,36] However, for the reasons discussed above, the cohabitation effects may have been overestimated. Thus, the Montreal Study,[16,18] the sibling part of the Quebec City Study,[19,22] the childhood part of the Danish Study,[27] and the Colorado Study[31] all suggested little or no effect of the rearing environment. The Danish and Iowa Studies of adult adoptees indicate that there are no sustained effects of the rearing environment.[20,21,24,26,30]

Gene-environment interaction implies that genetic effects are dependent on environmental conditions or exposures (and vice versa). Such interaction may occur despite the absence of effects of the shared environment, as indexed by the resemblance of nonrelated individuals. Gene-environment interaction was investigated in the Iowa Study[21] and the adult part of the Danish Study,[28] and no consistent effects were found. There are three major problems in detecting gene-environment interaction effects for a polygenic trait such as fatness: (1) the required statistical power of the study, (2) the inability to specify which genes are carried by which adoptees, and (3) the inaccuracy of measurement of relevant environmental exposures for both the adoptees and their biological relatives.[37]

VIII. MEASUREMENT AND CHARACTERISTICS OF FATNESS AND OBESITY

Direct measurement of the fat mass has been performed only in the Quebec Study.[19,22] The other studies have used surrogate measures such as various combinations of weight and height and skinfold thickness at various sites. The lack of direct measurement raises the question as to whether the genetic and shared environmental effects on the surrogate measures reflect effects on the fat mass. Two kinds of problems are posed. One is random, systematic, or correlated measurement error; the other is the heterogeneity of the surrogate measures, which are composed of disparate components that may be subject to different genetic and environmental influences.

The random errors in the surrogate measures of the fat mass will tend to reduce the familial correlations, whereas systematic or correlated errors could either reduce or increase them. In addition, the use of weight and height as reported by the subjects themselves or by their relatives instead of measured values may add to the errors.[10,15,21,26,31] It attests to the validity of the results, however, that the familial correlations based on reported weights and heights are quite similar to those obtained with measured values.

Weight-for-height measures are correlated with the fat-free mass, and according to the Quebec Study[19,22] the fat-free mass exhibits familial correlations which seem to be mainly of genetic origin. Different combinations of weight and height may differ in their correlations with the body components and therefore may produce different familial correlations, particularly in childhood.[18,31]

The use of skinfold thickness as a proxy for the fat mass may be confounded by special genetic or environmental influences on fat distribution. The results of the Quebec Study suggest that the extremity-to-trunk ratio of skinfolds and the ratio of the sum of subcutaneous skinfolds to total fat mass are subject to both genetic and shared familial environmental effects.[19,22] The latter ratio may be interpreted as an indirect measure of internal or visceral fat.[22] It should be noted that no adoption studies have as yet directly assessed the intraabdominal fat mass, a depot that is attracting increasing attention because of its relationship to the complications of obesity.

In addition to measuring obesity as such, it is of interest to measure genetic and environmental influences on predictors of obesity, such as the age at which adiposity rebound occurs. Adiposity rebound is the increase in the BMI of children around the age of 6 years.[38] It has been shown that the earlier the rebound takes place the more likely is the development of obesity.[38] The Colorado Study showed that the age of obesity rebound was subject to genetic control to about the same degree as BMI itself, and it was not influenced by shared family environmental factors.[31]

IX. CONCLUSIONS AND FUTURE TRENDS

All the complete and some of the partial adoption studies indicate that the familial resemblance in fatness from childhood through adulthood is mainly due to shared genes

(Table 1). All the complete and some of the partial adoptions studies found little or no influence of the shared family environment, particularly after the adoptee had left the home. The design features of the complete adoption studies suggest that their results are more valid.

Future adoption studies should include specific and accurate measurements of body fat components and body fat distribution as well as putative biochemical, physiological, behavioral, and psychosocial determinants of the amount and distribution of body fat. The studies should be large enough to characterize genetic effects with regard to nonadditivity and to address interaction between specific environmental factors and genetic predisposition as determined by the relationship between the adoptee and the biological relatives. Ideally, they should be designed as longitudinal studies or intervention experiments that include both adoptive and biological parents and siblings and cover the ages when the adoptees are still living in the rearing environment as well as later ages.

REFERENCES

1. **Davenport, C. B.,** *Body Build and Its Inheritance,* Publ. 329, Carnegie Institution, Washington D.C., 1923.
2. **Bouchard, C. and Perusse, L.,** Heredity and body fat, *Annu. Rev. Nutr.,* 8, 259, 1988.
3. **Friedlander, Y., Kark, J. D., Kaufmann, N. A., Berry, E. M., and Stein, Y.,** Familial aggregation of body mass index in ethnically diverse families in Jerusalem: The Jerusalem Lipid Research Clinic, *Int. J. Obes.,* 12, 237, 1988.
4. **Mueller, W. H.,** The genetics of human fatness, *Year. Phys. Anthropol.,* 26, 215, 1983.
5. **Garn, S. M. and Clark, D. C.,** Trends in fatness and the origins of obesity, *Pediatrics,* 57, 443, 1976.
6. **Feldman, M. W. and Lewontin, R. C.,** The heritability hang-up, *Science,* 190, 1163, 1975.
7. **Longini, I. M., Higgins, M. W., Hinton, P. C., Moll, P. P., and Keller, J. B.,** Genetic and environmental sources of familial aggregation of body mass in Tecumseh, Michigan, *Hum. Biol.,* 56, 733, 1984.
8. **Tambs, K., Moum, T., Eaves, L., Neale, M., Midthjell, K., Lund-Larsen, P. G., Næss, S., and Holmen, J.,** Genetic and environmental contributions to the variance of the body mass index in a Norwegian sample of first- and second-degree relatives, *Am. J. Hum. Biol.,* 3, 257, 1991.
9. **Langinvaino, H., Koskenvuo, M., Kaprio, J., and Sistonen, P.,** Finnish twins reared apart. II. Validation of zygosity, environmental dissimilarity and weight and height, *Acta Genet. Med. Gemellol.,* 33, 251, 1984.
10. **Withers, R. F. J.,** Problems in the genetics of human obesity, *Eugen. Rev.,* 56, 81, 1964.
11. **Shenker, I. R., Fisichelli, V., and Lang, J.,** Weight differences between foster infants of overweight and nonoverweight foster mothers, *J. Pediatr.,* 84, 715, 1974.
12. **Garn, S. M., Bailey, S. M., and Cole, P. E.,** Similarities between parents and their adopted children, *Am. J. Phys. Anthropol.,* 45, 539, 1976.
13. **Garn, S. M., Bailey, S. M., and Higgins, I. T. T.,** Fatness similarities in adopted pairs [Letter], *Am. J. Clin. Nutr.,* 29, 1067, 1976.
14. **Garn, S. M., Cole, P. E., and Bailey, S. M.,** Effects of parental fatness levels on the fatness of biological and adoptive children, *Ecol. Food Nutr.,* 6, 91, 1977.
15. **Hartz, A., Giefer, E., and Rimm, A. A.,** Relative importance of the effects of family environment and heredity on obesity, *Ann. Hum. Genet.,* 41, 185, 1977.
16. **Biron, P., Mongeau, J. G., and Bertrand, D.,** Familial resemblance of body weight and height in 374 homes with adopted children, *J. Pediatr.,* 91, 555, 1977.

17. **Garn, S. M., Cole, P. E., and Bailey, S. M.,** Living together as a factor in family-line resemblance, *Hum. Biol.,* 51, 565, 1979.
18. **Annest, J. L., Sing, C. F., Biron, P., and Mongeau, J. G.,** Family aggregation of blood pressure and weight in adoptive families. III. Analysis of the role of shared genes and shared household environment in explaining family resemblance for height, weight and selected height/weight indices, *Am. J. Epidemiol.,* 117, 492, 1983.
19. **Bouchard, C., Savard, R., Després, J.-P., Tremblay, A., and Leblanc, C.,** Body composition in adopted and biological siblings, *Hum. Biol.,* 57, 61, 1985.
20. **Stunkard, A. J., Sørensen, T. I. A., Hanis, C., Teasdale, T. W., Chakraborty, R., Schull, W. J., and Schulsinger, F.,** An adoption study of human obesity, *N. Engl. J. Med.,* 314, 193, 1986.
21. **Price, R. A., Cadoret, R. J., Stunkard, A. J., and Troughton, E.,** Genetic contributions to human fatness: an adoption study, *Am. J. Psychiatry,* 144, 1003, 1987.
22. **Bouchard, C., Perusse, L., Leblanc, C., Tremblay, A., and Theriault, G.,** Inheritance of the amount and distribution of human body fat, *Int. J. Obes.,* 12, 205, 1988.
23. **Sørensen, T. I. A., Price, R. A., Stunkard, A. J., and Schulsinger, F.,** Genetics of obesity in adult adoptees and their biological siblings, *Br. Med. J.,* 298, 87, 1989.
24. **Vogler, G. P., Srinivasan, M. R., Stunkard, A. J., Sørensen, T. I. A., and Rao, D. C.,** The significance of genetic and nonshared environmental influences on human obesity: the Danish adoption study [Abstract], *Am. J. Hum. Genet.,* 47(Suppl.), 81, 1990.
25. **Sørensen, T. I. A., Holst, C., and Stunkard, A. J.,** Recessive inheritance of a major gene for human obesity? Analysis of the Danish Adoption Study, in *Obesity in Europe 91,* Ailhaud, G., Guygrand, B., Lafontain, M., and Ricquier, D., Eds., John Libbey, London, 1992, 85.
26. **Sørensen, T. I. A., Holst, C., Stunkard, A. J., and Skovgaard, L. T.,** Correlations of body mass index of adult adoptees and their biological and adoptive relatives, *Int. J. Obes.,* 16, 227, 1992.
27. **Sørensen, T. I. A., Holst, C., and Stunkard, A. J.,** Childhood body mass index — genetic and familial environmental influences assessed in a longitudinal study, *Int. J. Obes.,* 16, 705, 1992.
28. **Sørensen, T. I. A., Holst, C., and Stunkard, A. J.,** Social and familial modifications of the genetic influences on body mass index of adult adoptees? (Abstract), *Int. J. Obes.,* 16(Suppl. 1), 21, 1992.
29. **Sørensen, T. I. A. and Stunkard, A. J.,** Does obesity run in families because of genes? An adoption study using silhouettes as a measure of obesity, *Acta Psychiatr. Scand.,* Suppl. 370, 67, 1993.
30. **Vogler, G. P., Sørensen, T. I. A., Stunkard, A. J., Srinivasan, M. R., and Rao, D. C.,** Genetic and nonshared environmental influences on body mass index in a Danish adoption study, 1993, submitted.
31. **Cardon, L. R. and Fulker, D. W.,** Genetic influences on body fat from birth to age 9, *Genet. Epidemiol.,* in press.
32. **Kety, S. S., Rosenthal, D., Wender, P. H., and Schulsinger, F.,** The types and prevalence of mental illness in the biological and adoptive families of adopted schizophrenics, *J. Psychiatr. Res.,* 6(Suppl. 1), 345, 1967/1968.
33. **Eldred, C. A., Rosenthal, D., Wender, P. H., Kety, S. S., Schulsinger, F., Welner, J., and Jacobsen, B.,** Some aspects of adoption in selected samples of adult adoptees, *Am. J. Orthopsychiatry,* 46, 279, 1976.
34. **Ravelli, G.-P., Stein, Z. A., and Susser, M. W.,** Obesity in young men after famine exposure in utero and early infancy, *N. Engl. J. Med.,* 295, 349, 1976.
35. **Charney, E., Goodman, H. C., McBride, M., Lyon, B., and Pratt, R.,** Childhood antecedents of adult obesity: do chubby infants become obese adults?, *N. Engl. J. Med.,* 295, 6, 1976.

36. **Khoury, P., Morrison, J. A., Laskarzewski, P. M., and Glueck, C. J.,** Parent-offspring and sibling body mass index associations during and after sharing of common household environments: The Princeton School District Family Study, *Metabolism,* 32, 82, 1983.
37. **Ottman, R.,** An epidemiologic approach to gene-environment interaction, *Genet. Epidemiol.,* 7, 177, 1990.
38. **Rolland-Cachera, M.-F., Deheger, M., and Guilloud-Bataille, M.,** Tracking of the development of adiposity from one month of age to adulthood, *Ann. Hum. Biol.,* 14, 219, 1987.

Chapter 5

Twin Studies of Human Obesity

Joanne M. Meyer and Albert J. Stunkard

TABLE OF CONTENTS

I. INTRODUCTION

The classical twin design was introduced more than a century ago by the pioneering research of Sir Francis Galton.[1,2] It still provides one of the most efficient methods of investigating the contribution of shared genes and shared environment to familial traits. The attraction of this design is clear: it not only controls for the effects of age within a pair of relatives, but it is simply the most powerful way to detect familial resemblance for a trait. After all, if identical (monozygotic [MZ]) twins show no similarity, it is doubtful that any other relatives will.

The basic principle underlying the twin study is straightforward. MZ twins share all of their genes and part of their rearing environment, while fraternal (dizygotic [DZ]) twins share all of their rearing environment, but, on average, only one half of their genes. Consequently, the difference in similarity between the members of MZ pairs vs. those of DZ pairs reflects the extent to which a trait is genetically determined. If there is no difference in similarity between MZ and DZ pairs, it suggests that the trait arises solely from environmental effects. On the other hand, any MZ/DZ difference strongly suggests that the trait is heritable within the population under study.

This classical twin design has been used extensively in studying the etiology of obesity per se as well as body mass, fat mass, and fat patterning in both children and adults. In this chapter, general analytic issues which arise in studying twins will first be discussed, and then the major findings of twin studies of obesity will be summarized.

0-8493-4880-3/94/$0.00+$.50

II. ANALYZING TWIN DATA

Methods for assessing twin similarity and comparing the similarity across zygosity groups vary in complexity and informativeness. One of the simplest calculations from continuous measures obtained on twin pairs (e.g., body mass index, percent fat mass, or skinfold thicknesses) is the mean absolute intrapair difference. If variation in a trait arises from genetic differences between individuals, then the mean difference between MZ twins should be less than that of DZ twins. The effect is illustrated in Figure 1, with body mass index data on female adult twins of the Virginia and American Association of Retired Persons Twin Registries.[3] The significance of the difference between MZ and DZ twins may be assessed with *t*-tests, and any difference suggests genetic control of the trait. In a comparable fashion, the twin similarity for a dichotomous trait (e.g., presence or absence of obesity) may be evaluated with the twin concordance rate.[4] Concordance rates for MZ and DZ twins are compared with a chi-square statistic, and if the MZ concordance exceeds the DZ concordance a genetic etiology is suggested.

Unfortunately, mean intrapair differences and concordance comparisons determine only whether MZ twin similarity exceeds DZ twin similarity. They do not allow quantification of the heritability of the trait or of the proportion of the variance which is due to genetic differences between individuals. This estimate is important since it facilitates assessment of the impact of biological inheritance on a trait and allows predictions to be made about the similarity expected in other types of relationships, such as parents and their offspring or sibling pairs. Testing such predictions is a vital step in confirming the results obtained in twin studies.

Several methods have been proposed to estimate the heritability of traits. The so-called "classical" estimate of heritability[4] is calculated as twice the difference between the MZ and DZ intraclass correlations. It is a simple calculation, has been popular for many years, and has been employed extensively in studies of obesity. In deriving this estimate, the assumption is made that only additive genetic effects and family (or common) environ-

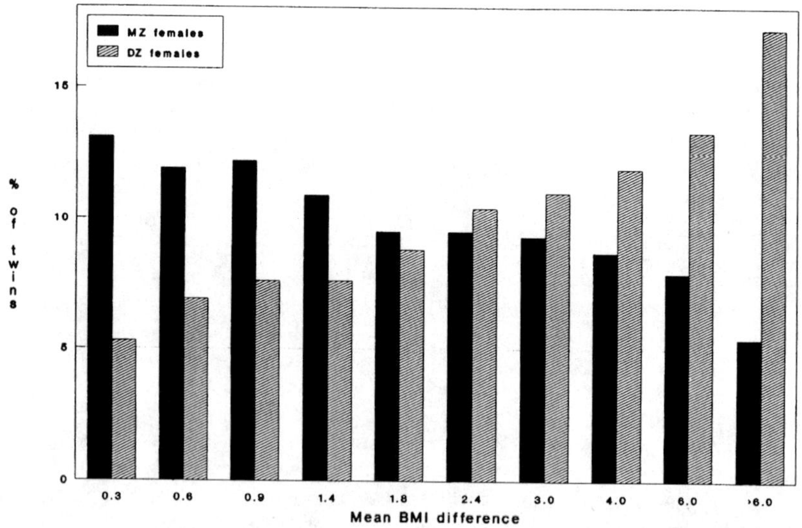

Figure 1. Absolute differences in the body mass index (BMI) of monozygotic (MZ) and dizygotic (DZ) twin pairs. Data are from adult females of the Virginia and American Association of Retired Persons Twin Registries.[3]

mental effects influence intrapair similarity. Additive genetic effects arise when alleles at a number of genetic loci contribute additively to the trait and there are no intraloci (dominance) or interloci (epistatic) interactions. Under such an assumption, the MZ twin correlation will be simply a function of the genetic variation within the population (denoted **H**) plus the common environmental variation (denoted **C**); thus,

$$r_{mz} = \mathbf{H} + \mathbf{C} \tag{1}$$

In contrast, the dizygotic twin correlation (r_{dz}) is a function of one half of the additive variation plus the common environmental effect, so that

$$r_{dz} = {}^{1}\!/_{2}\mathbf{H} + \mathbf{C} \tag{2}$$

The total population variation of the trait is simply a sum of the genetic variation, the common environmental variation, and the individual environmental variation (**E**).

To derive the "classical" heritability estimate, the rules of basic algebra are applied to the formula for MZ and DZ similarity in order to solve for **H** (Equation 3). An estimate of the influence of the individual environment on trait variation is provided by 1 – **H**.

$$\mathbf{H} = 2(r_{mz} - r_{dz}) \tag{3}$$

Although the computational simplicity of the classical heritability estimate has great appeal, there are limitations to this estimate. It is best suited for the comparison of like-sex MZ and DZ twins. When extended to the comparison of opposite-sex pairs it could result in an underestimate of heritability, particularly if different genes have different effects across gender. Further, classical heritability estimates cannot test competing hypotheses about twin similarity. For example, the classical approach does not allow the investigator to ask whether common environmental effects could explain twin similarity as well as the additive genetic model or whether both types of effects are required to account for the observed data. Finally, and significantly, this heritability estimate is subject to biases in the presence of genetic dominance or epistasis. These nonadditive genetic influences lower the DZ correlation to less than one half the MZ correlation, thereby spuriously inflating the classical heritability estimate.

A major methodological improvement over the classical heritability estimate has been the adoption of model-fitting approaches for twin data (see Reference 3). In these approaches, estimates of genetic and environmental effects are derived by "fitting" expectations in terms of these parameters to observed summary statistics (such as twin variances and intrapair covariances). Model fitting is typically carried out by the method of weighted least squares or maximum likelihood and results in chi-square statistics that can be used to assess the goodness of fit of the models. To select the best model for any given data set, alternative genetic and environmental models are fitted and the chi-square of each compared. Typically, two alternative reduced models (with **only** additive genetic and individual environmental effects **or** family and individual environmental effects) are compared against a "full" model with all three type of influences. An important feature of model-fitting approaches is that they are easily extended to accommodate data from types of relationships other than twins. Thus, nuclear family or extended pedigree data may be analyzed jointly with twin data to derive an optimal estimate of trait heritability which is based on several sources of information. Model-fitting methods also can be extended to test for differences across gender in the genetic and environmental control of a trait and to explain change and continuity in longitudinal data sets.

III. CRITICISMS OF THE CLASSICAL TWIN STUDY

The methods for analyzing twin data described above have important limitations. There exist a number of possible genotypic and environmental effects which the classical twin design cannot detect, but which nonetheless may result in biasing heritability estimates derived from such a design. For example, heritability estimates will be biased upward in the presence of genotype × environment correlations (such as obesity-prone individuals being reared in homes with plentiful fatty foods) and genotype × environment interactions (such as particular genotypes being more sensitive to high-fat diets). Further, special MZ twin environments (where MZ twins are treated more similarly than DZ twins) will also increase MZ intrapair correlations and, thus, result in an overestimate of heritability. In contrast, assortative mating (like marrying like) may produce spurious evidence for common environmental influences on obesity and at the same time reduce heritability estimates.

Fortunately, designs which depart somewhat from the classical twin approach address some of these criticisms. For example, data from twins reared apart will be free of genotype × family environment correlations and interactions, as well as MZ special twin environmental effects. Studies on human obesity which utilize such data are described below. Another method of assessing genotype × environment interactions has been experimental studies of feeding and exercise in identical twins. Such studies are also described below.

IV. EMPIRICAL FINDINGS

A. STUDIES OF TWIN CHILDREN

Studies of obesity in twin children are relatively few in number. They are, however, of great importance in understanding the etiology of obesity. Indeed, early-onset obesity is not only a good predictor of obesity in adult life;[5] it also appears to have strong genetic determinants.[6] Consequently, understanding the genetics of obesity in children may be an important step in understanding the genetics of obesity in adults.

In 1975, Brook et al.[7] conducted the first large twin study of fat distribution in children, utilizing the triceps and subscapular skinfolds of 222 pairs of like-sex twins aged 3 to 15. After correcting the data for linear age effects, they obtained classical heritability estimates of the skinfold thicknesses. Analyzing data from both boys and girls together, they found evidence for a higher heritability of trunk fat (0.98 ± 0.16) vs. limb fat (0.46 ± 0.17). Furthermore, when the data were separated into two different age groups (less than 10 years of age and 10 years of age and greater), significant heritability estimates for both measurements were obtained only in the older children. This finding may reflect differential genetic control of the skinfold thicknesses throughout early development or perhaps insufficient power of the study to detect significant heritable influences operating in the younger children. These two possibilities deserve further exploration.

Supporting the results of Brook et al. are those from a study conducted 1 year later by Borjeson[8] on a cohort of Swedish twins. Information on the height and weight at the time of school entry (typically age 7) were obtained from school records of all same-sex school-age twins in the country. From these pairs were selected those in which at least one member's weight (for height) exceeded the average by more than twice the standard deviation. The resulting sample of 40 MZ and 61 DZ pairs was therefore enriched with "obesity-prone" individuals. Triceps, subscapular, and abdominal skinfolds were measured and intrapair mean differences calculated. Results indicated a greater MZ than DZ similarity for all measures and, therefore, a genetic influence on fat patterning. However, since the design precluded the calculation of unbiased heritabilities of the skinfold thicknesses, the results of this study cannot be compared with those of the Brook study.

The largest and most carefully designed study of adiposity in twin children was that of Bodurtha and colleagues,[9] who collected anthropometric data on 259 11-year-old same-sex and opposite-sex twin pairs residing in the state of Virginia. All were examined in a laboratory on, or as near as possible to, their 11th birthdays. During the laboratory visits, measurements of height, weight, and skinfold thicknesses of the triceps, subscapular, and suprailiac areas were obtained. Pearson correlation coefficients, pooled over gender, are shown in Figure 2 for the skinfold thicknesses and the body mass index (BMI, weight in kilograms/height in meters squared). For all variables the MZ correlation was quite high, with a narrow range of 0.74 to 0.84. The DZ correlation, in contrast, ranged from 0.22 to 0.44. For all skinfold thicknesses the DZ correlation was less than one half the MZ twin correlation, suggesting a contribution of genetic nonadditivity. In contrast, for the BMI the DZ correlation exceeded one half the MZ correlation, suggesting a contribution of the common environment.

Maximum likelihood model-fitting methods were applied to the twin covariance matrices of Bodurtha and colleagues' anthropometric data. The best-fitting model for subscapular and triceps skinfolds and the BMI was one that included additive genetic and unique environmental effects. The possible effects of genetic dominance or common environment on these measures, which had been suggested by the correlational comparisons, were found to be nonsignificant. Under the best-fitting model, heritabilities (for both males and females) were equal to 0.75 and 0.77 for the triceps and subscapular skinfolds, respectively, and 0.87 for the BMI. Analysis of the suprailiac skinfolds indicated that heritability was significantly greater in girls (87%) than boys (81%).

The most striking feature of the Virginia data was the consistently high heritability estimates obtained on all measures. For these 11-year-olds, most of the variation in skinfold thickness and BMI was genetic in origin. Furthermore, in an analysis of longitudinal data from the same study, Meyer and colleagues[10] have recently shown that the high heritability of the BMI remains throughout the adolescence of these twins (up to age 17). Meyer and colleagues also found that the "tracking" of the BMI from age 11 to 17 was high and primarily due to genetic factors, with age-to-age genetic correlations

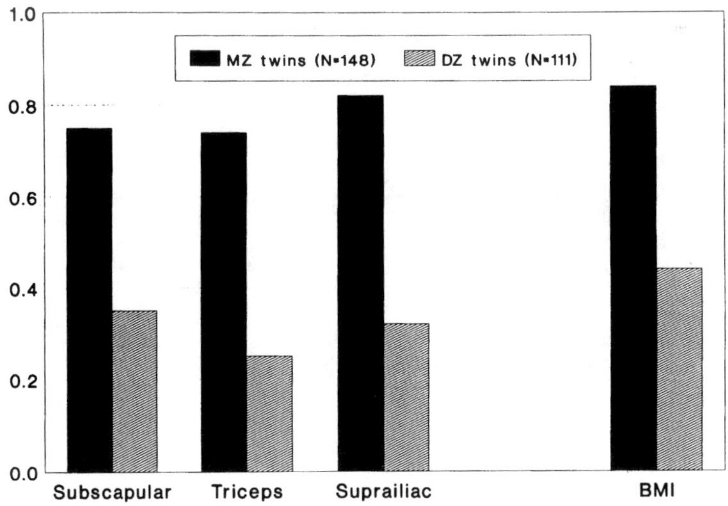

Figure 2. Twin correlations for skinfold thicknesses and body mass index (BMI) in 11-year-old twins, reported by Bodurtha and colleagues.[9] Data from same-sex and opposite-sex pairs have been pooled. MZ = monozygotic; DZ = dizygotic.

exceeding 0.79. However, some of the genetic and environmental variance during early adolescence (ages 11 and 12.5) dissipated over time, perhaps due to the variable onset of puberty in the twins.

B. STUDIES OF ADULT TWINS

1. The Body Mass Index of Twins Reared Together

a. The National Academy of Sciences-National Research Council Registry

The largest studies of the BMI of adults twins have been those conducted on male twin pairs who are members of the National Academy of Sciences-National Research Council (NAS-NRC) Twin Registry.[11] This registry was initiated in 1955 and at that time contained 15,924 twin pairs born between 1917 and 1927 who were ascertained through the Veterans Administration, each with prior military service. Weight and height measurements, obtained at induction into the military, were available on 13,376 of these pairs. In 1967, 4071 pairs responded to a questionnaire on current height and weight, as well as height and weight 25 years earlier. Three examinations of these twins were subsequently carried out between 1969 and 1986. During the first examination phase (1969 to 1973), 514 twin pairs were seen at clinics across the country. In 1980, 362 of these pairs returned for a second examination, and in 1986, 267 pairs returned for the third examination. On each of these three occasions height and weight measurements were obtained.

The NAS-NRC data have resulted in a number of publications[12-17] on the genetics of the BMI. Of these, the one based on the largest sample size is the study by Stunkard and colleagues,[14] who investigated the heritability of BMI at induction into service (average age 20) and after a 25-year follow-up (average age 45) in 4071 pairs of twins. Results, summarized in Table 1, show high heritabilities at both age 20 (0.77) and age 45 (0.84). Of further note is the marked decrease in the twin correlations over the 25 years, due either to an actual increase in the environmental variance in BMI over time or to the greater error inherent in the self-reported measures utilized at follow-up. It also should be pointed out that at age 20 the MZ correlation is approximately twice the DZ correlation, while at age 45 the DZ correlation is less than one half the MZ correlation. This latter finding suggests that nonadditive genetic variance has appeared during middle age and also that the heritability estimate is biased upward. This suggestion is supported by model-fitting analyses of other data sets described below.

Another analysis of the NAS-NRC data set was reported by Fabsitz and colleagues,[13] who investigated heritability changes of the BMI in 514 twin pairs who had both completed the mailed questionnaire in 1967 and participated in the 1969 to 1973 examination. Their analyses produced classical heritability estimates from four occasions of measurement: induction, retrospective report of height and weight at age 25, BMI assessed by the 1967 questionnaire, and BMI obtained at the 1969 to 1973 examination.

Table 1. **Correlations and heritability estimates for body mass index (BMI) obtained on National Academy of Sciences-National Research Council male veteran twin pairs**

BMI	r_{mz} (n = 1974)	r_{dz} (n = 2097)	Heritability[a]	SE
Age 20	0.81	0.42	0.77	0.04
Age 45	0.67	0.24	0.84	0.05

Note: mz = monozygotic, dz = dizygotic.

[a] Classical heritability estimate.

From Stunkard, A. J., Foch, T. T., and Hrubec, Z., *J. Am. Med. Assoc.*, 256(1), 51, 1986. With permission.

The heritability estimates ranged in magnitude from 0.80 at induction at age 20 to 0.51 for the 1967 questionnaire assessment at age 45. The authors also calculated the heritability of the **change** in BMI between induction at age 20 and the 1969 to 1973 examination and between the retrospective report at age 25 and the 1969 to 1973 examination. Their results indicated moderately high heritabilities for each change (0.60 and 0.71), suggesting that, even after maturation, increase in body size is influenced by genetic effects.

In 1992, Fabsitz and colleagues[17] published a second developmental analysis of the BMI data from 245 twin pairs measured at induction at age 20 and at the three subsequent examinations. A model fitted to these longitudinal data suggested that two independent genetic effects contributed to the BMI across the age span from 20 to 64. The first genetic effect occurred at or prior to age 20 and influenced the BMI through age 64. The second effect appeared during middle age, increased the total genetic variance of BMI, and persisted into old age. The schematic in Figure 3 illustrates these major results.

Although the findings of Fabsitz and colleagues[17] are limited to male veterans, they raise issues that must be considered in future genetic studies of the BMI. For example, the finding of age-dependent genetic influences (during middle age) suggests that heritability estimates derived from twin data in this age range will be greater than those estimated from parent-offspring data which span the period from youth through middle age, since the parent-offspring correlations reflect only those genetic effects common to both generations at the time of measurement. Thus, the impact of age-dependent genetic effects may, in part, explain the higher heritabilities of the BMI obtained in twin studies as compared to family studies.

b. Additional Studies of Adult Body Mass Index

Evidence supporting the relatively high heritability estimates obtained from the male twins in the NAS-NRC registry comes from several sources. Neale and Cardon[3] have recently described a model-fitting analysis of the (age-corrected) BMI of 5588 same-sex and opposite-sex twin pairs of the Virginia and the American Association of Retired Persons twin registries (average age 51). There were three major findings. First, there was a somewhat higher heritability for females (75%) than males (69%). Second, genetic nonadditivity influenced the male, but not the female, BMI. Thus, the age-corrected BMI correlations for the MZ and DZ males were 0.70 (n = 750) and 0.30 (n = 553), respec-

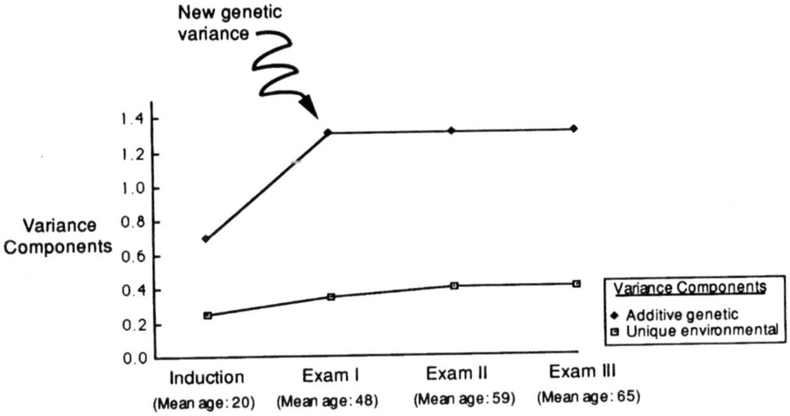

Figure 3. Changes in genetic and environmental variance components for the body mass index (BMI) across age. Data are from male twins of the NAS-NRC registry, age 20 to 64, reported by Fabsitz and colleagues.[17]

tively, figures quite similar to those found by Stunkard et al.[14] (0.67 and 0.24) in their analysis of the NAS-NRC male twins at age 45. Third, the DZ opposite-sex correlation (0.25; $n = 1341$) was lower than the same-sex correlations (0.35, females, $n = 1142$; 0.30, males, $n = 553$), suggesting the intriguing possibility that different genes might influence BMI across gender.

In another large twin study ($n = 7245$ pairs) of the BMI in Finnish same-sex pairs aged 18 to 54, Korkeila and colleagues[18] found that age accounted for 20% of the variance among men and 26% among women and that age-corrected heritability estimates were 0.72 for men and 0.68 for women. Model-fitting analyses conducted separately on 10-year age cohorts showed that heritability estimates differed significantly across cohorts, decreasing steadily with age.

Additional family studies of BMI which have included adult twin pairs (as well as other types of relative pairs) were conducted by Bouchard et al.,[19] Hunt et al.,[20] and Austin et al.[21] In the Quebec Family Study, Bouchard and colleagues[19] studied 69 DZ and 87 MZ young-adult twin pairs (mean age of 15 years for DZ twins and 17 years for MZ twins). Age- and gender-corrected correlations were 0.88 (MZ) and 0.34 (DZ), values which suggest a high heritability of BMI and which are quite similar to those obtained previously for NAS-NRC twins at induction into the armed services at age 20. These findings for BMI in young adults, taken together with those obtained for children, indicate a slightly higher heritability of this measure of body size in youth than at older ages.

Hunt and colleagues'[20] study of 308 adult male twins found MZ and DZ correlations of 0.65 and 0.43, respectively, after correcting the data for the effects of age and putative environmental mediators, including alcohol and coffee consumption and smoking status. The classical heritability estimate derived from these corrected correlations was 0.44. Austin and colleagues[21] conducted a similar analysis of BMI in 434 pairs of adult female twins. After correcting the BMI data for behavioral variables, they estimated a heritability of 0.55.

Overall, the twin studies of the adult BMI suggest a moderate to high heritability, with estimates ranging from 0.40 to 0.80. In general, there is higher heritability in younger twins and evidence for nonadditive effects in older twins. When the BMI data are corrected for putative behavioral mediators the heritability decreases, suggesting that some of the genetic variability in the BMI arises from the genetic effects on these mediating variables.

2. The Body Mass Index of Twins Reared Apart

Data from twins reared apart address some of the criticisms of the classical twin design, since twins reared apart, by definition, do not share any of their childhood rearing environment. For this reason, family environment effects, special twin environment effects, and genotype × family environment interactions or correlations cannot influence the similarity of twins.

Two studies of twins reared apart suggest that environmental influences exert only a modest effect on the BMI. The largest study from a reared-apart (and reared-together) sample of adult twins utilized the data of the Swedish Adoption/Twin Study of Aging.[22] In this study, Stunkard and colleagues obtained reports of height and weight from 93 MZ twins reared apart, 154 MZ twins reared together, 218 DZ twins reared apart, and 208 DZ twins reared together. Their mean age was 58.6 ± 13.6 years. Correlational findings are summarized in Table 2, for males and females separately.

The Swedish results show a marked similarity between the reared-together and reared-apart correlations, indicating that family rearing environment has at most a very modest effect on the BMI. For both men and women, and under both rearing conditions, a high heritability of the BMI is suggested. The availability of data on the 93 separated identical twins makes possible the most direct estimate of heritability yet obtained — the intrapair

Table 2. **Body mass index and intrapair correlations in monozygotic and dizygotic pairs of twins reared apart or together[22]**

Type	Men			Women		
	No. of pairs	Body mass index[a]	Intrapair correlation	No. of pairs	Body mass index[a]	Intrapair correlation
Monozygotic						
Reared apart	49	24.8 ± 2.4	0.70	44	24.2 ± 3.4	0.66
Reared together	66	24.2 ± 2.9	0.74	48	23.7 ± 3.5	0.66
Dizygotic						
Reared apart	75	25.1 ± 3.0	0.15	143	24.9 ± 4.1	0.25
Reared together	89	24.6 ± 2.7	0.33	119	23.9 ± 3.5	0.27

[a] Plus-minus values are means ± SD.

From Stunkard, A. J., Harris, J. R., Pederson, N. L., and McClearn, G. E., *N. Engl. J. Med.*, 322, 1483, 1990. With permission.

correlation for MZ twins reared apart. It is 0.70 for men and 0.66 for women, slightly lower than that from twins reared together. When all data were subjected to model-fitting analyses, results (shown in Figure 4) indicated that, in men, nonshared environmental effects contributed 26% of the variance — the remainder being due to nonadditive genetic effects (57%) and additive genetic effects (17%). For women, the comparable figures were 31% for individual environment, 37% for nonadditive genetic effects, and 32% for additive genetic effects. Once again, significant nonadditive variance is apparent in older persons.

The Swedish findings are supported by two studies of an English cohort of twins reared together and reared apart. In 1990, MacDonald and Stunkard[23] reported intraclass correlations for MZ adult twins in each situation. For men, the correlations were quite similar to those obtained from the Swedish data: $MZ_{together} = 0.68$ ($n = 38$) and $MZ_{apart} = 0.64$ ($n = 14$). For women, however, the reared-apart correlation ($MZ_{apart} = 0.39$; $n = 24$) was not only far lower than the reared-together correlation ($MZ_{together} = 0.76$), but also lower than that reported in the comparable Swedish sample (0.66). Price and Gottesman,[24] in an independent analysis of the English data, combined the MZ male and female BMI data and (after correcting for sex differences in the mean) reported a reared-apart correlation of 0.61.

3. Studies of Fat Mass, Patterning, and Distribution

One criticism of using the BMI to study genetic influences on obesity is that the measure does not directly index fat mass, nor does it provide any information about fat patterning or distribution of body fat. Instead, it represents a global measure of body size. Only the study of the genetics of actual measures of fat mass and fat distribution permits estimates of the heritability of these risk factors. Unfortunately, large studies of related individuals which incorporate such measures are few in number. Of these, the Quebec Family Study by Bouchard et al.[19] stands out.

The Quebec study assessed genetic influences not only on BMI, but also on subcutaneous fat (sum of six skinfolds), percentage body fat, and fat and fat-free mass as well as two measures of fat distribution — the ratio of trunk skinfolds to extremity skinfolds

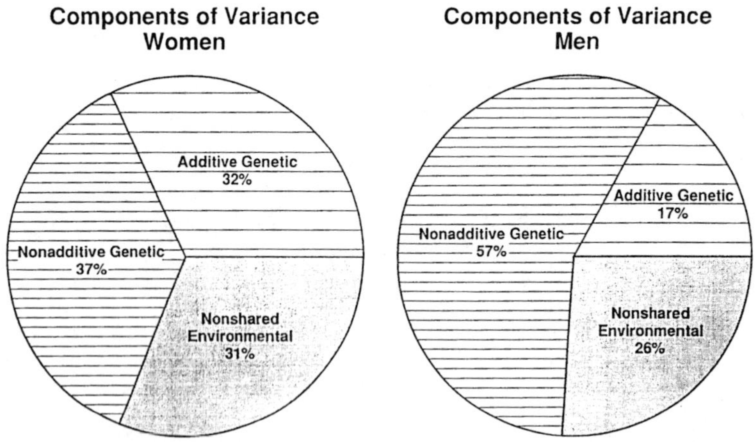

Figure 4. Genetic and environmental components of variance in body mass index. The contributions of shared and correlated environments each account for less than 1% of the variance among men and women. (From Stunkard, A. J., Harris, J. R., Pedersen, N. L., and McClearn, G. E., *N. Engl. J. Med.*, 322, 1483, 1990. With permission.)

and the ratio of total subcutaneous fat to total fat mass. Subjects included 87 MZ and 69 DZ twin pairs plus the following constellation of other relatives: foster parent-adopted children (322 pairs); adoptive siblings (120); first-degree cousins (95); uncles/aunts-nieces/nephews (88); biological parents-children (1239); and full siblings (370). The correlations for the twins are shown in Table 3. With the exception of the subcutaneous fat/fat mass ratio, the MZ correlations are quite high — at least 0.73. Also, except for fat-free mass and the extremity/trunk ratio, the MZ correlation exceeds the DZ correlation by more than a twofold difference, suggesting an absence of family environmental effects and possibly an influence of genetic nonadditivity. These results from the twin data alone indicate a high heritability for all measures of body composition and fat distribution. However, when Bouchard et al.[19] analyzed these twin data in conjunction with other family data, they found that the subcutaneous fat measures had a far lower heritability (5%) than the percentage of body fat, fat-free mass, and indicators of fat distribution (25 to 30%). Results such as these indicate the importance of extending the twin design to include other genetically informative relationships.

Selby and colleagues[25] have reported an additional twin study of fat distribution in 265 veteran pairs from the NAS-NRC registry. These individuals ranged in age from 59 to 70 years at the time of examination. Twin correlations for four skinfold measures are also shown in Table 3. With the exception of the subscapular/triceps ratio, all measures show high heritabilities, with classical estimates ranging from 0.63 (triceps) to 0.95 (sum of skinfolds). Of note is the fact that the MZ twin correlations are lower than those of Bouchard and colleagues,[19] perhaps a function of the greater age of the NAS-NRC twins.

4. Studies of Metabolic Rate

Although the studies described to this point indicate moderate to large genetic influences on various indices of human obesity, they have not elucidated a mechanism through

Table 3. **Twin correlations for measures of fat patterning and distribution**

Study	Variable	r_{MZ}	r_{DZ}
Bouchard et al.[19]			
(n_{mz} = 87, n_{dz} = 69)	Body mass index	0.88	0.34
	Sum of six skinfolds	0.83	0.39
	Percentage body fat	0.73	0.21
	Fat mass	0.76	0.31
	Fat-free mass	0.93	0.53
	Extremity/trunk ratio	0.80	0.40
	Subcutaneous fat/fat mass ratio	0.61	0.15
Selby et al.[25]			
(n_{mz} = 134, n_{dz} = 134)	Subscapular skinfolds	0.76	0.34
	Triceps skinfolds	0.70	0.38
	Triceps + subscapular skinfolds	0.73	0.25
	Subscapular/triceps ratio	0.67	0.55

Note: mz = monozygotic, dz = dizygotic.

which such genetic effects might operate. To this end, three investigations[26-28] have used the classical twin design to study the heritability of metabolic rate, a promising candidate. The study by Fontaine and colleagues[26] of 39 pairs of young-adult (average age 21) male twins indicated a high heritability (0.80) of resting metabolic rate (RMR). However, this value was reduced to 0.40 when RMR was adjusted for fat-free weight. Similarly, Bouchard and colleagues'[27] study of 37 MZ and 21 DZ like-sex pairs found a heritability of 0.40 for RMR after adjustments for gender, age, and fat-free mass. These results suggest that RMR and fat-free mass share a common genetic etiology, but there are also genetic influences on RMR which are independent of fat-free mass.

In contrast to these findings, Hewitt et al.[28] have reported a negligible heritability of metabolic rate in 80 pairs of adult male twins after adjusting for the BMI. A multivariate genetic analysis of height, weight, and metabolic rate found no genetic effects on metabolic rate which were not due to body weight. The authors propose an alternative to the traditional viewpoint that low metabolic rate is a mechanism giving rise to increased body weight. Instead, they suggest that low metabolic rate may index an instability in the equilibrium between body weight and energy expenditure. As weight is gained, they hypothesize, metabolic rate increases more sharply than body weight, bringing the system into a more stable equilibrium at an elevated body weight. Further study of these issues seems warranted.

5. Genotype × Environment Interactions

As noted previously, traditional analyses of data using the classical twin design cannot take into account genotype × environment interactions such as occur when genotypes differ in their sensitivity to environmental conditions. One way to study such interactions is through experiments, and Bouchard and colleagues have demonstrated the power of experiments in their controlled feeding studies of MZ twins.[29,30] In these investigations, 12 pairs of identical male twins were overfed by 1000 kcal/day (as compared to their established baseline energy intake) during 84 days of a 100-day period. Changes in body composition, topography of fat deposition, and adipose tissue lipolysis were assessed, and the twin similarity for these changes was quantified with the intraclass correlation coefficient. Significant MZ correlations (ranging from 0.40 to 0.60) were found for changes in the various indices of obesity. Furthermore, the heritability of body fat, fat-free mass, and abdominal visceral fat was higher than that of subcutaneous fat. Abdominal visceral fat has recently been shown to play a critical role in the complications of obesity, and this study suggests that this depot is the one that is most strongly determined genetically. The strong twin similarity for change in abdominal visceral fat, assessed by computed tomography (CT) scanning, is illustrated in Figure 5. These findings demonstrate a remarkable genetic control of the response to dietary intake and variability in the genetic control of body fat distribution.

V. FUTURE RESEARCH

The many achievements of twin research in obesity during the recent past provide a foretaste of future achievements. The directions of this future research are becoming apparent in three closely related and interactive areas — data analysis, experimentation, and substantive issues.

Data analysis — The rich contributions of the classical twin method are already being supplemented by more sophisticated methods that, as noted above, obviate old problems and provide information about new areas. Multivariate methods and model-fitting procedures make possible not only the testing of increasingly complex hypotheses, but also the estimation of important parameters. Already analytic methods are available that yield causal attributions from cross-sectional data. As data analytic measures increase in power

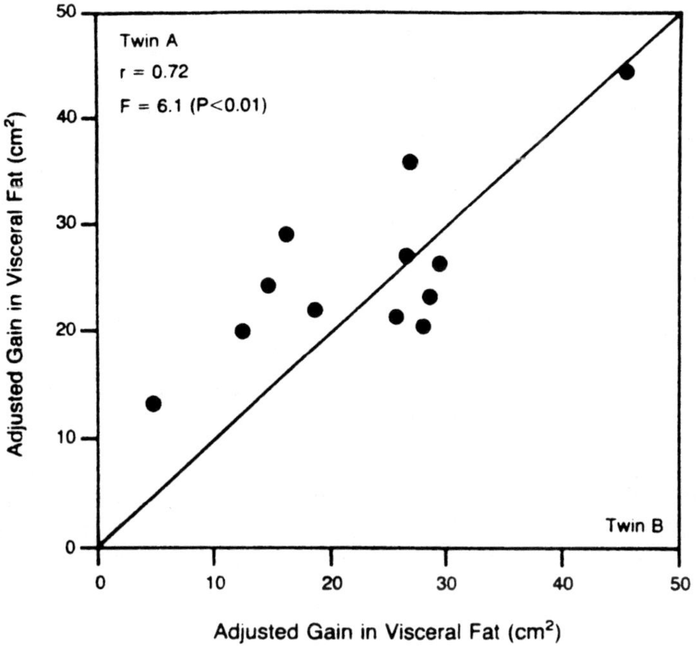

Figure 5. Similarity within twin pairs with respect to changing abdominal visceral fat in 12 pairs of male monozygotic twins in response to 100 days of overfeeding, after adjustment for gain in fat mass. (From Bouchard, C., Tremblay, A., Despres, J., Nadeau, A., Lupien, P. J., Theriault, G., Dusault, J., Moorjani, S., Pinault, S., and Fournier, G., *N. Engl. J. Med.,* 322(31), 1477, 1990. With permission.)

they will be able to contribute further to the study of issues that have already begun to be explored — the effects on obesity of gender, race, age, and various environmental determinants. They also will be useful in understanding the results of experimental approaches as these are developed.

Experimental methods — As noted above, experimental methods provide an unusual opportunity to obviate problems of traditional twin research and to investigate such important issues as gene × environment interactions and gene × environment correlations. The remarkable productivity of the Quebec study described above is a superb indication of the kind of experiments that will increasingly enrich twin research. Such methods can be applied to the wide variety of substantive issues noted below. A type of twin research not yet utilized in the study of obesity has great promise — the study of discordant identical twins. This method has been used with great success in the investigation of schizophrenia, showing evidence of deficits so limited that they could not have been detected by methods that utilized traditional control groups.[31,32] Finally, molecular genetic investigations can be greatly facilitated when applied to identical twins, as shown by recent studies of lipoprotein.[33,34]

Substantive issues — Improved data analytic and experimental methods make possible far more productive studies of substantive aspects of obesity than those that have been conducted to date. A major question in obesity is the origin of the various distributions of body fat with their radically different implications for health and disease. It already appears that genetic mechanisms play a key role in the distribution of body fat. Future studies, particularly experiments to increase and decrease body fat, could provide important information about the developmental, cellular, and humoral mechanisms that determine fat balance in these critical areas, particularly in the deep visceral fat. Two other fundamental questions with regard to obesity are the origins of the processes that determine energy output and energy intake. Of the two, genetic aspects of energy expenditure have been studied more extensively, but these studies can only hint at the discoveries to be made by the application of improved data analysis to creative experimentation. Genetic studies of energy intake, by contrast, have hardly begun. However, it is clear that sophisticated new twin studies could significantly advance our understanding of the genetic and environmental contributions to such promising measures as infant sucking behavior (an index of energy intake)[35,36] and the increasingly important area of nutrient partitioning.

VI. SUMMARY AND CONCLUSIONS

The study of twins, a method of genetic analysis introduced more than a century ago, has recently been applied to the study of human obesity and has provided strong evidence of the importance of genetic factors in this disorder. "Classical" twin studies have estimated very high heritabilities of various indices of obesity, particularly among younger persons. They also provide evidence of age-dependent genetic effects beginning during middle age. A limitation of the classical twin method is that it cannot detect gene × environment interactions or gene × environment correlations, thereby biasing estimates of heritability upward. Studies of twins reared apart obviate some of these problems. They show that the childhood rearing environment has no effect on body mass in adult life, but that heritability is still high. Another method of coping with these problems is to analyze twin data in conjunction with data from other genetically informative family relationships. When this is done, estimates of heritability are considerably lower. A third method of coping with problems of gene × environment interaction is by experiments designed to assess these interactions. An ambitious overfeeding experiment with twins has revealed considerable difference in genetic influence on the amount and distribution of fat gained by overfeeding.

REFERENCES

1. **Galton, F.,** *Hereditary Genius: An Inquiry into Its Laws and Consequences,* Macmillan, London, 1869.
2. **Galton, F.,** *Inquiries into Human Faculty,* Macmillan, London, 1883.
3. **Neale, M. C. and Cardon, L. R.,** *Methodology for Genetic Studies of Twins and Families,* Kluwer Academic Publishers, Dordrect, The Netherlands, 1992.
4. **Falconer, D. S.,** *Introduction to Quantitative Genetics,* 2nd ed., Ronald Press, New York, 1981.
5. **Mossberg, H. O.,** 40-Year follow-up of overweight children, *Lancet,* 2(8661), 491, 1989.
6. **Price, R. A., Stunkard, A. J., Ness, R., Wadden, T., Heshka, S., Kanders, B., and Cormillot, A.,** Childhood onset (age < 10) obesity has high familial risk, *Int. J. Obes.,* 14, 195, 1990.
7. **Brook, G. D., Huntley, R. M. C., and Slack, J.,** Influence of heredity and environment in determination of skinfold thickness in children, *Br. Med. J.,* 28, 719, 1975.
8. **Borjeson, M.,** The aetiology of obesity in children, *Acta Paediatr. Scand.,* 65, 279, 1976.
9. **Bodurtha, J. N., Mosteller, M., Hewitt, J. K., Nance, W. E., Eaves, L. J., Moskowitz, W. B., Katz, S., and Schieken, R. M.,** Genetic analysis of anthropometric measures in 11-year-old twins: The Medical College of Virginia Twin Study, *Pediatr. Res.,* 28, 1, 1990.

10. **Meyer, J. M., Bodurtha, J. N., Eaves, L. J., Hewitt, J. K., Mosteller, M., Nance, W. E., Neale, M. C., and Schieken, R. M.,** Tracking genetic and environmental effects on adolescent BMI: The MCV Twin Study, *Am. J. Hum. Genet.*, in review.
11. **Jablon, S., Neel, J. V., and Gershowitz, H.,** The NAS-NRC Twin Panel: methods of construction of the panel, zygosity diagnosis, and proposed use, *Am. J. Hum. Genet.*, 19, 133, 1967.
12. **Feinleib, M., Garrison, R. J., Fabsitz, R., Christian, J. C., Hrubec, Z., Borhani, N. O., Kannel, W. B., Rosenman, R., Schwartz, J. T., and Wagner, J. O.,** The NHLBI Twin Study of cardiovascular disease risk factors: methodology and summary of results, *Am. J. Epidemiol.*, 10(4), 284, 1977.
13. **Fabsitz, R., Feinleib, M., and Hrubec, Z.,** Weight changes in adult twins, *Acta Genet. Med. Gemellol.*, 29, 273, 1980.
14. **Stunkard, A. J., Foch, T. T., and Hrubec, Z.,** A twin study of human obesity, *J. Am. Med. Assoc.*, 256(1), 51, 1986.
15. **Newman, B., Selby, J. V., Quesenberry, C. P., King, M.-C., Friedman, G. D., and Fabsitz, R. R.,** Nongenetic influences of obesity on other cardiovascular disease risk factors: an analysis of identical twins, *Am. J. Public Health,* 80(6), 675, 1990.
16. **Selby, J. V., Reed, T., Newman, B., Fabsitz, R. R., and Carmelli, D.,** Effects of selective return on estimates of heritability for body mass index in the National Heart, Lung and Blood Institute Twin Study, *Genet. Epidemiol.*, 8, 371, 1991.
17. **Fabsitz, R. R., Carmelli, D., and Hewitt, J. K.,** Evidence for independent genetic influences on obesity in middle age, *Int. J. Obes.*, 16, 657, 1992.
18. **Korkeila, M., Kaprio, J., Rissanen, A., and Koskenvuo, M.,** Effects of gender and age on the heritability of body mass index, *Int. J. Obes.*, 15(10), 647, 1991.
19. **Bouchard, C., Perusse, L., Leblanc, C., Tremblay, A., and Theriault, G.,** Inheritance of the amount and distribution of human body fat, *Int. J. Obes.*, 12, 205, 1988.
20. **Hunt, S. C., Hasstedt, S. J., Kuida, H., Stults, B. M., Hopkins, P. N., and Williams, R. R.,** Genetic heritability and common environmental components of resting and stressed blood pressures, lipids, and body mass index in Utah pedigrees and twins, *Am. J. Epidemiol.*, 129(3), 625, 1989.
21. **Austin, M. A., King, M.-C., Bawol, R. D., Hulley, S. B., and Friedman, G. D.,** Risk factors for coronary heart disease in adult female twins, *Am. J. Epidemiol.*, 125, 308, 1987.
22. **Stunkard, A. J., Harris, J. R., Pedersen, N. L., and McClearn, G. E.,** The body-mass index of twins who have been reared apart, *N. Engl. J. Med.*, 322, 1483, 1990.
23. **MacDonald, A. and Stunkard, A. J.,** Body-mass index of British separated twins, *N. Engl. J. Med.*, 322, 1530, 1990.
24. **Price, R. A. and Gottesman, I. I.,** Body fat in identical twins reared apart: roles for genes and environment, *Behav. Genet.*, 21(1), 1, 1991.
25. **Selby, J. V., Newman, B., Quesenberry, C. P., Fabsitz, R. R., Carmelli, D., Meaney, F. J., and Slemenda, C.,** Genetic and behavioral influences on body fat distribution, *Int. J. Obes.*, 14, 593, 1990.
26. **Fontaine, E., Savard, R., Tremblay, A., Despres, J. P., Poehlman, E., and Bouchard, C.,** Resting metabolic rate in monozygotic and dizygotic twins, *Acta Genet. Med. Gemellol.*, 34, 41, 1989.
27. **Bouchard, C., Tremblay, A., Nadeau, A., Despres, J. P., Theriault, G., Boulay, M. R., Lortie, G., Leblanc, C., and Fournier, G.,** Genetic effect in resting and exercise metabolic rate, *Metabolism,* 38, 364, 1989.
28. **Hewitt, J. K., Stunkard, A. J., Carroll, D., Sims, J., and Turner, J. R.,** A twin study approach towards understanding genetic contributions to body size and metabolic rate, *Acta Genet. Med. Gemellol.*, 40, 133, 1991.

29. **Bouchard, C., Tremblay, A., Despres, J., Nadeau, A., Lupien, P. J., Theriault, G., Dussault, J., Moorjani, S., Pinault, S., and Fournier, G.,** The response to long-term overfeeding in identical twins, *N. Engl. J. Med.,* 322(31), 1477, 1990.
30. **Mauriege, P., Despres, J., Marcotte, M., Tremblay, A., Nadeau, A., Moorjani, S., Lupien, P., Dussault, J., Fournier, G., Theriault, G., and Bouchard, C.,** Adipose tissue lipolysis after long-term overfeeding in identical twins, *Int. J. Obes.,* 16, 219, 1992.
31. **Goldberg, T. E., Ragland, J. D., Torrey, E. F., Gold, J. M., Bigelow, L. B., and Weinberger, D. R.,** Neuropsychological assessment of monozygotic twins discordant for schizophrenia, *Arch. Gen. Psychiatry,* 47(11), 1066, 1990.
32. **Weinberger, D. R., Berman, K. F., Suddath, R., and Torrey, E. F.,** Evidence of dysfunction of a prefrontal-limbic network in schizophrenia: a magnetic resonance imaging and regional blood flow study of discordant MZ twins, *Am. J. Psychiatry,* 149(7), 890, 1992.
33. **Berg, K., Kondo, I., Drayna, D., and Lawn, R.,** "Variability gene" effect of cholesteryl ester transfer protein (CETP) genes, *Clin. Genet.,* 35(6), 437, 1989.
34. **Pedersen, J. C. and Berg, K.,** Interaction between low density lipoprotein receptor (LDLR) and apolipoprotein E (apo E) alleles contributes to normal variation in lipid level, *Clin. Genet.,* 35(5), 331, 1989.
35. **Agras, S. W., Kraemer, H. C., Berkowitz, R. I., Korner, A. F., and Hammer, L. D.,** Does a vigorous feeding style influence early development of adiposity?, *J. Pediatr.,* 110, 799, 1987.
36. **Agras, S. W., Kraemer, H. C., Berkowitz, R. I., and Hammer, L. D.,** Influence of early feeding style on adiposity at 6 years of age, *J. Pediatr.,* 116, 805, 1990.

Chapter 6

Genetics of Obesity: Family Studies

Claude Bouchard and Louis Pérusse

TABLE OF CONTENTS

I. INTRODUCTION

The present chapter deals with the genetics of body fat content, regional fat distribution, and nutrient partitioning phenotypes. Additive genetic effects, major gene and single gene effects, and genotype-environment interaction effects are considered. The field was reviewed by us 5 years ago[1] and more recently in several publications.[2-4] The emphasis of the review is on familial data, but it will also incorporate some of the more important findings from adoption studies and twin study designs. Complete exposés of adoption study data and twin data are, however, presented elsewhere in this volume (Chapters 4 and 5, respectively).

II. HERITABILITY OF BODY FAT CONTENT

Although the familial nature of obesity is well established,[1,5,6] there is still some disagreement among researchers regarding the importance of genetic factors in this familiality. Most studies on the genetics of obesity used the body mass index (BMI) or skinfold thicknesses at a few sites as measures of body fat content or obesity. Heritability estimates ranging from almost zero to values as high as 90% have been reported for BMI.[1,7] With the use of different designs (twin, family, and adoption studies), with large variation in age of subjects, and with only a few types of relatives and, very often, small sample sizes, such wide variation in the reported heritabilities within and between populations is not unexpected. With few exceptions, these studies could not separate the effects of genes from those of the environment shared by relatives living together in the same household. Moreover, only a handful of studies have included the full range of BMI values to ensure that the obese phenotypes are adequately represented.

0-8493-4880-3/94/$0.00+$.50

A. TWIN AND ADOPTION DATA

The comparison of monozygotic (MZ) twins reared apart with MZ twins reared together represents an interesting design to assess the role of heredity with some control over some of the confounding influences of shared environment. The correlations of MZ twins reared apart are generally similar to those of MZ twins reared together, as shown by three studies[7-9] suggesting that shared familial environment does not contribute much to the variation in BMI. The correlations of MZ twins reared apart provide a direct estimate of the genetic effect if it is assumed that members of the same pair were not placed in a similar environment, that twins were not, for some undefined reasons, behaving similarly despite the fact that they were living apart, and that intrauterine factors did not influence long-term variation in BMI. According to these studies, the heritability of BMI would be in the range of 40 to 70%. Other twin study designs also tend to generate similar heritability estimates and often even higher values (see Chapter 5).

Five recent adoption studies,[10-14] in which BMI data were available in both the biological as well as the adoptive relatives of the adoptees, reported that the effects of shared family environment on BMI were negligible. In a recent review of behavioral genetic studies relevant to obesity, Grilo and Pogue-Geile[15] also concluded that experiences shared among family members appeared largely irrelevant in determining individual differences in body weight and obesity. These findings are somewhat at odds with the strong familiality of some of the major affectors of energy balance and body fat content — energy intake[16] and energy expenditure.[17] The whole issue deserves further investigation by genetic epidemiologists. The heritability estimates for the BMI derived from the adoption studies tend to cluster around 30% or less (see Chapter 4).

B. FAMILY STUDIES

During the last 60 years or so, a large number of authors have reported that obese parents have a higher risk of having obese children than lean parents. This does not constitute a clear demonstration that obesity of the offspring is determined by the so-called "obesity" genes of the parents since both generations share not only genes, but also household milieu and many other environmental conditions. The data of these early studies nonetheless suggest that having an obese mother or one obese parent means a greater risk of becoming obese.[18]

These series of investigations were complemented by studies comparing the resemblance in pairs of spouses, parent-child, and brothers and sisters (sibs) for body weight, BMI, and selected skinfold measurements. These studies have been reviewed by Mueller,[19] Bouchard and Lortie,[20] and Bouchard and Pérusse.[1,4] From computations performed on a variety of published studies it was found that the weighted mean correlation for skinfolds reached 0.23 in about 8800 parent-child pairs and 0.28 in more than 3300 full-sib pairs. Mean sib-sib correlations were always slightly higher than, or equal to, the mean parent-child correlations. It should also be noted that sister-sister coefficients were consistently higher than the brother-brother values.[20]

Table 1 summarizes some of the correlations reported in four rather large family-based studies of the BMI. These results were obtained from the Framingham Heart Study,[21] the Canada Fitness Survey,[22] the Quebec Family Study,[23] and the Nord-Trøndelag Norwegian National Health Screening Service Family Study.[24]

In the Framingham Heart Study, adult levels of BMI were used in both the parental and the offspring generations.[21] The authors reported that their results provided little support for a genetic effect on BMI. In the more recent study of the BMI obtained on 74,994 persons of both genders, 20 years of age and older, from the population of Nord-Trøndelag, Norway, correlations were available for many types of relatives; some of these

Table 1. **Familial correlations for body mass index derived from four large family studies[a]**

Relationship	FHS[21]	CFS[22]	QFS[32]	Norway[24]
Spouses	0.19 (1,163)	0.12 (3,183)	0.10 (248)	0.12 (23,936)
Parent-offspring	0.23 (4,027)	0.20 (7,194)	0.23 (1,239)	0.20 (43,586)
Siblings	0.28 (992)	0.34 (3,924)	0.26 (370)	0.24 (19,157)
Uncle/aunt-nephew/niece	0.08 (1,970)	–0.11 (34)	0.14 (88)	0 (1,146)
Grandparent-grandchild	NA	0.05 (32)	NA	0.07 (1,251)
Dizygotic twins	NA	NA	0.34 (69)	0.20 (90)
Monozygotic twins	NA	NA	0.88 (87)	0.58 (79)

[a] The family studies are the Framingham Heart Study (FHS), the Canada Fitness Survey (CFS), the Quebec Family Study (QFS), and the Norwegian Family Study (Norway). Number of pairs are given in parentheses. NA = no data available.

are summarized in Table 1. Fitting a path model for genetic and environmental transmission to their data, a broad heritability of about 40% was obtained.[24] They concluded that a simple model with only an additive genetic effect and an individual environmental effect could be rejected.

Two of our own studies considered the transmission effects and heritability of the BMI and subcutaneous fat as assessed by the sum of several skinfolds. The first was based on a stratified sample of the Canadian population and included the BMI and the sum of five skinfold measurements on 18,073 subjects living in thousands of households, yielding 4825 pairs of spouses, 8881 parent-child pairs, 3929 pairs of siblings, 43 uncle/aunt-nephew/niece pairs, and 85 grandparent-grandchild pairs.[22] The total transmission effect across generations for the age- and gender-adjusted phenotypes reached about 35%. The second study relied on 1698 members of 409 families, which included nine types of relatives by descent or adoption.[23] Under these conditions there was a total transmissible variance across generations for the BMI and the sum of six skinfold measurements of about 35%, but a genetic effect of only 5% (Figure 1).

Only one report has dealt with fat mass and percent body fat measured with one of the commonly accepted direct methods for determining body composition.[23] Underwater weighing measurements of body density were performed on a relatively large number of individuals representing nine different kinds of relatives. About one half of the variance, after adjustment for age and gender, in fat mass or percent body fat was associated with a transmissible effect, and 25% of the variance was compatible with an additive genetic effect (Figure 1).

Taken as a whole, these family studies indicate that the heritability of body mass for height or body fat content is not particularly high. These results are well supported by the results of several adoption studies. It is the opinion of these authors that the heritability level does not exceed 30 to 40% of the age- and gender-adjusted phenotype in Caucasian populations and that the value may be significantly less than that.

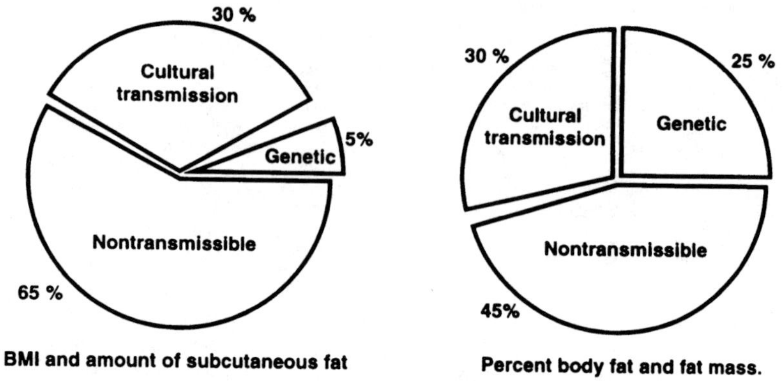

Figure 1. Total transmissible variance and its genetic component for the body mass index and indicators of subcutaneous and total body fat. (Reproduced from Bouchard, C., Perusse, L., Leblanc, C., Tremblay, A., and Thériault, G., *Int. J. Obes.*, 12, 205, 1988. With permission.)

III. NUTRIENT PARTITIONING

Nutrient partitioning can be defined in terms of the pattern of deposition of the ingested energy in the form of fat (lipid) or lean (protein) tissue. Nutrient partitioning can be visualized by following the processes of dietary carbon utilization in the body. In adult human beings, the prime metabolic fate of the ingested energy is to sustain ATP synthesis for the maintenance of cells, tissues, and a variety of essential functions. Most of the dietary energy is used to meet these needs, particularly in mature individuals. By some estimates, about 99% of the food energy serves for maintenance in the broad sense.[25]

When the basic maintenance needs have been met, the excess dietary energy can be used to support the metabolic processes leading to protein synthesis or fat deposition. Thus, nutrient partitioning becomes an even more important metabolic property when nutrients are ingested in excess of maintenance dietary carbon needs. Nutrient partitioning in animal husbandry has been shown to be a trait that can be altered by a variety of factors, including dietary means and variation in energy expenditure.[25] It is also influenced by genetic differences.

Moreover, as argued by Reeds et al.,[25] an increase in deposition of 1 g of protein carbon is equivalent to a reduction in lipid carbon deposition of about 1.4 g because of the differences in the energetic efficiencies of protein and lipid deposition.[26] Thus, a nutrient partitioning phenotype resulting in greater protein deposition should result in a decrease in efficiency of energy storage in comparison to a nutrient partitioning profile favoring lipid accretion. These considerations are of considerable importance for the understanding of the etiology of excess body fat content in humans.

A nutrient partitioning profile favoring lipid accretion over protein deposition is likely to contribute to a chronic state of positive energy balance for two main reasons: first, because of the higher energy efficiency of energy storage in the form of lipid deposition; and second, because when nutrient partitioning favors lipid accretion, fat-free mass is likely to progressively contribute a decreasing proportion of total body mass. In turn, resting metabolic rate will not increase at the same rate as body mass does, thus setting the stage for a state of chronic positive energy balance. The latter scenario is illustrated in Figure 2. One could also envisage a scenario whereby the rate of lipid deposition is slightly more elevated than normal early in life, perhaps even during the intrauterine period, or during childhood. Such a predisposition to fat accretion would likely be a major risk factor for the subsequent development of an obese state.

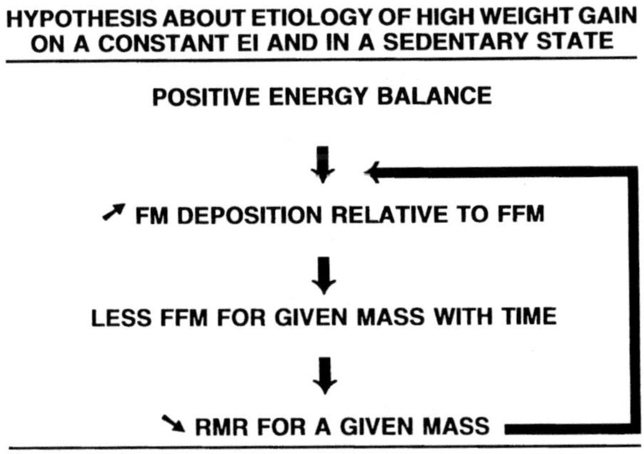

Figure 2. Hypothesis about etiology of high weight gain on a constant EI and in a sedentary state. FM = fat mass; FFM = fat-free mass; RMR = resting metabolic rate.

Cells and tissues of the body are exposed to the same profile of blood substrates and humoral factors. One may entertain the notion that variation in nutrient partitioning characteristics is likely to depend on end organ sensitivity and responsiveness to a variety of circulating regulatory factors as well as on gene expression. The mechanisms associated with the regulation of nutrient partitioning have been discussed recently,[25,27] and the topic is beyond the scope of this chapter. However, the issue of the contribution of DNA sequence variation to individual differences in nutrient partitioning is of particular interest. From animal literature it is known that there are strain differences in nutrient partitioning characteristics, an indication that genes are an important determinant of the phenotype.

The genetic epidemiology of the nutrient partitioning phenotype has not been considered to any extent in humans. Only one report has dealt with the heritability of nutrient partitioning characteristics, and it is based on data from the Quebec Family Study.[28] A total transmission effect of about 50% was found, with a genetic transmission of approximately 20% after adjustment for the proper concomitants.

IV. REGIONAL FAT DISTRIBUTION

Part of the increased interest in the genetics of human obesities observed in the last few years is attributable to the fact that regional fat distribution has been shown to be an important determinant of the relationship between obesity and health and an independent risk factor for various morbid conditions, like cardiovascular diseases or non-insulin-dependent diabetes. The topic of the genetics of fat topography phenotypes has recently been reviewed more extensively.[29]

A. TRUNCAL-ABDOMINAL SUBCUTANEOUS FAT

Upper body obesity is more prevalent in males than in females, and it increases in frequency with age in males and after menopause in females. It is moderately correlated with total body fat and appears to be more prevalent in individuals habitually exposed to stress. In females it is also associated with the levels of plasma androgens and cortisol. In addition, the activity of abdominal adipose tissue lipoprotein lipase is elevated with higher levels of truncal-abdominal fat.[2] Important correlates of upper body obesity are listed in Table 2.

Evidence for familial resemblance in body fat distribution has been reported.[30] Based on skinfold measurements obtained in 173 monozygotic and 178 dizygotic pairs of male

Table 2. **Correlates of truncal-abdominal subcutaneous fat**

Age	Increasing from puberty onward
Gender	Males have more than females
Total body fat	Correlated with the component, but not perfectly: about 50% common variance
Positive energy balance	An important condition, probably essential for its development
AT-LPL activity	High activity in relevant depots
AT-lipolytic activity	High α-2 effect in relevant depots
Androgen levels	Augmented levels of free androgens in plasma (women)
Cortisol levels	Augmented plasma levels and high tissue receptor levels
Undetermined genetic characteristics	Probably affecting AT-LPL and α-2 balance, fat cell number in relevant depots, and hormonal status and sensitivity; lasting effects of genomic imprinting or pubertal events also need to be considered

twins, Selby et al.[31] recently reported heritability estimates of 0.77 (p<0.0001) for subscapular skinfold, 0.29 ($p < 0.05$) for the difference between subscapular and triceps skinfolds, and 0.17 ($p > 0.05$) for the subscapular to triceps skinfolds ratio. After adjustment for BMI, heritability levels were reduced and remained significant only for subscapular skinfold ($h^2 = 0.44$, p=0.002). Based on these results, the authors concluded that there was a significant genetic influence on central deposition of body fat.

Using data from the Canada Fitness Survey and the strategy of path analysis, it has been shown[22] that the across-generation transmissible effect reached about 40% for trunk skinfolds (sum of subscapular and suprailiac skinfolds), limb skinfolds (sum of biceps, triceps, and medial calf skinfolds), and the trunk to limb skinfolds ratio and 28% for the waist to hip ratio. Assuming that all transmissible effects are genetic, these results suggest that heredity accounts for a maximum of 40% of the phenotypic variance for various indicators of fat topography. The biological and cultural components of transmission in regional fat distribution were assessed with data from the Quebec Family Study.[32] Two indicators of regional fat distribution were considered. The trunk to limb skinfold ratio and the ratio of subcutaneous fat to fat mass obtained by dividing the sum of the six skinfolds by fat mass derived from body density measurements. A genetic effect of 25% was found for the trunk to limb skinfold ratio, with a slightly higher genetic effect of 30% for the ratio of subcutaneous fat to fat mass. These results suggest that the pattern of subcutaneous fat distribution is partly determined by the genotype. When the influence of total body fat was taken into account, the profile of subcutaneous fat deposition was found to be characterized by higher heritability estimates, reaching about 40 to 50% of the residual variance.[33,34] These results imply that, for a given level of fatness, some individuals store more fat on the trunk or in abdominal area than others.

It is not surprising that the pattern of subcutaneous fat distribution is influenced by some genetically controlled mechanisms given the heritability levels of collagenase isolated adipocyte lipolysis and heparin-releasable adipose tissue lipoprotein lipase activity from tissues obtained from the suprailiac depot.[35] It is also consistent with the significant identical twin intrapair resemblance seen in the response of adipose tissue lipolysis and lipoprotein lipase activity when the twins are challenged by overfeeding, acute exercise, or exercise training.[36-39] Of considerable significance is the observation that the profile of subcutaneous fat is characterized by slightly higher heritability coefficients when total body fat is taken into account. These results imply that, for a given level of fatness or fat mass gain, some individuals are storing more fat on the trunk or abdominal area while others are storing primarily on the lower body segments.[34,40]

B. ABDOMINAL VISCERAL FAT

Abdominal visceral fat is the type of obesity with the most critical metabolic and health implications. Less is known about the causes of individual differences in abdominal visceral fat level than for the other types of obesity. Visceral fat increases with age, in both genders, in lean as well as obese individuals.[41] Males have on the average more visceral fat than females, and the obese have more than lean persons. However, the level of visceral fat is only moderately correlated with total body fat, with a common variance level ranging from about 30 to 50% and perhaps lower.[40,42] In women, high plasma androgen and cortisol concentrations are commonly seen. In addition, high lipoprotein lipase and lipolytic activities in the visceral adipose depot are observed, but it is not known whether these characteristics are causes or effects of visceral obesity. No data have been reported on the heritability of abdominal visceral fat levels, and the population data needed to deal with this issue are difficult to generate with the present methodology since visceral fat can be assessed only by computerized tomography (CT) or nuclear magnetic resonance. In addition, the visceral fat draining in the portal circulation seems to be the visceral depot of greatest importance from a metabolic point of view, but no simple method is available to quantify the size of that depot.

The only indication that the genotype may be an important determinant of abdominal visceral fat comes from a long-term overfeeding experiment with identical twins.[40] About six times more variance was found between pairs than within pairs for the increases with overfeeding in CT-assessed abdominal visceral fat after controlling for gains in total fat. These data strongly suggest that when the energy intake surplus is clamped at the same level for every individual, some genotypes are more likely to store fat in the visceral compartment than others. Given the fact that there was a twofold range between the low gainers and the high gainers for abdominal visceral fat, this effect may be of considerable significance.

V. GENETIC-ENVIRONMENT INTERACTIONS

Some individuals are susceptible to excessive accumulation of fat and are always trying to lose these extra pounds, while others seem relatively well protected against the extra calories they ingest. Recently an attempt was made to test whether genetic factors could explain such differences by comparing the intrapair (within-genotype) and interpair (between-genotype) resemblances in the response of MZ twins to overfeeding and negative energy balance or, in other words, by testing for the presence of genotype-environment interaction effects.

A. RESPONSE TO OVERFEEDING

Two experiments were undertaken to study individual differences when subjects were exposed to a positive energy balance protocol. In both experiments, subjects had to eat a 4.2 MJ (1000 kcal)/day caloric surplus during periods of 22 days (in a short-term overfeeding experiment[32,38]) and 100 days (in a long-term overfeeding experiment[40]). Both experiments resulted in significant changes in the various obesity phenotypes, but considerable interindividual differences in the adaptation to the extra calories were observed. In the long-term overfeeding experiment,[40] the mean body mass gain of the 24 subjects (12 pairs of MZ twins) was 8.1 kg, but the range of weight gain was from 4 to 13 kg. However, the variation observed was not randomly distributed; there was about three times more variance in response between pairs than within pairs for gains in body

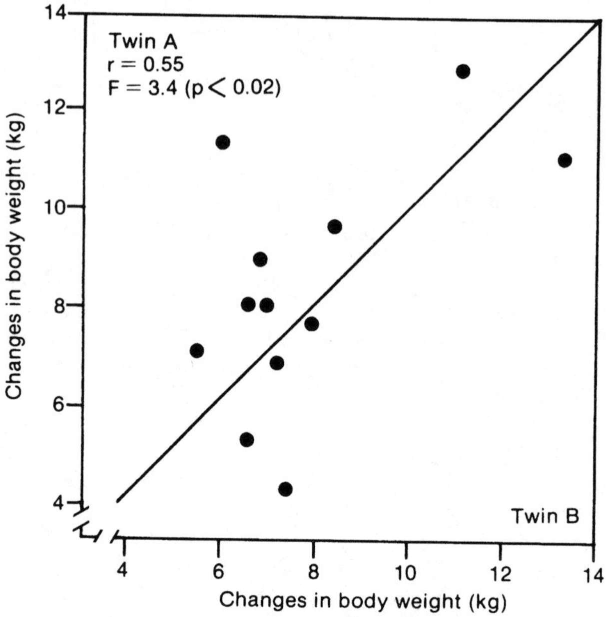

Figure 3. Changes in body weight during a 100-day overfeeding treatment in 24 young-adult males (12 pairs of identical twins). (Reproduced from Bouchard, C. et al., *N. Engl. J. Med.*, 322, 1477, 1990. With permission.)

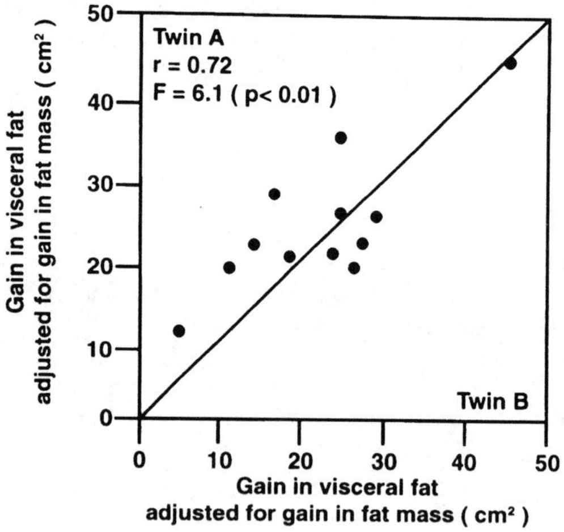

Figure 4. Response of computerized tomography-assessed abdominal visceral fat to a 100-day overfeeding treatment in 24 young-adult males (12 pairs of identical twins). Gains in visceral fat are adjusted for gains in total fat mass. (Reproduced from Bouchard, C. et al., *N. Engl. J. Med.*, 322, 1477, 1990. With permission.)

weight and fat mass and about six times more variance between pairs than within pairs for changes in visceral fat (assessed by CT) after adjustment for gains in fat mass.[40] Figure 3 illustrates the within-pair resemblance in weight gain and Figure 4 the changes in abdominal visceral fat under the influence of the 100-day overfeeding protocol. These results suggest that the amount of weight gained or fat stored in response to a caloric surplus is significantly influenced by the genotype of the individual. This genotype-overfeeding interaction effect appears to be more important for fat topography than for the amount of body weight or fat gained, as indicated by a higher F ratio for the amount of abdominal visceral fat gained. These findings suggest that genes may determine not only the gain in fat mass of body energy when an individual subjected to a positive energy balance, but also the pattern of fat deposition among the various fat depots of the body. This has important implications for health since truncal-abdominal fat and, particularly, visceral fat are associated with greater health risks than total amount of body fat.

B. RESPONSE TO NEGATIVE ENERGY BALANCE

In two other experiments, exercise was used to induce an energy deficit in MZ twins in order to test for the contribution of the genotype in the response to a negative energy balance sustained for 22 days[43] or 100 days.[44] In both experiments, the energy deficit was obtained by exercising twins on a cycle ergometer twice a day for about 50 min per session. The exercise prescription was designed to induce an extra energy expenditure of about 4.2 MJ (1000 kcal) over the resting metabolic rate while maintaining energy intake at the baseline level throughout the study. Results from the long-term experiment revealed a significant within-pair resemblance for the reduction in body weight and fat mass as well as for the changes in regional fat distribution phenotypes, while results from the short-term study revealed that only fat-free mass changes were characterized by a significant MZ twin resemblance.

Thus, results from both overfeeding and negative energy balance experiments generally suggest that undetermined genetic characteristics specific to each individual are associated with the response to changes in energy balance. The stage has now been reached where the use of the measured genotype approach could be helpful in the identification of some of the genes involved in determining variation in responsiveness.

VI. MAJOR GENE EFFECTS

The genetic effect reported above for the various obesity phenotypes was assumed to be polygenic, meaning that it resulted from the additive effects of a large number of genes, with each having small effects on the phenotypes. Recent research reported over the last few years has provided evidence that, in addition to a polygenic component, some obesity phenotypes are influenced by major gene effects. Most of the evidence for the contribution of major genes in measures of body fat comes from commingling and segregation analyses. Commingling analysis is used to obtain preliminary evidence of major gene effects by testing the hypothesis that the distribution of a variable is best fitted by a mixture of two or three distributions rather than one. Although evidence of commingling or mixture of distributions is compatible with a major gene effect on the phenotype, it is not sufficient to conclude that a major locus genotype exists, since commingling can also result from the influence of nongenetic factors. More direct evidence for a major gene effect can be obtained with segregation analysis, a method used by geneticists to evaluate alternate models of genetic transmission by analysis of pedigree data (see Chapters 7 and 8 for a more complete treatment of these issues).

A summary of the current evidence for major gene effects in body fat phenotypes is presented in Chapters 7 and 8 of this book. Results for BMI are conflicting, since some studies have provided support for a major gene effect whereas others have not. However, the results will likely be more homogeneous and supportive of a major locus if age- or generation-associated effects are taken into account in the analysis. As for percent body fat, results from a recent study provided evidence for a major locus genotype accounting for 45% of the phenotypic variance, with another 22 to 26% of the variance attributable to a multifactorial component.[45] Results from two studies also suggest the influence of major genes for regional fat distribution phenotypes. In one study Hasstedt et al.[46] reported a major gene effect explaining 42% of the variance in a relative fat pattern index defined as the ratio of the subscapular skinfold to the sum of the subscapular and suprailiac skinfold thicknesses, while recent results from the Quebec Family Study suggest major gene effects for the amount of subcutaneous fat (sum of six skinfolds) as well as for the trunk to extremity skinfolds ratio, both adjusted for total fat mass, accounting for about 35% of the phenotypic variance.[47]

VII. CONTRIBUTION OF SINGLE GENES: A BEGINNING

The definition of the genetic architecture of excess body fat in humans has just begun. It is likely that the human obesity genotypes will be complex multigenic systems with networks of gene-gene and gene-environment interactions.[48] There are already some promising data, primarily derived from animal models, that are highly suggestive of significant contributions from single gene mutations.

Some studies had suggested that allelic variation at the class I loci of the human lymphocyte antigen (HLA) system (chromosomal assignment: 6p21.3) is associated with the BMI as a marker of obesity.[49-51] However, a study with relatively large samples of males and females and more elaborate assessments of body fat has not confirmed these results.[52]

Based on sib-pair linkage analysis data obtained in four large families, it was suggested that there were significant associations between a subcutaneous fat pattern index and the adenylate kinase 1 locus (9q34) as well as the glutamic-pyruvate transaminase locus (8q24).[53] It was also reported that erythrocyte acid phosphatase (locus 1; 2p25) phenotypes exhibiting low enzyme activity levels (ACP_1 A and BA) were associated with excess body mass for age, height, and gender among 75 children, 3 to 14 years of age.[54] On the other hand, mitochondrial DNA sequence variation also was found to be nonrandomly related to body fat content and fat topography in 42 women.[55] Thus, carriers of the morph 1 generated by the KpnI restriction enzyme in the D-loop were markedly fatter than the noncarriers.

The augmented expression of adipocyte genes was studied in overfed primates and rats in an attempt to identify candidate genes that could be used in genetic studies of body weight regulation and obesity.[56] A subtractive cDNA cloning strategy allowed the identification of a 5-kilobase (kb) message expressed preferentially in the adipose tissue of overfed macaques and rats. The 5-kb mRNA was also found in human subcutaneous fat.

The relationship between rodent obesity genes and human obesity is being considered by several investigators. Friedman et al.[57] have reported that five mouse mutations which are all causing obesity in the animals are encoded on five different mouse chromosomes. However, these mouse obesity genes seem to be part of coding regions that have homologous counterparts on human chromosomes. These human homologous regions are also located on five different human chromosomes (1p31-ter; 7q31; 11p15.1; 16q22-24; 20q13). Interestingly, the mouse *db* gene may be homologous to the rat *fa* obesity gene,[58] and they both appear to have a human counterpart on chromosome 1p31.[59]

Two putative loci of interest for excessive body fat content have been identified in backcross mice by quantitative trait loci mapping with restriction fragment length polymorphism.[60] Backcross progeny from crosses between mouse strains C57BL/6J and *Mus spretus* exhibit a body fat content ranging from almost zero to 50%.[61] A transgenic mouse with impaired corticosteroid receptor function was created by partially knocking out gene expression with type II glucocorticoid receptor (5q31-32) antisense RNA.[62] The transgenic animals had increased fat deposition with a body mass that was twice as high by about 6 months of age in comparison to controls. An elevated body fat content was observed despite the fact that transgenic animals ate about 15% less than the normal mice.

The results reported thus far suggest that several genes have the potential to cause obesity in humans. It seems likely that the obesity genotype will be a complex multigenic system, perhaps with the more severe cases carrying mutations at several loci and the less affected individuals carrying one or only a few of the mutant genes. Each of the putative single gene effects reviewed here seems to be encoded on a different human chromosome region. Moreover, it is also known that another putative obesity gene, of the necessary type, causing the paternally imprinted Prader-Willi syndrome, is encoded on human chromosome 15q11–13.[63] Other loci are associated with some of the other Mendelian conditions resulting in obesity as well as a score of other disorders.[1]

The growing number of genes does not bode well for the single gene hypothesis. It implies, however, that genetic heterogeneity is likely to become a major difficulty in future genetic studies of this complex phenotype. Thus far, no single gene polymorphism has been consistently associated with the regional fat distribution phenotypes.

VIII. SUMMARY

From a population perspective, large family studies reveal that the heritability of body mass for stature or body fat content reaches 40% and less of the age- and gender-adjusted phenotypic variance. The profile of subcutaneous fat distribution after adjustment for age, gender, and total fat mass is also characterized by significant heritability estimates. Future studies also must consider the role of heredity in the changes observed in these phenotypes over time. The investigation of the nutrient partitioning characteristics has just begun in humans, but it seems that some people may have inherited a greater susceptibility to storage of excess energy in the form of lipids than others. There are individuals who are more likely than others to gain body fat or to store excess energy in the upper-body fat depots when challenged by chronic overfeeding; this susceptibility is partly dependent on undefined genetic factors, as revealed by experimental studies with identical twins.

Current research on the molecular markers of body fat content strongly suggests that a good number of loci may be involved in determining the susceptibility genotypes. A combination of animal experimentation using the quantitative trait loci mapping strategy and human molecular studies will be required to identify all the loci that may contribute to individual differences in the proneness to become obese, in the resistance to weight loss regimens, and in the development of an atherogenic and diabetogenic fat distribution profile.

REFERENCES

1. **Bouchard, C. and Pérusse, L.,** Heredity and body fat, *Annu. Rev. Nutr.*, 8, 259, 1988.
2. **Bouchard, C., Després, J. P., Mauriège, P., Marcotte, M., Chagnon, M., Dionne, F. T., and Bélanger, A.,** The genes in the constellation of determinants of regional fat distribution, *Int. J. Obes.*, 15, 9, 1991.
3. **Bouchard, C.,** La génétique des obésités humaines, *Ann. Med. Intern.*, 143(7), 463, 1992.
4. **Bouchard, C. and Pérusse, L.,** Genetics of obesity, *Annu. Rev. Nutr.*, 8, 259, 1993.
5. **Garn, S. M., Sullivan, T. V., and Hawthorne, V. M.,** Fatness and obesity of the parents of obese individuals, *Am. J. Clin. Nutr.*, 50, 1308, 1989.
6. **Price, R. A., Stunkard, A. J., Ness, R., Wadden, T., Heshka, S., Kanders, B., and Cormillot, A.,** Childhood onset (age < 10) obesity has high familial risk, *Int. J. Obes.*, 14, 185, 1990.
7. **Stunkard, A. J., Foch, T. T., and Hrubec, Z.,** A twin study of human obesity, *JAMA*, 256, 51, 1986.
8. **MacDonald, A. and Stunkard, A. J.,** Body mass indexes of British separated twins, *N. Engl. J. Med.*, 322, 1530, 1990.
9. **Price, R. A. and Gottesman, I. I.,** Body fat in identical twins reared apart: roles for genes and environment, *Behav. Genet.*, 21, 1, 1991.

10. **Price, R. A., Cadoret, R. J., Stunkard, A. J., and Troughton, E.,** Genetic contributions to human fatness: an adoption study, *Am. J. Psychiatry,* 144, 1003, 1987.
11. **Sørensen, T. I. A., Holst, C., and Stunkard, A. J.,** Childhood body mass index — genetic and familial environmental influences assessed in a longitudinal adoption study, *Int. J. Obes.,* 16, 705, 1992.
12. **Sørensen, T. I. A., Holst, C., Stunkard, A. J., and Theil, L.,** Correlations of body mass index of adult adoptees and their biological relatives, *Int. J. Obes.,* 16, 227, 1992.
13. **Sørensen, T. I. A., Price, R. A., Stunkard, A. J., and Schulsinger, F.,** Genetics of obesity in adult adoptees and their biological siblings, *Br. Med. J.,* 298, 87, 1989.
14. **Stunkard, A. J., Sørensen, T. I. A., Hannis, C., Teasdale, T. W., Chakraborty, R., Schull, W. J., and Schulsinger, F.,** An adoption study of human obesity, *N. Engl. J. Med.,* 314, 193, 1986.
15. **Grilo, C. M. and Pogue-Geile, M. F.,** The nature of environmental influences on weight and obesity: a behavior genetic analysis, *Psychol. Bull.,* 110, 520, 1991.
16. **Pérusse, L. and Bouchard, C.,** Genetics of energy intake and food preferences, in *Genetics of Obesity,* Bouchard, C., Ed., CRC Press, Boca Raton, FL, 1994, chap. 9.
17. **Bouchard, C., Pérusse, L., Dériaz, O., Després, J. P., and Tremblay, A.,** Genetic influences on energy expenditure in humans, *Crit. Rev. Food Ser. Nutr.,* 33, 345, 1993.
18. **Bray, G. A.,** The inheritance of corpulence. in *The Body Weight Regulatory System: Normal and Disturbed Mechanisms,* Cioffi, L. A., James, W. P. T., and Van Itallie, T. B., Eds., Raven Press, New York, 1981, 185.
19. **Mueller, W. H.,** The genetics of human fatness, *Yearb. Phys. Anthropol.,* 26, 215, 1983.
20. **Bouchard, C. and Lortie, G.,** Heredity and endurance performance, *Sports Med.,* 1, 38, 1984.
21. **Heller, R., Garrison, R. J., Havlik, R. J., Feinleib, M., and Padgett, S.,** Family resemblances in height and relative weight in the Framingham Heart Study, *Int. J. Obes.,* 8, 399, 1984.
22. **Pérusse, L., Leblanc, C., and Bouchard, C.,** Inter-generation transmission of physical fitness in the Canadian population, *Can. J. Sport Sci.,* 13, 8, 1988.
23. **Bouchard, C., Pérusse, L., Leblanc, C., Tremblay, A., and Thériault, G.,** Inheritance of the amount and distribution of human body fat, *Int. J. Obes.,* 12, 205, 1988.
24. **Tambs, K., Moum, T., Eaves, L., Neale, M., Midthjell, K., Lund-Larsen, P. G., Naess, S., and Holmen, J.,** Genetic and environmental contributions to the variance of the body mass index in a Norwegian sample of first- and second-degree relatives, *Am. J. Hum. Biol.,* 3, 257, 1991.
25. **Reeds, P. J., Fiorotto, M. L., and Davis, T. A.,** Nutrient partitioning: an overview, in *The Science of Food Regulation: Food Intake, Taste, Nutrient Partitioning, and Energy Expenditure,* Bray, G. A. and Ryan, D. H., Eds., Louisiana State University Press, Baton Rouge, 1992, 103.
26. **Pullar, J. D. and Webster, A. J. F.,** The energy cost of fat and protein deposition in the rat, *Br. J. Nutr.,* 37, 355, 1977.
27. **Bray, G. A.,** Obesity, a disorder of nutrient partitioning: the Mona Lisa hypothesis, *J. Nutr.,* 12, 1146, 1991.
28. **Bouchard, C., Tremblay, A., Després, J. P., Dériaz, O., and Dionne, F. T.,** The genetics of body energy content and energy balance: an overview, in *The Science of Food Regulation: Food Intake, Taste, Nutrient Partitioning and Energy Expenditure,* Bray, G. A. and Ryan, D. H., Eds., Louisiana State University Press, Baton Rouge, 1992, 3.
29. **Bouchard, C., Després, J. P., and Mauriège, P.,** Genetic and nongenetic determinants of regional fat distribution, *Endocr. Rev.,* 14(1), 72, 1993.

30. **Donahue, R. P., Prineas, R. J., Gomez, O., and Hong, C. P.,** Familial resemblance of body fat distribution: the Minneapolis Children's blood pressure study, *Int. J. Obes.,* 16, 161, 1992.
31. **Selby, J. V., Newman, B., Quesenberry, C. P., Jr., Fabsitz, R. R., King, M.C., and Meaney, J. M.,** Evidence of genetic influence on central body fat in middle-aged twins, *Hum. Biol.,* 61, 179, 1989.
32. **Bouchard, C., Tremblay, A., Després, J. P., Poehlman, E. T., Thériault, G., Nadeau, A., Lupien, P. J., Moorjani, S., and Dussault, J.,** Sensitivity to overfeeding: the Québec experiment with identical twins, *Prog. Food Nutr. Sci.,* 12, 45, 1988.
33. **Bouchard, C.,** Inheritance of human fat distribution, in *Fat Distribution during Growth and Later Health Outcomes,* Bouchard, C. and Johnson, F. E., Eds., Alan R. Liss, New York, 1988, 103.
34. **Bouchard, C.,** Variation in human body fat: the contribution of the genotype, in *Obesity: Towards a Molecular Approach,* Bray, G. A., Ricquier, D., and Spiegelman, B. M., Eds., Alan R. Liss, New York, 1990, 17.
35. **Bouchard, C.,** Inheritance of human fat distribution and adipose tissue metabolism, in *Metabolic Complications of Human Obesities,* Vague, J., Björntörp, P., Guy-Grand, B., Rebuffé-Scrive, M., and Vague, P., Eds., Elsevier, Amsterdam, 1985, 87.
36. **Després, J. P., Bouchard, C., Savard, R., Prud'homme, D., Bukowiecki, L., and Thériault, G.,** Adaptive changes to training in adipose tissue lipolysis are genotype dependent, *Int. J. Obes.,* 8, 87, 1984.
37. **Mauriège, P., Després, J. P., Marcotte, M., Tremblay, A., Nadeau, A., Moorjani, S., Lupien, P., Dussault, J., Fournier, G., Thériault, G., and Bouchard, C.,** Adipose tissue lipolysis after long-term overfeeding in identical twins, *Int. J. Obes.,* 16, 219, 1992.
38. **Poehlman, E. T., Després, J. P., Marcotte, M., Tremblay, A., Thériault, G., and Bouchard, C.,** Genotype dependency of adaptation in adipose tissue metabolism after short-term overfeeding, *Am. J. Physiol.,* 250, E480, 1986.
39. **Savard, R. and Bouchard, C.,** Genetic effects in the response of adipose tissue lipoprotein lipase activity to prolonged exercise: a twin study, *Int. J. Obes.,* 14, 771, 1990.
40. **Bouchard, C., Tremblay, A., Després, J. P., Nadeau, A., Lupien, P. J., Thériault, G., Dussault, J., Moorjani, S., Pineault, S., and Fournier, G.,** The response to long-term overfeeding in identical twins, *N. Engl. J. Med.,* 322, 1477, 1990.
41. **Enzi, G., Gasparo, M., Biondetti, P. R., Flor, D., Semisa, M., and Zurlo, F.,** Subcutaneous and visceral fat distribution according to sex, age, and overweight, evaluated by computed tomography, *Am. J. Clin. Nutr.,* 44, 739, 1986.
42. **Ferland, M., Després, J. P., Tremblay, A., Pinault, S., Nadeau, A., Moorjani, S., Lupien, P. J., Thériault, G., and Bouchard, C.,** Assessment of adipose tissue distribution by computed axial tomography in obese women: association with body density and anthropometric measurements, *Br. J. Nutr.,* 61, 139, 1989.
43. **Poehlman, E. T., Tremblay, A., Marcotte, M., Pérusse, L., Thériault, G., and Bouchard, C.,** Heredity and changes in body composition and adipose tissue metabolism after short-term exercise-training, *Eur. J. Appl. Physiol.,* 56, 398, 1987.
44. **Bouchard, C., Tremblay, A., Després, J. P., Thériault, G., Nadeau, A., Lupien, P. J., and Moorjani, S.,** The response to exercise with constant energy intake in identical twins, *FASEB J.,* 6(Abstr.), A1647, 1992.
45. **Rice, T., Borecki, I. B., Bouchard, C., and Rao, D. C.,** Segregation analysis of fat mass and other body composition measures derived from underwater weighing, *Am. J. Hum. Genet.,* 52, 967, 1993.
46. **Hasstedt, S. J., Ramirez, M. E., Kuida, H., and Williams, R. R.,** Recessive inheritance of a relative fat pattern, *Am. J. Hum. Genet.,* 45, 917, 1989.

47. **Borecki, I. B., Rice, T., Pérusse, L., Bouchard, C., and Rao, D. C.,** Segregation analysis of regional fat distribution measures: the Québec Family Study, *Am. J. Hum. Genet.,* (revision pending review).
48. **Bouchard, C.,** Human obesities: chaos or determinism?, in *Obesity in Europe 91. Proc. 3rd Eur. Congr. Obesity,* Ailhaud, G., Guy-Grand, B., Lafontan, M., and Ricquier, C., Eds., John Libbey, Paris, 1992, 7.
49. **Digy, J. P., Raffoux, C., Pointel, J. P., Perrier, P., Drouin, P., Mejean, L., Streiff, F., and Debry, G.,** HLA and familial obesity: evidence for a genetic origin, in *Recent Advances in Obesity Research,* Hirsch, J. and Van Itallie, T., Eds., John Libbey, London, 1985, 171.
50. **Fabsitz, R. R., Nam, J. M., Gart, J., Stunkard, A., Price, A. R., and Wilson, P. W. F.,** HLA associations with obesity, *Hum. Hered.,* 39, 156, 1989.
51. **Fumeron, F. and Apfelbaum, M.,** Association between HLA-B18 and the familial obesity syndrome, *N. Engl. J. Med.,* 305, 645, 1981.
52. **Bouchard, C., Pérusse, L., Rivest, J., Morissette, J., Allard, C., Thériault, G., Leblanc, C., and Tremblay, A.,** HLA system, body fat and fat distribution in children and adults, *Int. J. Obes.,* 9, 411, 1985.
53. **Siervogel, R. M., Wilson, A. F., Baumgartner, R. N., and Elston, R. C.,** Evidence of possible genetic linkage for a postulated fat patterning gene and marker genes using the robust sib-pair method, *Am. J. Hum. Biol.,* 3, 67, 1991.
54. **Lucarini, N., Finocchi, G., Gloria-Bottini, F., Macioce, M., and Borgiani, P.,** A possible genetic component of obesity in childhood. Observations on acid phosphatase polymorphism, *Experientia,* 46, 90, 1990.
55. **Truchon, J., Dionne, F. T., Song, T. K., Després, J. P., and Bouchard, C.,** Kpn1 mitochondrial DNA sequence polymorphism and obesity, submitted.
56. **Wilson, B. E., Meyer, G. E., Cleveland, J. C., and Weigle, D. S.,** Identification of candidate genes for a factor regulating body weight in primates, *Am. J. Physiol.,* 259, R1148, 1990.
57. **Friedman, J. M., Leibel, R. L., and Bahary, N.,** Molecular mapping of obesity genes, *Mamm. Genome,* 1, 130, 1991.
58. **Truett, G. E., Bahary, N., Friedman, J. M., and Leibel, R. L.,** Rat obesity gene fatty (fa) maps to chromosome 5: evidence for homology with the mouse gene diabetes (db), *Proc. Natl. Acad. Sci. U.S.A.,* 88, 7806, 1991.
59. **Friedman, J. M. and Leibel, R. L.,** Tackling a weighty problem, *Cell,* 69, 217, 1992.
60. **Warden, C. H., Fisler, J. S., Pace, M. J., Diep, A., He, K. Y., and Lusis, A. J.,** Identification of two loci underlying polygenic obesity in mice, *Int. J. Obes.,* 15(Suppl. 3), 54 (Abstr.), 1991.
61. **Fisler, J. S., Pace, M. J., Warden, C. H., and Lusis, A. J.,** Spretus/B6: a new mouse model of polygenic obesity, *Int. J. Obes.,* 15(Suppl. 3), 54(Abstr.), 1991.
62. **Pépin, M. C., Pothier, F., and Barden, N.,** Impaired type II glucocorticoid-receptor function in mice bearing antisense RNA transgene, *Nature,* 235, 725, 1992.
63. **McKusick, V. A.,** *Mendelian Inheritance in Man. Catologs of Autosomal Dominant, Autosomal Recessive, and X-Linked Phenotypes,* Johns Hopkins University Press, Baltimore, 1992.

Chapter 7

The Case for Single Gene Effects on Human Obesity

R. Arlen Price

TABLE OF CONTENTS

I. INTRODUCTION

Evidence has accumulated from a variety of sources in support of single gene effects on human obesity — from animal models,[1,2] human syndromes,[3] analyses of pooled family data,[4,5] twin and adoption data,[6-8] analysis of distribution characteristics through commingling analysis,[9-14] segregation analysis of families including very young children,[13,15] and segregation analysis of adults and older children.[11,12,16] Finally, a recessive inheritance pattern has been found consistently in diverse human populations — including, for example, Brazilians,[15] Scandinavians,[7] American blacks,[12] and a variety of Americans of European ancestry.[11,13,16]

The pattern of inheritance is clearly pervasive. Furthermore, several research groups are using a variety of approaches to identify single gene effects on obesity in humans. Whether explicitly or naively, all these approaches assume that obesity-predisposing genes exist and that their effects, either alone or in combination with other causal factors, can be identified using currently available epidemiological and molecular methods. Ultimately, the only way to unambiguously confirm the existence of obesity-predisposing genes is by the identification

0-8493-4880-3/94/$0.00+$.50

of the assumed genes using molecular methods. This chapter examines the strength of the evidence that such genes exist, and, if so, how many genes there are, what their effect sizes are, and what strategies will be appropriate for finding them.

II. INDIRECT EVIDENCE FROM ANIMAL MODELS OF OBESITY

Animal models for genetic obesity are discussed in Chapter 12 and will not be presented in this chapter except to note that animal models may be good ones for some types of human obesity. Genes involved in metabolism and energy storage are likely to have been highly conserved in mammalian evolution; thus, there probably are many human homologs of genes identified in other species. In rodents, for example, the majority of obesity syndromes are due to recessively expressed mutations[1] — *obese mouse, diabetic-obese mouse, fat mouse, tubby mouse*, and *Zucker fatty rat.* At least two other mutations are dominantly expressed — yellow obese and adipose. Obesity in several other rodent strains selected for this trait or large body size is most likely due to polygenic inheritance.

Animal models also demonstrate some of the complications that are likely to exist for human obesity. First, expression of single obesity-predisposing genes commonly depends on background genotype. This phenomenon has been demonstrated in the case of differences in insulin resistance when the *ob* and *db* mutations in mouse and the *fa* mutation in rats are expressed in different congenic strains.[2,17] Given these differences in gene expression between closely related strains of the same species, it is to be expected that homologous human genes may be expressed very differently than in rodents. Another complication is that diet mediates gene expression in both mutant and wild-type animal strains as well as in humans. Finally, there has been some recent evidence that strain differences in weight gain on high-fat diets may be mediated in part by major gene differences among some strains.[18] Such findings in animal species are consistent with evidence for similar genetically mediated susceptibility to weight gain on high-fat diets noted in human studies (see, for instance, Reference 19).

III. GENETIC SYNDROMES

There are several genetic syndromes in humans for which obesity is a prominent symptom. These include the Prader-Willi, Börjeson-Forssman-Lehmann, Bardet-Biedl, Biemond, Pickwickian, and Cohen syndromes.[3] Prader-Willi syndrome is one of the best understood in terms of its genetic causes. It is commonly due to deletions in chromosome region 15q11–12, although in some cases no deletions may be detected cytogenetically. Deletions visible under a light microscope probably involve the loss of at least 2 to 5 million base pairs of DNA. Disorders caused by such deletions are called contiguous gene syndromes because their phenotypes are probably due to the deletion of three to ten genes and regulatory sequences. Deletions associated with Prader-Willi syndrome suggest that genes in chromosome region 15q11–12 may affect appetite and/or satiety cues that mediate food intake. A variety of other genes involved in carbohydrate metabolism, lipid metabolism and storage, and endocrine function may be deleted in other human syndromes. The existence of genetic obesity syndromes is important because it indicates that altering one or a few genes can cause obesity in humans. Once the obesity-relevant genes from these syndromes are identified, it will be possible to determine whether normal variation in the same genes causes obesity in people with a normal chromosome complement.

IV. TWIN AND ADOPTION STUDIES

A few studies have noted indirect evidence for the effects of single obesity-predisposing genes. The evidence is indirect in the sense that inheritance patterns in families differ from what would be expected under simple polygenic models. Inferences about mode of inheritance are made that are consistent with the observed deviations. For example, Sørensen et al.[7] reported a greater difference in similarity of adoptees with their full siblings than with their parents and a greater difference in similarity between full and half siblings than would be predicted on the basis of shared additive polygenic effects. (The expectations are that parent-offspring and full sibling correlations should be the same and that the half sibling correlation should be about one half that of siblings.) They suggested nonadditive genetic variance shared with full siblings, but not with parents or half siblings, as one possible explanation for the observed differences in similarity. The nonadditive effects could be due to one or many genes. Stunkard et al.[6] and Price and Gottesman[8] made similar interpretations of differences between correlations of identical and fraternal twins reared apart. Identical twin correlations are typically more than double those for fraternal twins, the predicted magnitude under an additive polygenic model. Of course the apparent nonadditive genetic effects observed in these studies could be due either to major genes, polygenes, or both.

V. POOLED FAMILY DATA

Studies of pooled family data do not examine specific relationships within the families. Instead, interpretations are made and at times models are fitted to obesity rates, correlations, or variance-covariances matrices that are derived as an aggregate of all families. Studies that have examined pooled data in order to evaluate single gene models of transmission of human obesity have produced mixed results.[4,5,20] All these studies are limited in that they do not examine segregation patterns directly.

VI. EVIDENCE BASED ON DISTRIBUTION CHARACTERISTICS

Another approach to evaluating whether single gene effects exist is to examine the frequency distribution of a quantitative measure of obesity such as the BMI. Departures from normality both with and without transformation suggest that additive polygenic inheritance alone cannot explain the distribution pattern. Single genes or environmental factors with major effects may cause the shape of a continuous distribution, e.g., the BMI, to be skewed because of the admixture of two or more component subgroups that differ in genetic predisposition, environmental exposure, or both (see Figure 1 and References 9 and 21). Such analyses of commingled distributions have been undertaken by several investigators as a first step in determining whether single genes may be segregating for obesity. These studies have shown that it is possible to separate the distribution of the BMI into multiple (usually two or three), components.[9-12,14,16,22-24] Generally speaking, younger samples tend to provide evidence for three distributions and middle-aged samples for two distributions. While consistent with single gene effects, such studies cannot unambiguously confirm them because environmental factors, genetic and environmental interactions, and even scaling effects may produce departures from normality.

VII. SEGREGATION ANALYSIS OF NORMAL-WEIGHT FAMILIES

Segregation analysis differs from analyses of pooled data because each family is examined separately (see, for instance, Reference 25). The term derives from Mendel's first law, which states that maternally and paternally derived genes separate or segregate in the formation of gametes. Segregation patterns, which are ratios of phenotypes in offspring, are determined by the mode of inheritance and gene expression. For example, a single gene causing a rare recessive trait is usually detected in the offspring of matings of two heterozygous carriers, which on average yield one quarter homozygous affected individuals, one quarter homozygous normals, and one half heterozygous carriers.

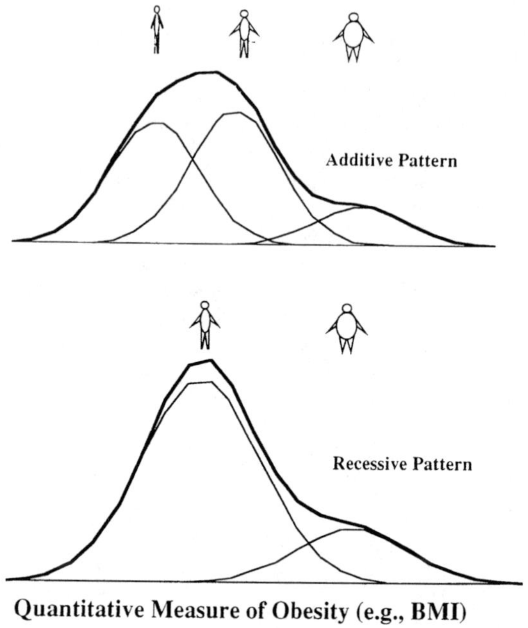

Figure 1. This figure depicts the way in which a quantitative measure of obesity, such as the body mass index (BMI), may be divided into components using commingling or segregation analysis. The X axis represents a quantitative measure of obesity and the height of the curve (Y axis not shown) represents frequency. The stick figures denote components made up of individuals with lean, average-weight, or obesity-prone genotypes. The two panels show distribution patterns that would be expected from segregation of a single obesity gene. That is, individuals with zero gene copies (homozygotes) would have a lean phenotype, those with one gene copy would have a normal-weight phenotype, and those with two gene copies would have an obese phenotype. Note that genotype at the single locus is not fixed, but determines a range of phenotypes. The actual phenotype observed depends on polygenic background genotype and environmental effects such as diet and exercise. The upper panel shows a three-distribution pattern expected from segregation of an additive or codominant gene. This is the pattern found for segregation analyses of Pima Indian siblings within birth cohorts. The lower panel shows the two-distribution pattern associated with recessive inheritance. This is the pattern found most consistently from commingling analyses and from segregation analyses of a number of nuclear family samples.

One of the first applications of segregation analysis to body weight was by Rao et al.,[15] who found evidence for major gene transmission within a mixed model only when very young children (under age 3) were included in the analysis, and the investigators felt that their data did not support major gene transmission. However, their methods of analysis were somewhat different from those that followed. For example, the analyses did not allow for estimating major gene influence, polygenic heritability, and transmission probabilities within the same model. They also used a transformation of weight (cube root) that is generally not independent of height, which is known to be influenced primarily by polygenic inheritance and the environment (see, for example, Reference 15). Furthermore, the investigators did not control for confounding variables such as social class and nonlinear effects of age, which affect patterns of familial resemblance. Even so, this was the first study of its type, and the overall pattern of results found by Rao et al.[15] was similar to those of investigators who have followed.

Several studies applying segregation analysis to family data have been completed, and most have examined the BMI. The studies have consistently found some evidence for recessively expressed single gene inheritance (see Figure 1). In fact, the pattern of results is so consistent that even many of the model parameter estimates have been similar. For example, most studies have reported a very common obesity-prone variant, with a frequency of one quarter to one third. The studies have included segregation analyses of families including very young children[13,15] and segregation analyses of adults and older children.[11,12,16]

Considering evidence from all sources, a recessive inheritance pattern consistently has been suggested from studies of diverse human populations — including, for example, Brazilians,[15] Scandinavians,[7] American blacks,[12] and a variety of Americans of European ancestry.[11,13,16] Later sections in this chapter will examine the meaning of this pattern.

VIII. GENETIC HETEROGENEITY

The development and clinical expression of obesity is so heterogeneous that it seems unlikely that any one gene could account for all cases of obesity in the aggregate. Indeed, there is apparent heterogeneity even for some narrowly defined genetic syndromes. The number of separate mutants in other mammalian species also suggests heterogeneity. On the other hand, while polygenic factors are obviously important in obesity, the reviewed studies suggest that not all relevant genes fit the polygenic model, that is, have small additive effects. Thus, single genes with major effects may account for most cases of obesity within individual families.

IX. HOW MANY GENES ARE INVOLVED?

If it is assumed for illustrative purposes that single obesity genes are common, from the existing literature it is not clear whether there is one gene or a few of them. However, the complexity of the obesity phenotype in humans and animals suggests that there may be several major single gene effects, i.e., individual genes with large effects in individual families. Results from several segregation studies place gene frequency estimates between one quarter and one third. The combined frequencies of several individual genes could make the apparent frequency of a "single gene" inferred from segregation analysis appear quite high. One way to differentiate these alternatives (one vs. a few genes) would be to examine the offspring of matings between two very obese parents. If overweight, as with, say, deafness, were due to several recessive genes, then assortative mating would increase the risk of homozygosity in offspring only slightly. An increase in overweight in this group of offspring would be primarily due to polygenic inheritance or other factors. In the analysis reported by Price and others[11] there were only 8 such matings among the 473 from which full information was available on both parents and all offspring. While the risk to the 21 offspring was higher than that for those from other mating types, the risk in this group was relatively low — 14%. The 60% predictive power for identifying homozygous parents (based on parameters from this study) leads to an estimate of more than double (36%) the number of obese offspring that were observed. Whereas the amount of data on these informative matings in this study was small, the relatively low risk to offspring of two obese parents having a 60% chance of being homozygous suggests that several recessively inherited genes may account for the pattern of transmission observed.

Data published by Garn[26] and data from this author's laboratory[27] on larger numbers of obese and lean mating types also suggest that the increase in risk from having two obese parents is too high to fit a single-gene recessive model. Moreover, the increase in risk associated with having one or two obese parents is roughly additive, a finding that is not consistent with the segregation of one recessively expressed obesity-predisposing gene.

Overall, the data suggest that there are likely to be several relatively rare genes that have large effects in particular families. Common genes are likely to have smaller effects, and the inherited polygenic background against which single obesity genes segregate suggests that there are also numerous genes with small quantitative effects. Such quantitative trait loci are discussed in detail in Chapter 13 of this volume.

X. GENE EFFECT SIZES

To date there have been no studies aimed specifically at estimating effect sizes for obesity-predisposing genes. Presumably, the effect sizes will vary considerably. In extreme obesity there may well be genes with large effects that account for most of the risk for obesity in the families in which they are segregating. More common genes are likely to have smaller effects, and genes accounting for variation of body fatness in the normal range are likely to be numerous and to have very small individual effects. Whereas it is impossible to know at the present time just how many genes with each magnitude of effect are present, genetic research strategies can be designed which will be robust in the presence of this complexity.

XI. SEGREGATION ANALYSES OF EXTREME OBESITY

All of the segregation and other analyses reviewed thus far have focused on the full range of body fat; thus, it is fair to ask how such studies may be generalized to extreme obesity. Recently, Price et al.[29] reported segregation analyses of one extreme group. The Pima Indians in southern Arizona have a very high prevalence of obesity and diabetes.[28] Segregation analyses of the BMI in Pima Indian nuclear families[29] identified the same pattern of transmission that has been found by different investigators in studies of several other populations, recessive major gene inheritance.[11-13,16] However, there were also notable differences. Mean BMI values were larger for Pima Indians, variances appeared to be greater, polygenic models were uniformly rejected, and tests of all models applied to nuclear families rejected Mendelian transmission.

XII. ENVIRONMENTAL DISTORTIONS OF SEGREGATION PATTERNS

Whereas Chapter 8 discusses temporal trends in detail, some aspects of such trends are particularly relevant to inferences regarding mode of inheritance and so will be presented in this chapter. During the past half century there have been large increases in the prevalence of obesity in developed countries.[30] Such short-term changes in prevalence must be environmentally determined, but genes may mediate phenotypic response to environmental change, e.g., through variable gene penetrance and expression. Obesity increases of varying degrees have been observed in white and black American women[31,32] and children of both sexes,[33] in native Americans of both sexes and all ages,[28,34] and in several other groups from around the world.[35,36] Especially large increases have been reported in the level and prevalence of obesity in the Pima Indian population, particularly among individuals born after World War II.[30]

The recent increases in obesity can incorrectly suggest a recessive pattern, since the prevalence of obesity is higher in offspring than in parents (as would be the case if most parents were normal-weight heterozygous carriers). For example, analyses of Pima Indian nuclear families attempted to control for generation differences by adjusting the data for effects of sex, generation, and subgroup and for linear, quadratic, and cubic effects of age and birth year.[29] The same types of adjustments were made to data from earlier analyses of white[11] and black[12] families, and other investigators took similar approaches to data adjustment.[13,16] The types of effects controlled by such statistical adjustments are shown in the upper and middle portions of Figure 2.

Segregation analyses of Pima Indian siblings within birth cohort avoided the shortcomings of statistical corrections.[29] The results uniformly supported a codominant major gene model with no polygenic heritability. For the untransformed data, transmission was Mendelian in cohorts born in 1945 or later. After transformation to remove skewness, codominant major gene inheritance continued to be supported, but transmission was Mendelian only in the cohort born prior to 1945.

These differences in results suggest that the cultural changes bringing about the large increase in the prevalence of obesity could have affected certain genotypes differently. Such a gene-environment interaction would have the effect of changing gene penetrance in a way that would not have been controlled for in previous statistical analyses. For

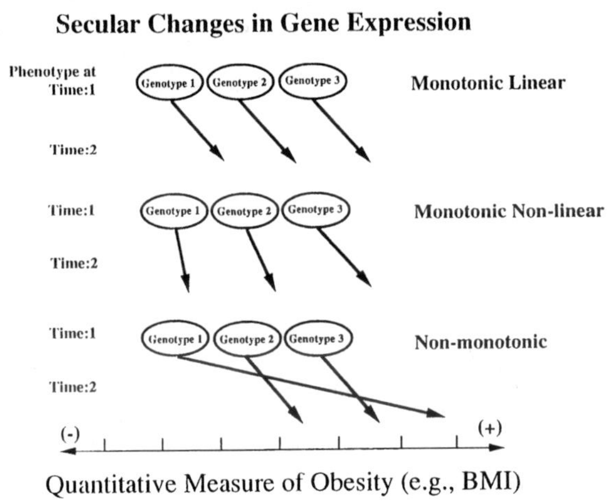

Figure 2. This figure shows three types of changes in phenotypic expression of major obesity-predisposing gene loci in the presence of environmental changes in patterns of diet and exercise. In the upper panel, all genotypes are affected to the same extent and, thus, maintain their relative positions at two time points. That is, phenotypic changes brought about by the environment are linear with major genotype. In the middle panel, genotypes are affected differently such that phenotypes that are more extreme at time one also have a greater response to the environment so that the differences between genotypes grow between the two time points. This is a nonlinear change in phenotypic expression of the obesity-prone genotype. Statistical adjustments of data prior to segregation analyses control for the first two types of increases because both assume monotonic changes. The lower panel depicts the pattern of change that would occur if some genotypes are expressed only in an obesity-promoting environment and not in others. Note that the changes are nonmonotonic and that the relationships among genotypes change across the two time points. Differences in segregation patterns found for nuclear families and siblings examined within birth cohorts suggest that environmental changes in diet and exercise have brought about nonmonotonic changes in gene expression that mimic recessive inheritance. BMI, body mass index.

example, if some genes have large effects only in the post-World War II obesity-predisposing environment (with high-fat diet and limited exercise), then the correspondences of phenotypes with genotypes will not be the same at different time points (see the lower portion of Figure 2). Price et al.[37] reported changes in the shape of the BMI distribution of Danish young men that were consistent with an increased penetrance of obesity-predisposing genes in cohorts born after World War II. The occurrence of similar trends in such geographically and culturally different groups suggested that an environmentally influenced penetrance increase could be a worldwide phenomenon. The type of genetic variability suggested by these studies is analogous to the concept of preadaptation (or pre-maladaption!) in that gene polymorphisms ("mutations") contribute to phenotypic variability only in the changed environment. Statistical controls that have been applied previously cannot adjust for such changes in gene penetrance and expression. Lack of information on parental phenotypes restricts the amount of information available for the segregation analysis of siblings, and this factor alone could be responsible in part for differences in results.

Taken together, the results of these studies suggest that the recessive pattern identified in the Pima Indian nuclear families may be accounted for by temporal changes in penetrance of obesity-predisposing genes. By implication, more modest temporal changes in other populations could account in part for the recessive pattern of inheritance that has been described by several investigators. Molecular studies will be needed to resolve this question. However, the complications due to temporal increases which have been detected provide important considerations that may guide the selection of families to be used in genetic linkage studies. Appropriately selected families will assure that families are in fact segregating genes and not merely exhibiting effects of birth-cohort-associated environmental influences.

XIII. THE ROLE OF IDIOSYNCRATIC ENVIRONMENTAL EFFECTS IN GENE EXPRESSION

Studies of identical twins provide one of the clearest demonstrations of how a genetically mediated response to the environment can affect the obesity phenotype. In these studies, different twin pairs overfed by the same number of calories gained quite different amounts of weight.[19] However, within-pair weight gains were strikingly similar. The genetic proneness to obesity that produces twin similarities in weight gain in response to these controlled "laboratory" diets may result in large twin differences when only one of the twins adopts obesity-promoting habits of diet and exercise during adult life. For example, Price and Stunkard[9] noted that while twin concordance for presence of obesity was high (perhaps representing proneness to genetic obesity), the correlation in extent of obesity was lower for obese twins than for normal-weight twins (perhaps because of differing environmental exposures). These results suggest that, for humans, genotype determines response to obesity-promoting environments. Idiosyncratic dietary and exercise habits can result in quite large differences in two individuals having identical levels of genetic risk for obesity.

Since human obesity genotypes must be inferred rather than measured, extreme obesity phenotypes provide more information about underlying genotypes than do normal-weight phenotypes. That is, an extremely obese individual probably has both genetic and environmental risk factors for obesity. A normal-weight relative may possess neither predisposing factor or else may possess only one without the other.

XIV. APPROACHES TO IDENTIFYING SINGLE GENE EFFECTS

Currently, several research groups are beginning to apply molecular genetic and linkage methods to identify specific genes involved in risk for extreme obesity and complex diseases with which obesity is associated. These genetic methods are very alluring because of their successful application to diseases with simple modes of inheritance and their potential for elucidating mechanisms of diseases with complex inheritance. Although virtually everyone now accepts the importance of broadly defined genetic factors in obesity, and some have even suggested plausible candidate genes, no one has identified specific genetic mechanisms for common forms of extreme obesity. Furthermore, there is controversy as to which aspects of the obesity phenotype have genetic relevance. Thus, the identification of single obesity-predisposing genes is likely to be a long and difficult undertaking.

XV. DEFINING THRESHOLDS FOR GENE SEGREGATION

The availability of weight-for-height thresholds that would guarantee segregation of obesity-predisposing genes would be of great value in genetic studies, and several approaches have been taken to identify them. It makes intuitive sense to select extreme cases, but there is no unambiguous way of deciding just how extreme obesity must be. For example, defining levels of obesity that are associated with health risk is controversial, but some consensus has emerged, at least regarding white men. Burton and colleagues[38] used the revised Metropolitan Life tables of "ideal weight" as a standard. They found that being as little as 20% over this standard conveys some increase in risk for several diseases and that being 40% overweight conveys substantial risks in white men. However, there is no certainty that these levels of obesity will assure gene segregation.

One empirical means of defining obesity thresholds is to examine population distributions of weight for height or other measures of obesity. For example, commingling and segregation analyses have been used to define obesity thresholds that may reflect increased genetic susceptibility[9-12,14,29] and have identified obese subgroups of men and women among Danish whites,[10] American whites,[9,11] American blacks,[12] and Pima Indians.[14,29]

Obesity is highly prevalent in many human populations, but there are substantial differences in prevalence rates depending on the ethnicity, sex, age, and birth cohort of the particular group. The presence and extent of differences among groups have tended to be based on a common standard of overweight. Biological and genetic studies require obesity thresholds with high positive predictive power to ensure selection of families in which obesity susceptibility genes segregate. For example, based on the studies reviewed, it appears that appropriate thresholds for the Pima Indian group are likely to be much higher than those for other groups studied previously. Whereas a BMI of about 31 kg/m^2 (40% over Metropolitan Life standard weight) may be a sufficiently high threshold for many populations, it appears that a BMI of at least 40 kg/m^2 (80% over Metropolitan Life standard weight) may be needed for such studies of Pima Indians.

XVI. CANDIDATE GENE APPROACHES TO IDENTIFYING OBESITY-PREDISPOSING GENES

Molecular geneticists tend to use the term "candidate gene" rather restrictively to refer to an identified DNA sequence for a specific gene.[39] However, as applied to complex traits such as obesity, candidate genes usually represent biological variables associated with obesity phenotypes for which genes presumably exist. When the biological defect is specific enough, then that knowledge can be used to identify the causal gene. Phenylketonuria (PKU) is one of the best-known examples of a candidate gene approach. This approach to mapping obesity-related genes has strong intuitive appeal since it may be seen as an extension of biological and physiological studies of obesity phenotypes. However, there are several problems with this strategy. Many biological variables are plausible because of their associations with obesity, but the biological candidate variable may have no known causal gene or else many possible causal genes. For example, the number of hormones, enzymes, receptors, transport proteins, regulatory sequences, and transcriptional factors that are plausibly involved in mediating the effect of insulin on obesity could result in a large number of "insulin candidate genes". Other "candidates" include adipsin, lipoprotein lipase, apolipoproteins, glucocorticoids, adrenergic receptors, insulin, insulin receptors, insulin-like growth factor, cholecystokinin, mitochondrial uncoupling protein, adipocyte growth hormones, glucose transport proteins, and genes involved in fat oxidation such as carnitine palmitoyl transferase, to name but a few. Another shortcoming of this approach is that if a specific gene has been well characterized its DNA sequence may vary little or not at all among obese and lean individuals, although polymerase chain reaction technology makes nearly all genes informative. In summary, candidate gene approaches to mapping human obesity genes usually turn out to be much less specific and to have much less power than intuition would suggest. Thus, other gene mapping approaches are likely to be more effective. A possible exception is that obesity genes identified from other species sometimes may be tested for linkage to human obesity in a straightforward manner.

XVII. RANDOM GENE MAPPING APPROACHES

Random gene mapping approaches, also called positional cloning, involve the identification of causal genes exclusively through the association of random DNA markers with the obesity phenotype. Currently, nearly all parts of the human genome have markers spaced no more than 5 to 10 million base pairs apart, and many parts of the human genome are more densely mapped. A large number of these markers are highly polymorphic, that is, have substantial individual differences in DNA sequences. For example, some di- to tetranucleotide repeats differ between virtually every pair of unrelated individuals, ensuring the segregation of these marker genotypes in nearly all families. The genome map has been used to identify genes for several diseases caused by single gene mutations, such as cystic fibrosis, Duchenne muscular dystrophy, and neurofibromatosis. Random gene mapping approaches appear to be the most practical for identifying genes for obesity and other complex phenotypes for several reasons. The required genetic markers are available. The markers are highly polymorphic. The number of markers required to screen the genome (about 300) is much less than the sum of plausible candidate genes.

XVIII. QUANTITATIVE TRAIT LOCI APPROACHES

Chapter 13 presents approaches to identifying quantitative trait loci (QTL) that have small but measurable effects on the obesity phenotype. What level of effect constitutes a major single gene effect, as opposed to a QTL effect, is arbitrary. Ultimately, larger samples of families and relative homogeneity provide the power necessary to identify smaller gene effects. These QTL approaches are usually applied to random gene mapping methods, but it may well be that some candidate genes that are currently under investigation have only small QTL levels of effects on the obesity phenotype.

XIX. SELECTING THE "BEST" OBESITY PHENOTYPE

Most epidemiologic studies of obesity have used indices of obesity that are derived from weight corrected for height, e.g., the BMI. Other estimates of total obesity can be made from skinfold measures, both individually and in combination, bioelectrical impedance, underwater weighing, and whole-body imaging with computerized tomography (CT) and magnetic resonance imaging (MRI). Although all such indices of obesity are highly correlated, there appear to be unique variances associated with individual measures which may be genetically based.[13] Some investigators have advocated the study of fat distribution because of its specific health risk for cardiovascular disease. Still others have advocated the study of metabolic rate or other biological measures. All these phenotypes are appropriate ones for identifying obesity genes, and there is no way of predicting in advance which are likely to have the strongest relationship with specific obesity genes. When possible it will be important to examine several alternative phenotypes in attempting to map obesity genes. However, care should be taken to adjust statistical criteria for the multiple phenotypes examined. Such an approach will increase the probability of finding true genetic effects and minimize spurious reports of linkage.

XX. CONSTRUCTIVE USE OF GENETIC HETEROGENEITY

Many levels of obesity occur in the same families, and a given normal or obesity-prone genotype may have a broad range of expression. Thus, it is probably true that many clinical heterogeneous forms of obesity have common etiologies, i.e., are genetically homogeneous. On the other hand, several different single gene mutations may result in quite similar obesity phenotypes. Thus, it is also likely that clinically homogeneous obesity phenotypes are genetically heterogeneous. This complex relationship between genotypes and phenotypes creates a dilemma for genetic research.

The understanding of the genetic basis of other complex disorders has progressed by splitting common conditions like breast cancer or diabetes into subsets based on some clinical or biological characteristic shared by some, but not all, individuals affected with the disease. Using this approach, gene locations have recently been identified for early-onset familial breast cancer[40] and for a non-insulin-dependent childhood form of diabetes[41] (maturity-onset diabetes of the young, or MODY). The study of these complex disorders may provide a useful analogy for obesity. Continuity of symptoms across all ill individuals (e.g., breast tumors and glucose intolerance, respectively) helped researchers understand the epidemiology of breast cancer and diabetes (e.g., population base rates). However, clues about the genetic basis of these diseases were discovered only by focusing on individual patient differences that breed true in families. Such a shift of emphasis away from global explanations for obesity is likely to be an important step in reducing etiological complexity to manageable proportions.

XXI. SELECTING FAMILIES SEGREGATING OBESITY GENES

Quantitative studies alone cannot resolve the question as to the number and type of genes involved in common forms of obesity. However, such analyses provide hypotheses that are necessary to guide linkage, biochemical, and molecular genetic studies. Genetic linkage studies of obesity are justified, but care should be exercised that the sampling and analytic methods selected are compatible and that the approaches chosen maximize the efficiency of the search for human obesity genes.

As much as feasible, approaches should take into account all of the information reviewed in this chapter. Figure 3 depicts one possible sampling design. Selecting families with extreme obesity (for example, at least 80% overweight in one individual and 50% overweight in another) and some normal-weight individuals (for example, at least one parent who is no more than 20% overweight) will optimize the probability of gene segregation within families and will minimize heterogeneity within families. Focusing only on the obese siblings within such families will avoid problems associated with reduced gene penetrance and expression due to genetic background and environmental conditions. Utilizing a sibling design also makes it feasible to use analytic methods that do not require genetic homogeneity among families. This family sampling design should be useful for identifying genes with a wide range of effect sizes from major genes to QTL, since power will depend on sample size and not on idiosyncracies of specific family structures.

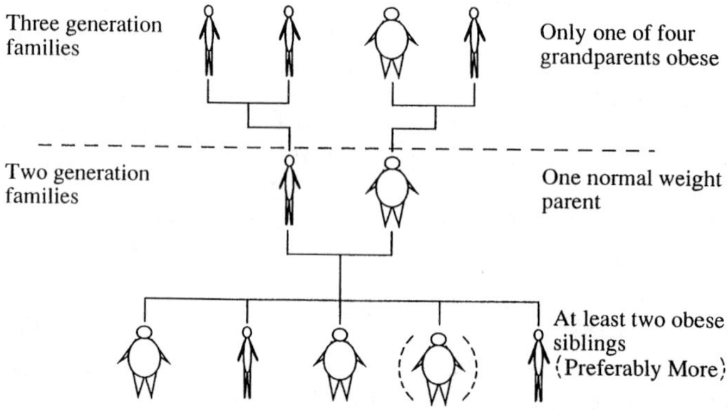

Figure 3. This pedigree structure shows a sampling design that may be used to identify families which are segregating obesity genes. Two-generation families (below the dashed line) would include at least two obese siblings (preferably more) and at least one normal-weight parent. The extent of obesity required is somewhat arbitrary since thresholds for genetic obesity can only be estimated. Based on segregation analyses, it appears that an obese person should have a body mass index of at least 31 to 40 kg/m^2 (40 to 80% over ideal weight according to revised Metropolitan Life tables[38]). Such a sampling design is model independent in the sense that it should work for recessively expressed or dominantly expressed major genes, but also for additively expressed major genes and quantitative trait loci (genes with small effects). Extensions of such families to three generations (above dashed line) may be justified if only one of the four grandparents is obese. However, genetic heterogeneity within families is increased when larger pedigree structures are used. Thus, a three-generation sampling design is likely to be most powerful when families are drawn from groups with relatively limited genetic variability, e.g., population isolates and clinically homogeneous subgroups of families.

In some highly stable populations with large family sizes, extended pedigree structures also may be of value in mapping obesity genes. These structures will be most useful when they are drawn from population isolates with limited genetic variability and, possibly, inbreeding. Furthermore, the most informative families will be those with obesity descending from a single branch, i.e., from only one of the four grandparents in the case of three-generation families.

XXII. SUMMARY

Overall, the data suggest that there are likely to be several relatively rare genes that have large effects in particular families. Common genes are likely to have smaller effects, and the inherited polygenic background against which single obesity genes segregate suggests that there are also numerous genes with smaller quantitative effects. Studies aimed at identifying obesity-predisposing genes should adopt strategies that take into account genetic heterogeneity, varying gene effect sizes, and environmentally mediated gene penetrance and expression. One design which appears to be robust in the face of such complexities requires the sampling of families with at least two extremely obese siblings and one normal-weight parent. Finally, random gene mapping approaches to identifying obesity-predisposing genes appear to have greater efficiency than more biologically intuitive candidate gene approaches.

ACKNOWLEDGMENTS

This work has been supported in part by National Institutes of Health Grant R01-DK44073 to Dr. Price. Dr. Danielle Reed made useful suggestions on earlier drafts.

REFERENCES

1. **Bray, G. A. and York, D. A.,** Hypothalamic and genetic obesity in experimental animals: an autonomic and endocrine hypothesis, *Physiol. Rev.,* 59, 719, 1979.
2. **Friedman, J. M., Leibel, R. L., and Bahary, N.,** Molecular mapping of the mouse ob mutation, *Mamm. Genome,* 1, 130, 1991.
3. **McKusick, V. A.,** *Mendelian Inheritance in Man,* The Johns Hopkins University Press, Baltimore, 1983.
4. **Karlin, S., Williams, P. T., Jensen, S., and Farquhar, J. W.,** Genetic analysis of the Stanford LRC family study data. I. Structured exploratory data analysis of height and weight measurements, *Am. J. Epidemiol.,* 113, 307, 1981.
5. **Zonta, L. A., Jayakar, S. D., Bosisio, M., Galante, A., and Pennetti, V.,** Genetic analysis of human obesity in an Italian sample, *Hum. Hered.,* 37, 129, 1987.
6. **Stunkard, A. J., Harris, J. R., Pedersen, N. L., and McClearn, G. E.,** The body mass index of twins who have been reared apart, *N. Engl. J. Med.,* 322, 1483, 1990.
7. **Sørensen, T. I. A., Price, R. A., Stunkard, A. J., and Schulsinger, F.,** Genetics of obesity in adult adoptees and their biological siblings, *Br. Med. J.,* 298, 87, 1989.
8. **Price, R. A. and Gottesman, I. I.,** Body fat in Shields' cohort of identical twins reared apart, *Behav. Genet.,* 21, 1, 1991.
9. **Price, R. A. and Stunkard, A. J.,** Commingling analysis of obesity in twins, *Hum. Hered.,* 39, 121, 1989.
10. **Price, R. A., Stunkard, A. J., Sørensen, T. I. A., and Schulsinger, F.,** Component distributions of body mass index defining moderate and extreme overweight in Danish women and men, *Am. J. Epidemiol.,* 130, 193, 1989.
11. **Price, R. A., Ness, R., and Laskarzewski, P.,** Common major gene inheritance of extreme overweight, *Hum. Biol.,* 62, 747, 1990.
12. **Ness, R., Laskarzewski, P., and Price, R. A.,** The inheritance of obesity in black families, *Hum. Biol.,* 63, 39, 1991.
13. **Moll, P. P., Burns, T. L., and Lauer, R. M.,** The genetic and environmental sources of body mass index variability: the Muscatine ponderosity family study, *Am. J. Hum. Genet.,* 49, 1243, 1991.
14. **Price, R. A., Lunetta, L., Ness, R., Charles, M. A., Saad, M. F., Ravussin, E., Bennett, P. H., Pettitt, D. J., and Knowler, W. C.,** Obesity in Pima Indians: distribution characteristics and possible thresholds for genetic studies, *Int. J. Obes.,* 16, 851, 1992.
15. **Rao, D. C., MacLean, C. J., Morton, N. E., and Yee, S.,** Analysis of family resemblance. V. Height and weight in Northeastern Brazil, *Am. J. Hum. Genet.,* 27, 509, 1975.
16. **Province, M. A., Arnqvist, P., Keller, J., Higgins, M., and Rao, D. C.,** Strong evidence for a major gene for obesity in the large, unselected, total Community Health Study of Tecumseh, *Am. J. Hum. Genet.,* 47(Suppl.), A143, 1990.
17. **Johnson, P. R., Greenwood, M. R. C., Horwitz, B. A., and Stern, J. S.,** Animal models of obesity: genetic aspects, *Ann. Rev. Nutr.,* 11, 325, 1991.
18. **Schemmel, R., Mickelsen, O., and Gill, J. L.,** Dietary obesity in rats: body weight and body fat accretion in seven strains of rats, *J. Nutr.,* 100, 1041, 1970.
19. **Bouchard, C., Tremblay, A., Despres, J.-P., Nadeau, A., Lupien, P. J., Theriault, G., Dussault, J., Moorjani, S., Pinault, S., and Fournier, G.,** The response to long-term overfeeding in identical twins, *N. Engl. J. Med.,* 322, 1477, 1990.

20. **Fain, P. R.,** Characteristics of simple sibship variance tests for the detection of major loci and application to height, weight and spatial performance, *Ann. Hum. Genet.,* 42, 109, 1978.
21. **MacLean, C. J., Morton, N. E., Elston, R. C., and Yee, S.,** Skewness in commingled distributions, *Biometrics,* 32, 695, 1975.
22. **Morton, N. E., MacLean, C. J., Kagan, A., Gulbrandsen, C. L., Rhoads, C. G., Yee, S., and Lew, R.,** Commingling in distributions of lipids and related variables, *Am. J. Hum. Genet.,* 29, 52, 1977.
23. **Sharma, K., Byard, P. J., and Rao, D. C.,** Commingling in the distributions of fat-related measures in Punjabi families, *Hum. Hered.,* 34, 278, 1984.
24. **Borecki, I. B., Rice, T., Bouchard, C., and Rao, D. C.,** Commingling analysis of generalized body mass and composition: the Québec family study, *Int. J. Obes.,* 15, 763, 1991.
25. **Morton, N. E., Rao, D. C., and Lalouel, J. M.,** *Methods in Genetic Epidemiology,* S. Karger, New York, 1983.
26. **Garn, S. M.,** Continuities and changes in fatness from infancy through adulthood, *Curr. Probl. Pediatr.,* 15, 1, 1985.
27. **Reed, D. R., Bradley, E., and Price, R. A.,** Obesity in families of extremely obese women, *Obes. Res.,* 1, 167, 1993.
28. **Knowler, W. C., Pettitt, D. J., Saad, M. F., Charles, M. A., Nelson, R. G., Howard, B. V., Bogardus, C., and Bennett, P. H.,** Obesity in the Pima indians: its magnitude and relationship with diabetes, *Am. J. Clin. Nutr.,* 53, 1543S, 1991.
29. **Price, R. A., Charles, M. A., Pettitt, D. J., and Knowler, W. C.,** Obesity in Pima Indians: genetic segregation analysis of human obesity complicated by temporal increases in obesity, *Human Biology,* 66, in press.
30. **Price, R. A., Charles, M. A., Pettitt, D. J., and Knowler, W. C.,** Obesity in Pima Indians: large increases among post-World War II birth cohorts, *Am. J. Physiol. Anthropol.,* 1993, in press.
31. **Flegal, K. M., Harlan, W. R., and Landis, J. R.,** Secular trends in body mass index and skinfold thickness with socioeconomic factors in young adult women, *Am. J. Clin. Nutr.,* 48, 535, 1988.
32. **Harlan, W. R., Landis, J. R., Flegal, K. M., Davis, C. S., and Miller, M. E.,** Secular trends in body mass in the United States, 1960–1980, *Am. J. Epidemiol.,* 128, 1065, 1988.
33. **Shear, C. L., Freedman, D. S., Burke, G. L., Harsha, D. W., Webber, L. S., and Berenson, G. S.,** Secular trends of obesity in early life: the Bogalusa heart study, *Am. J. Public Health,* 78, 75, 1988.
34. **Sugarman, J. R., White, L. L., and Gilbert, T. J.,** Evidence for a secular change in obesity, height, and weight among Navajo Indian schoolchildren, *Am. J. Clin. Nutr.,* 52, 960, 1990.
35. **Chinn, S. and Rona, R. J.,** Secular trends in weight, weight-for-height and triceps skinfold thickness in primary school children in England and Scotland from 1972 to 1980, *Ann. Hum. Biol.,* 14, 311, 1987.
36. **Sørensen, T. I. A. and Price, R. A.,** Secular trends in body mass index among Danish young men, *Int. J. Obes.,* 14, 411, 1990.
37. **Price, R. A., Ness, R., and Sørensen, T. I. A.,** Changes in commingled body mass index distributions associated with secular trends in overweight among Danish young men, *Am. J. Epidemiol.,* 133, 501, 1991.
38. **Burton, B. T., Foster, W. R., Hirsch, J., and Van Itallie, T.,** Health implications of obesity: an NIH consensus development conference, *Int. J. Obes.,* 9, 155, 1985.
39. **Williamson, R.,** Human gene mapping, in *Molecular Approaches to Human Polygenic Disease,* Williamson, R., Ed., John Wiley & Sons, Chichester, U.K., 1987.

40. **Hall, J. M., Lee, M. K., Newman, B., Morrow, J. E., Anderson, L. A., Huey, B., and King, M. C.,** Linkage of early-onset breast cancer to chromosome 17q21, *Science,* 250, 1684, 1990.
41. **Bell, G. I., Xang, K. S., Newman, M. V., Wu, S. H., Wright, L. G., Fajans, S. S., Spielman, R. S., and Cox, N. J.,** Gene for non-insulin-dependent diabetes mellitus (maturity onset diabetes of the young subtype) is linked to DNA polymorphism on chromosome 20q, *Proc. Natl. Acad. Sci. U.S.A.,* 88, 1484, 1991.

Chapter 8

Genetics of Obesity: Etiologic Heterogeneity and Temporal Trends

Ingrid B. Borecki, Michael A. Province, Claude Bouchard, and D. C. Rao

TABLE OF CONTENTS

I. INTRODUCTION

A. FAMILIAL RESEMBLANCE FOR OBESITY

Phenotypes devised to quantitate the degree of obesity have been the subject of many recent investigations, motivated by the increased risk of cardiovascular morbidity and mortality,[1-3] largely through increased risk of diabetes, hypertriglyceridemia, changes in plasma lipoprotein profile and composition, and hypertension.[4,5] Specifically of interest are the identification and characterization of both genetic and environmental determinants of obesity so as to foster an understanding of the heterogeneous processes leading to human obesity and to provide an opportunity to devise rational intervention strategies aimed at reducing health risks.

Obesity can be considered as a complex phenotype that is multifactorially determined, involving genes, environmental exposures, and gene by environment interactions.[6] Perhaps the most widely studied phenotype is the body mass index [BMI = weight (kg)/height (m)^2]. The BMI is a measure of "heaviness"[7,8] rather than "fatness", reflecting the combined effects of body build, proportions, and lean body mass as well as body fat;[6] however, it exhibits substantial correlations with fat mass on the order of 0.81 and 0.83 in adult males and females, respectively,[9] and has been validated as a risk factor for cardiovascular disease.[3]

Genetic studies of the BMI have produced some conflicting results, although it is generally agreed that there is a significant degree of familial resemblance, with low to moderate correlations among first-degree relatives. However, to what degree the resemblance is due to shared genes remains a point of contention. Some family and adoption studies suggest low polygenic effects relative to familial environmental effects,[10-13] and in one adoption study[8] the midparent-natural child correlation did not differ significantly

0-8493-4880-3/94/$0.00+$.50

from the foster midparent-adopted child correlation, providing no evidence to support a role for genetic factors at all. In contrast, accumulating evidence from recent studies of adoptive families and twins reared together and apart suggests that genetic factors are more important than environmental ones.[14-21] For example, data from the Danish adoption study suggest that there is a clear absence of effects of the familial environment, and all familial resemblance is attributed to genetic effects yielding a polygenic heritability of about 34%.[17,22,23] Aside from genetic effects, examination of the evidence regarding environmental influences also has raised the suggestion that only environmental experiences that are not shared among family members appear to be important.[23-25]

B. TEMPORAL VARIATIONS IN OBESITY PHENOTYPES

The observation that the prevalence of obesity has been increasing in developed countries over the last half century[26] is consistent with studies suggesting the importance of nonshared environmental influences. While the frequency and magnitude of precipitating factors may be rising, the phenotypic response at the individual level possibly could be a function of genetic predisposition. Direct evidence to support this hypothesis has been presented recently for various obesity phenotypes by measuring the response in identical twins to a 100-day overfeeding regimen.[27] The changes in absolute and relative fat mass to the homogeneous, controlled environment were significantly more similar within each monozygotic twin pair than among nonrelated subjects and additionally suggested that gene by environment interaction effects also might account for an appreciable amount of the variance in obesity phenotypes. The presence of secular environmental effects could be manifest in an analysis of cross-sectional data as intergenerational differences in heritability or shared environmental effects for individuals close in age belonging to the same cohort, depending on the age structure of the families. Thus, unaccounted temporal trends in environmental factors could explain some of the variability in the conclusions regarding the relative importance of genetic and environmental factors.

In addition to the complication of secular trends, there are developmental trends for most obesity phenotypes studied to date. That is, the absolute and relative amounts of fat mass and fat-free mass and the amount of fat in regional depots change through early childhood and the growth spurts that characterize adolescence before attaining more stable adult values.[28] For example, the absolute and relative amounts of fat in truncal-abdominal subcutaneous depots increase progressively with time until about 60 to 70 years of age, particularly and more frequently in males.[29] In recognition of this variability, it is common practice to adjust obesity phenotypes for the effects of age, usually by multiple regression, prior to analysis. While this statistical procedure can correct adequately for age trends in the mean, and optionally in the variance as well, there may remain temporal trends in the covariance structure within families that reflect these developmental phases. Consideration of these sorts of temporal trends is motivated by the first-order question of whether the genetic component exerts the same degree of influence on the phenotype throughout life or, rather, whether there is some age (range) at which the genetic effect is maximized. A common assumption made in most studies is that the effects of the relevant determinants remain constant over all ages, with variations being attributed to random or unique environmental effects. Failure to take account of temporal trends in either the genetic or environmental components can be another factor contributing to the heterogeneity of results, besides being a well-motivated biological question.

II. TEMPORAL TRENDS UNDER A MULTIFACTORIAL MODEL

A. THE STATISTICAL MODEL

A model to assess temporal trends in familial correlations under multifactorial inheritance has been developed in the context of path analysis,[30,31] using a simple tau model.[32] The model is depicted in Figure 1 for a nuclear family with two children. The quantitative phenotype (P) is determined by a linear regression on a transmissible factor (T) with a residual factor (R) for each of the fathers, mothers, and children (subscripted F, M, and 1 or 2, respectively). Since they do not appear in the equations for the expected correlations between any pair of phenotypes, the residual factors for parents are not shown. It is important to note that in this case the transmissible component includes both polygenic and familial environmental factors, and the relative contributions of genes vs. shared environment will not be distinguished here. The effect of T on the phenotype (a standardized partial regression coefficient) is denoted t(A), a function of the individual's age (A). The effect of the residual is denoted by e(A), which is constrained by the relation $e^2(A) = 1 - t^2(A)$ since the correlation of P with itself is 1. The residuals for siblings are potentially correlated, which allows for additional sibling resemblance above and beyond that which is transmitted from the parents. The correlation is a function of the absolute age difference (ΔA) of the sib pair, denoted by ρ(ΔA). The transmissible factor of a child is assumed to be given by a linear regression on the transmissible factors of his or her parents with uncorrelated residuals. It is further assumed that effects of parental transmissible factors on those of their children (τ_F, τ_M) are the same for each child, regardless of age. Finally, marital resemblance is assumed to be a constant, regardless of parental ages or their duration of cohabitation, and is represented by a copath p.

Thus, the transmissibility (or generalized heritability) and the residual sibling correlation are potentially functions of age, absolute age in the case of the former and age difference in the case of the latter. The functional forms available for modeling the age trends were chosen such that they were simple and practical (with few parameters), with asymptotes on both ends. An ample variety of functional forms have been implemented such that practically any shape of trend can be modeled. It is possible to choose a function that permits the heritability to increase or decrease monotonically from childhood to adulthood, and different functional forms can be combined such that the heritability may increase (decrease) up to a certain age and then decrease (increase) again to a different value. In this analysis, t(A) and ρ(ΔA) were allowed to vary according to a logistic function and a (right-half of a) Gaussian function, respectively. The observed parent-child correlations based on longitudinal studies of weight appear to justify the logistic formulation for t(A),[33] which starts at t(0) at birth and asymptotes to t(25) at 25 years of age. Similarly, let ρ(ΔA) decrease over the age difference between sibs (ΔA) according to a (right-half) Gaussian function that starts at ρ_0 for twins (ΔA = 0) and decreases to ρ_{20} at ΔA = 20 years. It should be noted that the choices for the ages at which the functions asymptote were based on some exploration of the data and are taken to be known. In general, these points may be set to different values for other applications or may be estimated along with other parameters of

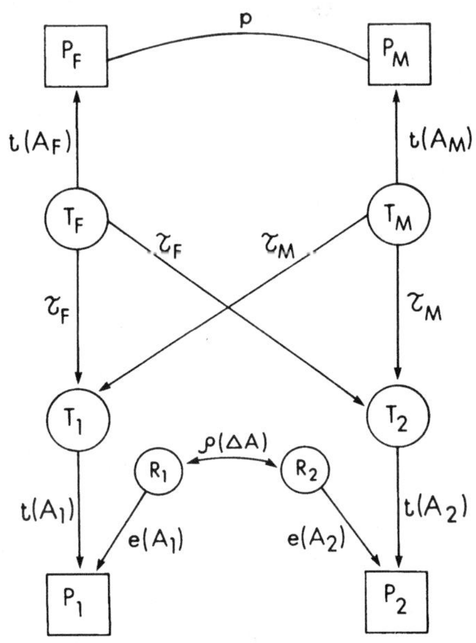

Figure 1. Tau model with temporal trends for familial transmission in nuclear families. See text for parameter definitions.

the model. A detailed discussion of the available functional forms and the justification for their parameterization can be found elsewhere.[30,31]

All parameters of the model are estimated by maximum likelihood using the FORTRAN program TAUTREND, and tests of hypotheses are carried out using the likelihood ratio criterion.

B. ANALYSIS OF THE BODY MASS INDEX IN FAMILIES FROM NORTHEASTERN BRAZIL

Evidence for temporal trends in the heritability and residual sibship correlation for BMI was assessed using data from a Brazilian family study which was based on 6750 individuals in 1067 nuclear families.[34] The BMI first was standardized (i.e., z-scores) in several age-sex classes, and the resulting phenotype was then normalized using an inverse normal transformation of the ranks. Thus, the final phenotype used in the analysis is normalized; the effects of age and sex on both the means and the variances have been eliminated. Therefore, any remaining trends should be in the correlations (covariances) only.

As a first step in the analysis, the maximum likelihood estimates of the familial correlations were obtained; these are shown in Table 1. It is clear that, in the absence of trends, not all five basic parameters (p, t, τ_F, τ_M, and ρ) can be resolved from nuclear family data alone, which generate only four correlations (marital, father-child, mother-child, and sibling). Either ρ has to be fixed or eliminated or at least one of the τ values has to be fixed. Since the sample sibling correlations are greater than the pooled parent-child correlations, the sibling residual correlation appears to be important. Thus, the constraint $\tau_F = \tau_M = 1/2$ was employed, which is the assumption underlying the polygenic/multifactorial model; i.e., fathers and mothers each contribute one half of the transmissible factors to their offspring. Therefore, $t^2(A)$ may be considered the pseudopolygenic heritability at age A.

The results of the analysis of the BMI with temporal trends are shown in Table 2. For each hypothesis tested, minus twice the log likelihood (denoted "likelihood") is shown along with the marital correlation (p), the generalized heritability t^2 at age 0 (birth) and age 25 years (adulthood), and the sibship correlation ρ for sib-pairs whose age differences are 0 (twins), 5, and 20 years. The model in which trends were entertained for both t and ρ requires the estimation of five parameters. This model yields a substantial improvement in the log-likelihood value when compared to the result without trends, that is, when all of the parameters are constant over time and only three parameters are estimated (χ^2 = 57.71, 2 df). The test of the hypothesis that there are no trends in t yields a $\chi^2 = 4.70$, with 1 df, leading to rejection of this hypothesis at the $P = 0.03$ level. This result is significant using the conventional $\alpha = 5\%$; however, the test is conditional on the chosen age asymptote. Thus, it should be noted that the evidence for temporal trends in heritability is perhaps of marginal significance. Testing the hypothesis that there are no trends in ρ yields $\chi^2 = 52.09$, which is clearly significant. Thus, it appears that the primary source of temporal variation is in the correlation between the siblings' residual factors as a function of their proximity in age, while the pseudopolygenic heritability increases from 0.32 at birth to 0.51 at adulthood.

The parent-child and sibling residual correlations as predicted from

Table 1. **Maximum likelihood estimates of family correlations and estimated sample sizes for the BMI in the Brazilian sample**

Type of correlation	r	*n*
Spouse-spouse	0.149	1066
Father-child	0.243	2085
Mother-child	0.250	2131
Sib-sib	0.301	2966
Pooled parent-child	0.249	4216

Table 2. **Path analysis of normalized BMI under the temporal trend model**

Hypothesis	Likelihood	p	t^2 (0)	t^2 (25)	ρ (0)	ρ (5)	ρ (20)
Trends in both t and ρ	5658.09	0.148	0.318	0.510	0.287	0.185	–0.005
No trends	5715.80	0.148	0.437	0.437	0.123	0.123	0.123
No trend in t	5662.79	0.148	0.431	0.431	0.261	0.149	–0.059
No trend in ρ	5710.18	0.147	0.300	0.535	0.176	0.176	0.176

Note: See text for details and definitions.
From Province, M. A. and Rao, D. C., *Am. J. Hum. Genet.*, 37, 178, 1985. With permission.

the model are displayed graphically in Fig. 2. Since parents have generally reached the asymptotic value of t, the predicted parent-child correlation primarily varies with the age of the child and increases as does t to about 0.3. For the sibling correlations, the expected correlation depends on the ages of both sibs; for simplicity, the correlation is shown here in reference to a newborn sib. As the age difference between the one sib and the newborn increases, the effect of ρ dominates and produces a drop in the predicted sibling correlation. That is, there remains the portion of the sibling correlation that is generated by virtue of the familial factors transmitted from parents to children, but there appears to be no *additional* sibling resemblance due to shared residual environmental factors when the sibs are over 20 years apart in age. As time progresses, any observed pair of sibs will always have a constant age difference, but in addition there is a predicted increase over time in sib-sib resemblance due to the effect of increasing t. When both members of the pair have reached adulthood (defined here as over 25 years of age), their age difference is no longer as critical in determining their correlation, and the effect of t is assumed to be constant in adulthood.

C. DISCUSSION

The data from the Brazilian family study suggest that the effect of the transmissible component, potentially including both polygenes and familial environmental factors, increases from birth to adulthood. A parallel finding has been reported recently using data from the Colorado Adoption Project, where BMI was investigated in 247 adoptive families and 246 control families.[35] Longitudinal measurements were made on all children from birth to age 12. Longitudinal factor and time-series models were designed to examine possible developmental changes in genetic and environmental effects over time. The main finding was that the phenotypic stability over time was largely attributable to genetic influences rather than familial environmental factors, and there was evidence that the effect of the genetic component increased during early development. Again, there was evidence that the only parental effect on offspring adiposity was genetic,

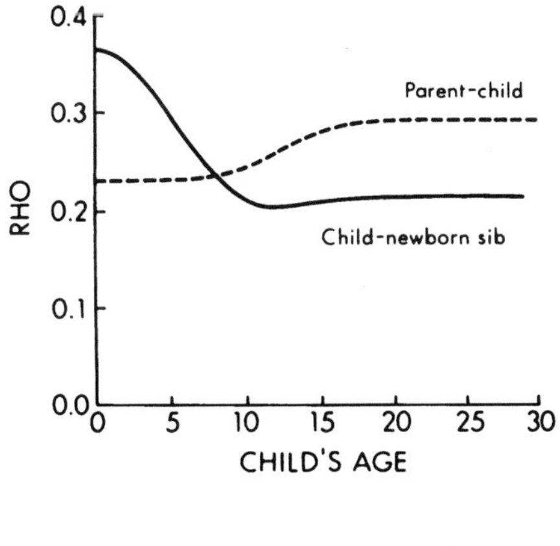

Figure 2. Predicted parent-child (broken line) and sib-sib (solid line) correlations for body mass index, based on the full model with temporal trends in both t and ρ. (From Province, M. A. and Rao, D. C., *Am. J. Hum. Genet.*, 37, 178, 1985. With permission.)

and the effect of the home environment was slight at all ages; neither of these factors contributed to parent-offspring resemblance. While this study is focused on childhood and the Brazilian study includes offspring of a wide age range, the findings in both cases suggest the importance of inherited factors and further suggest that the effect of these factors on the resulting phenotype increases as individuals grow and mature.

One other recently published study deals with age trends in heritability estimates.[25] These investigators utilized information on the BMI in 7245 same-sexed monozygotic (MZ) and dizygotic (DZ) twin pairs drawn from the Finnish Twin Cohort. The represented age range was 18 to 54 years — hence, the question is focused on possible trends in adulthood. In the analysis of the Brazilian data presented here, heritability was assumed to be constant after the attainment of adult status (over 25 years of age). It should be noted from the first that, typically, twin studies yield higher estimates of heritability than family studies. For example, data from the Finnish twin study suggest that genetic effects account for 72 and 68% of the total variance in men and women, respectively, as compared to the approximate range of 30 to 40% heritability estimated from family studies. Nonetheless, while there remains concern regarding whether estimates from twin studies are applicable to families in the general population, it is still instructive to consider the qualitative results presented with regard to age trends.

Using a variance components approach such as that available in LISREL, a model including additive genetic effects and shared and nonshared environmental components was tested. There was no evidence to support a role for shared environmental effects. Although not stated explicitly, it is likely that these adult-aged twins were not cohabitating at the time of the study; thus, the conclusion of a lack of shared environmental effects probably reflects the lack of an effect of childhood rearing environment, which is supported also by adoption studies[16,23] and other twin studies.[20,21] The remaining variance is therefore attributable to unique environmental factors experienced by individual members of the twin pairs. Heritabilities and the effect of residual environment were estimated in four age groups: 18 to 24, 25 to 34, 35 to 44, and 45 to 54 years. In both sexes, the estimated heritability decreased from 72, 74, 67, to 67% in males and, more dramatically, from 72, 69, 68, to 53% in females for each of the four advancing age groups, respectively. These results suggest that accumulation of unique environmental experiences dilutes the additive genetic effect as individuals age.

A related observation from the Brazilian data was that residual sibling resemblance (that is, the extent to which sibling phenotypes are correlated after accounting for the transmitted familial factors) decreases as a function of the age difference of the sibs. These are the environmental effects that individuals experience which are not provided or fostered by parents. It stands to reason that sibs close in age would probably share, for example, more similar dietary and physical activity habits than sibs with a large age difference. By the time sibs are nominally 20 years apart in age, these environmental factors essentially are unique for each member of the sib pair and do not contribute at all to sibling resemblance. Nonetheless, the resemblance between two sibs of a pair increases as time goes on because of the increasing effect of the heritable component. Considering the results of the twin study described above, the heritability might begin a slow decrease in about the fourth decade of life with the accumulation of unique environmentally based experiences.

Additional data consistent with this hypothesis have been reported by Mueller,[36] who proposed that transient environmental effects should be associated with a decrease in the sibling correlation with increasing age difference between members of a pair of adult sibs. Contrasting the correlations for various adiposity measures in adult sib pairs whose age difference was <7 years ($n = 58$) with those whose age difference was ≥7 years ($n = 53$) revealed that the group with greater age difference consistently exhibited lower correlations than the former group, although the differences were not statistically significant. Following up on this suggestion, Bouchard[37] showed that, indeed, shared environmental factors (specifically, socioeconomic status indicators in this case) were responsible for higher sibling correlations than in cases where the environmental factors were statistically controlled.

III. BODY MASS INDEX AND THE MAJOR GENE HYPOTHESIS

While the majority of genetic studies have investigated the BMI under a multifactorial model, there have been a few investigations testing a major gene hypothesis — that is, after allowing for the possibility of many genes and environmental factors, is there evidence that a single gene has a major effect on the distribution of BMI values? Earlier studies using structured exploratory data analysis (SEDA) concluded that there was no evidence to support a major gene hypothesis,[38,39] although there was the suggestion of possible dominance effects. Several recent studies using large samples and parametric mixed-model segregation analysis have provided support for a recessive major gene with transmission patterns conforming to the Mendelian hypothesis.[40-42] The case for the major gene hypothesis is reviewed in detail by Price in Chapter 7 of this volume.

A. EVIDENCE FOR MAJOR GENE EFFECTS IN THE QUÉBEC FAMILY STUDY

Analysis of the BMI has been carried out recently using data on 1630 individuals in 375 randomly sampled French-Canadian families living in the environs of Québec City to determine whether the major gene finding could be replicated. Prior to analysis, raw BMI values were adjusted for the effects of age on the mean and variance within four groups (fathers, mothers, sons, and daughters) by multiple regression. There was minimal heteroscedasticity. Commingling analysis carried out on the adjusted BMI values revealed that the parents and offspring were distributed identically under any distributional model, although under parsimony there was an admixture of normal components in the parental distribution, while only residual skewness under a single distribution was found in the offspring.[9] Thus, while there was no significant indication of distributional heterogeneity by generation, the differing parsimonious models was consistent with a developmental hypothesis.

Segregation analysis was carried out[43] using the mixed model as implemented in the computer program POINTER.[44] The phenotype is assumed to be determined by the independent and additive contributions of a biallelic major gene, a multifactorial background, and a unique residual component. There are seven parameters that can be estimated: the overall variance (V), the overall mean (u), the frequency of the allele associated with higher BMI values (q), the displacement between the means of the two homozygote distributions (t), the relative position of the heterozygote distribution or dominance (d), the multifactorial heritability (H), and a factor to distinguish the multifactorial effect in adults from that in children (Z). In order to detect violations of model assumptions and verify that the transmission patterns of the putative gene conform with Mendelian expectations, the transmission probabilities also can be estimated and tested. They comprise three additional parameters: τ_1, τ_2, and τ_3 are the probabilities that an *A* allele is transmitted from a parent whose genotype is *AA*, *Aa*, or *aa*, respectively. Under Mendelian transmission, $\tau_1 = 1$, $\tau_2 = 1/2$, and $\tau_3 = 0$. Estimation of the parameters and testing of hypotheses are carried out using maximum likelihood methods.

The main results of segregation analysis are displayed in Table 3. The null hypothesis of no major gene (d = t = q = 0) was rejected ($\chi^2 = 65.37$, 3 df), as was that of no multifactorial effect (H = Z = 0; $\chi^2 = 21.19$, 2 df). Thus, the mixed model, in which the estimated d indicated a recessive mode of inheritance, is favored. Other tests on d indicated that dominant and additive models were untenable (data not shown). Finally, there was no evidence that the multifactorial effects differed by generation (Z = 1; χ^2 =

0.35, 1 df). Tests on the transmission parameters were carried out to assess the tenability of the major gene model. After freeing the three transmission probabilities it was possible to reject the Mendelian hypothesis ($\chi^2 = 8.33$, 3 df), while the environmental hypothesis where all the τ values are constrained to be equal was not rejected ($\chi^2 = 2.27$, 2 df). This was a somewhat perplexing result since not only was the Mendelian major gene hypothesis not confirmed, but it appeared that the major effect was not transmitted within families and was probably of environmental origin. In addition, the major effect does not appear to be in equilibrium between the parental and the offspring generations, since the equal τ values do not approximate the quantity $1 - q$.

B. A MAJOR GENE MODEL WITH GENOTYPE-SPECIFIC AGE EFFECTS

The suggestion of possible intergenerational differences in the major effect came from the observation that the parsimonious distributional models in parents and children differed and that while there was solid statistical evidence of a major effect from segregation analysis, the transmission did not apparently depend on parental type and, again, suggested a lack of intergenerational equilibrium. Thus, it was hypothesized that evidence for a Mendelian major gene could be affected by possible developmental trends. A reanalysis of the data was undertaken using a model which allowed the estimation of genotype-specific age effects. This provided the opportunity to entertain the hypothesis that genotypes might respond differently to developmental effects — that is, gene by environment interaction.[45]

Segregation analysis with genotype-dependent covariate effects was carried out using REGRESS, which is based on the regressive models of Bonney.[46] The extension including the simultaneous estimation of covariate effects (with or without genotypic dependencies) is easily carried out in this context and has been done for another application.[47] The quantitative phenotype is denoted Y (e.g., BMI). The penetrance function takes the form $P(Y \mid g, Y_A, X)$, where the probability of observing the phenotypes is conditional on the underlying major genotypes (g), phenotype observations on relevant ancestors (Y_A), and adjustment for an arbitrary number of covariates (X). In general, since the underlying trait genotypes (g) are unobserved, their prior probabilities are taken to be in Hardy-Weinberg proportions for individuals with no parents in the pedigree and are based on segregation probabilities from parental mating types for individuals with ancestors in the pedigree, formulated by using transmission probabilities as described above. The dependency on phenotypes of ancestors (Y_A) is modeled under class A assumptions,[46] which essentially posits that sibs are conditionally independent, given their parents' genetic contribution.

The quantitative penetrance can be modeled by a normal density function $\Phi(z,w)$ whose mean, z, is given by $z = (Y - \mu_g) - b_S(Y_S - \mu_{gS}) - b_F(Y_F - \mu_{gF}) - b_M(Y_M - \mu_{gM}) - \Sigma\, b_{gj}X_j$, where μ_g is the genotype-specific mean, b is a regression coefficient, b_g is a genotype-specific regression coefficient, S refers to the spouse of this individual, F refers to the father, M refers to the mother, C refers to a child, and the covariate adjustment is summed over all j covariates. It should be noted that the dependencies are modeled on residual phenotypes, after the mean effects of the major locus are taken into account. The variance can be written as $w = \sigma_g^2 (1 - b_S\, \rho_{FM} - b_F\, \rho_{FC} - b_M\, \rho_{MC})$, with no adjustment for the covariates since they are treated here as fixed effects.

The parameters of the model are as follows: the mean of the overall distribution or, under a major gene model, the mean of low homozygotes is m; the within-genotype variance is v; q, t, and d are parameters of the remaining genotypic distributions as described above in POINTER; r_{PC} is the residual parent-child correlation; and regression coefficients for age up to third-order terms are entertained, which can be subscripted by the homozygous low (LL), heterozygous (LH), or homozygous high (HH) genotypes. Again, parameter estimation and tests of hypotheses are carried out using the maximum likelihood method.

Although covariate adjustments can be carried out readily in the context of the genetic model, the same age- and sex-adjusted phenotypes used in the POINTER analysis were

Table 3. **Segregation analysis results for BMI in the Québec Family Study**

Model	d	t	q	H	Z	τ_1	τ_2	τ_3	–2 ln L+c
General Mendelian	0[a]	3.07	0.14	0.40	0.74	[1]	[½]	[0]	8.33
No major effect (d = t = q = 0)	[0]	[0]	[0]	0.45	0.86	—	—	—	73.70
No multifactorial effect (H = Z = 0)	0.25	2.60	0.27	[0]	[0]	[1]	[½]	[0]	29.52
No generation difference (Z = 1)	0[a]	2.99	0.15	0.35	[1]	[1]	[½]	[0]	8.68
Free τs, d = 0, and Z = 1	[0]	2.58	0.04	0.41	[1]	0.85	0.14	0.17	0.00
Equal τs, d = 0, and Z = 1	[0]	2.55	0.01	0.42	[1]	0.79	0.79	0.79	2.27

Note: Parameters in square brackets were fixed at the value indicated. See text for details and definitions.

[a] Parameter went to boundary value indicated during iteration.

From Rice, T., Borecki, I. B., Bouchard, C., Rao, D. C., *Obes. Res.*, 1, 288, 1993. With permission.

utilized here. In this way, remaining age trends are probably of developmental significance since simple age effects on the phenotypic mean or variance have been removed. The results of hypothesis testing are shown in Table 4. Testing for the presence of family resemblance by allowing a parent-child correlation showed a significant improvement in the fit of the model ($\chi^2 = 64.8$, 1 df), as did allowing for an additional major gene effect ($\chi^2 = 130.3$, 3 df). There was a good fit to a recessive mode of inheritance ($d = 0$; $\chi^2 = 0.51$, 1 df), similar to the POINTER analysis. As expected, allowing for simple age effects independent of the genotype did not improve the fit ($\chi^2 = 1.58$, 2 df) since the data were adjusted prior to analysis. However, allowing for residual age effects for the phenotypically indistinguishable LL and LH genotypes to differ from those for the HH genotypes did yield a significant test ($\chi^2 = 9.08$, 3 df). Higher-order terms above linear genotype-specific age effects were not supported by the data. At this point, an attempt was made to check Mendelian transmission in the context of this model. In contrast to the results using the POINTER model (which only differed in the lack of genotype-specific age effects), Mendelian transmission was not rejected ($\chi^2 = 2.67$, 3 df).

C. DISCUSSION

The final model included a recessive major gene effect where the frequency of the HH genotype was 4.8%, similar to previous reports.[40-42] There was a residual parent-child correlation of 0.18, with no evidence of spouse correlation.

The genotypic means are shown as a function of age in Figure 3. On the standardized scale, the mean was –0.198 for the LL/LH group and 3.797 for the HH group at birth. It should be recalled that age effects in the mean that are common to all genotypes have been removed prior to analysis, so trends (e.g., most people tend to get heavier as they get older) no longer exist in the data. For the most part it appears that individuals of the LL or LH genotypes do not exhibit much difference from the general population trend, since the phenotypic mean does not change much over the course of time, showing only a slight increase. The more pronounced trend can be observed in relation to the HH genotype, where the difference with respect to the other genotypes is the largest at birth, when environmental influences are at a minimum, and decreases over time. The specific reason for this is not immediately apparent. These data would seem to suggest that the unique environmental variations experienced by these HH individuals act in a such a way as to systematically decrease the degree of obesity over time. This could be the case if genetically obese individuals were systematically dieting or taking some other measures to reduce their heaviness with some degree of success. In any case, it also suggests that

Table 4. **Results of hypothesis tests in the analysis of BMI with genotype-specific age effects in the Québec Family Study**

Terms in model	Likelihood	χ^2 (df)
m, v	1294.11	
m, v, r_{PC}	1229.31	64.80 (1)
m, v, q, t, d, r_{PC}	1099.01	130.30 (3)
m, v, q, t, $d = 0$, r_{PC}	1099.52	0.51 (1)
m, v, q, t, $d = 0$, r_{PC}, age, age^2, age^3	1097.94	1.58 (3)
m, v, q, t, $d = 0$, r_{PC}, $age_{LL/LH}$, age_{HH}	1090.44	9.08 (2)
m, v, q, t, $d = 0$, r_{PC}, $age_{LL/LH}$, age_{HH}, τ_1, τ_2, τ_3	1087.77	2.67 (3)

Note: See text for details and definitions.

From Borecki, I. B., Bonney, G. E., Rice, T., Bouchard, C., Rao, D. C., *Am. J. Hum. Genet.*, 53, 676, 1993. With permission.

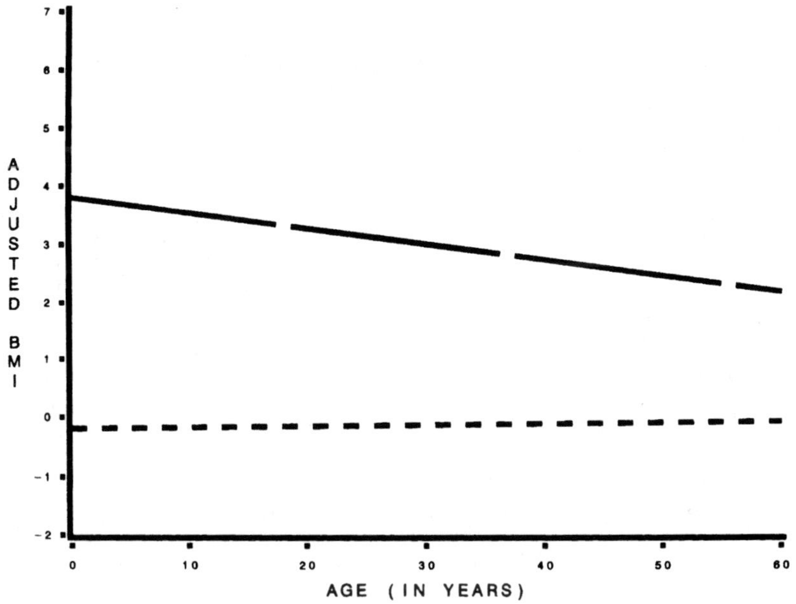

Figure 3. Predicted mean BMI for individuals in the Québec Family Study with HH or "high" recessive genotype (long dashed line) and individuals with the LL or LH "low" genotype (short dashed line) as a function of age. From Borecki, I. B., Bonney, G. E., Rice, T., Bouchard, C., Rao, D. C., *Am. J. Hum. Genet.,* 53, 676, 1993. With permission.

the strategy of selecting families through obese children for the identification of specific genes relevant to obesity or heaviness is a sound one.

IV. SUMMARY

Identification of the determinants of human obesity is a complex problem and poses numerous research challenges. It is clear that each of polygenic, shared environmental, unique environmental, and major gene factors all have been implicated in various studies, and the evidence for the presence and magnitude of each is not entirely consistent across all studies. All of this supports the notion of etiologic heterogeneity — that is, there are probably several (many?) heterogeneous processes that could lead to the same obesity phenotype. Thus, one important challenge is to identify specific families or groups of families in which the determinants appear to be homogeneous such that specific measurable factors can be identified. One approach to the identification of homogeneous patterns of determination is to relax some of the assumptions of traditional analysis models when it is justified and feasible. This chapter has focused on possible temporal and developmental trends and has summarized efforts toward incorporating these effects into the analysis models, thereby relaxing the assumption that the effects of genes and environment are invariant over time.

Two different approaches have been reviewed. The first allows for temporal trends in familial correlations in the context of a multifactorial model, which allows a preliminary assessment. In the second approach, age trends in the penetrance under a major gene model are explored, allowing for a constant multifactorial background. The choice of approach will depend on the question being posed.

The data on BMI from a large Brazilian study indicate that generalized heritability, including both polygenic and familial environmental factors, increases from birth to adulthood. Taken with the evidence from other adoption[16,23] and twin studies[20,21] suggesting that early rearing environment has no effect on the resulting phenotype, the increasing heritability could indicate that it is the expression of the genotype that evolves over time, with familial predispositions becoming realized to their fullest extent by adulthood. Further studies of changes in heritability during adulthood suggest the importance of unique environmental factors and may precipitate a decline in familial resemblance.[25] On the other hand, suggestion of possible single gene effects in the Québec families prompted an analysis of the BMI with genotype-specific temporal trends. After correcting for age trends in the mean and variance in the general population, the data suggested that individuals with the "high" recessive genotype showed the greatest degree of heaviness at birth, with a subsequent trend toward lower values throughout life. It should be noted that this conclusion is based on cross-sectional data, and longitudinal measurements would be desirable to confirm this trend. Whether this observed major gene effect is the same as that reported previously[40-42] is not clear, although the genotype frequency for the "high" individuals is similar to the estimates obtained in those studies. However, this analysis is the first to entertain genotype-specific age effects on the BMI. The decrease in the nonadditive effect of a major genotype is consistent with the observed increase in heritable effect up to early adulthood. Again, a role for unique environmental factors is implicated. It appears that the treatment of temporal variation in the context of genetic models for the etiology of obesity can lend some insight and perhaps even resolve some of the conflicting reports.

Another approach to disentangling heterogeneous processes is to utilize phenotypic measures that are more homogeneous themselves. This paradigm has met with some success in the realm of cardiovascular disease research, where measurements of total cholesterol have given way to subphenotypes such as low- and high-density lipoprotein cholesterol and further refinement by use of quantitative apoprotein phenotypes. Analogous to total cholesterol, the BMI is a relatively heterogeneous phenotype reflecting the contributions of both fat and lean mass in unknown proportions. The BMI also is greatly affected by the overall energy balance, varying as a function of habitual energy intake relative to the level of physical activity. Fat mass,[13,48] fat-free mass,[13] energy intake,[49] and habitual level of physical activity[50] have all been shown to exhibit familial resemblance as well as to be affected by unique environmental determinants, suggesting that from a biological standpoint the BMI is a heterogeneous phenotype with a truly multifactorial determination. However, use of the BMI has some advantages, among them being its ease of measurement in large epidemiological studies, and in view of its correlation of about 0.8 with fat mass in adults[9] it serves as an index of overall fatness. Nonetheless, the development and use of subphenotypes will advance efforts at defining genetic and environmental determinants of human obesity and likely will be useful in resolving etiologic heterogeneity.

ACKNOWLEDGMENTS

This work was partly supported by National Institutes of Health grants GM28719 and HD18281, National Institute of Mental Health grant MH31302, and Medical Research Council of Canada grant MA-10499.

REFERENCES

1. **Burton, B. T., Foster, W. R., Hirsch, J., and van Itallie, T. B.,** Health implications of obesity: an NIH consensus development conference, *Int. J. Obes.*, 9, 155, 1985.

2. **Kral, J. G.,** Morbid obesity and related health risks, *Ann. Intern. Med.,* 103, 1043, 1985.
3. **van Itallie, T. V. and Abraham, S.,** Some hazards of obesity and its treatment, in *Recent Advances in Obesity Research,* Vol. 4, Hirsch, J. and van Itallie, T. B., Eds., J. Libbey, London, 1985.
4. Royal College of Physicians, Obesity, *J. R. Coll. Phys.,* 17, 5, 1983.
5. **Bray, G.,** Complications of obesity, *Ann. Intern. Med.,* 103, 1052, 1985.
6. **Bouchard, C.,** Genetic factors in obesity, *Med. Clin. North Am.,* 73, 67, 1989.
7. **Garn, S. M., Leonard, W. R., and Hawthorne, V. M.,** Three limitations of the body mass index, *Am. J. Clin. Nutr.,* 44, 996, 1986.
8. **Bouchard, C. and Pérusse, L.,** Heredity and body fat, *Annu. Rev. Nutr.,* 8, 259, 1988.
9. **Borecki, I. B., Rice, T., Bouchard, C., and Rao, D. C.,** Commingling analysis of generalized body mass and composition measures: the Québec family study, *Int. J. Obes.,* 15, 763, 1991.
10. **Hartz, A., Giefer, E., and Rimm, A. A.,** Relative importance of the effect of family environment and heredity on obesity, *Ann. Hum. Genet.,* 41, 185, 1977.
11. **Annest, J. L., Sing, C. F., Biron, P., and Mongeau, J. G.,** Familial aggregation of blood pressure and weight in adoptive families. III. Analysis of the role of shared genes and shared household environment in explaining family resemblance for height, weight and selected weight/height indices, *Am. J. Epidemiol.,* 117, 492, 1983.
12. **Longini, I. M., Jr., Higgins, M. W., Hinton, P. D., Moll, P. P., and Keller, J. B.,** Genetic and environmental sources of familial aggregation of body mass in Tecumseh, Michigan, *Hum. Biol.,* 56, 733, 1984.
13. **Bouchard, C., Pérusse, L., Leblanc, C., Tremblay, A., and Thériault, G.,** Inheritance in the amount and distribution of human body fat, *Int. J. Obes.,* 12, 205, 1988.
14. **Biron, P., Mongeau, J.-G., and Bertrand, D.,** Familial resemblance of body weight and weight/height in 374 homes with adopted children, *J. Pediatr.,* 91, 555, 1977.
15. **Heller, R., Garrison, R. J., Havlik, R. J., Feinleib, M., and Padgett, S.,** Family resemblances in height and relative weight in the Framingham heart study, *Int. J. Obes.,* 8, 399, 1984.
16. **Stunkard, A. J., Foch, T. T., and Hrubec, Z.,** A twin study of human obesity, *J. Am. Med. Assoc.,* 256, 51, 1986.
17. **Stunkard, A. J., Sørenson, T. I. A., Hanis, C., Teasdale, T. W., Chakraborty, R., and Schull, W. J.,** An adoption study of human obesity, *N. Engl. J. Med.,* 314, 193, 1986.
18. **Price, R. A., Cadoret, R. J., and Stunkard, A. J.,** Genetic contributions to human fatness: an adoption study, *Am. J. Psychiatry,* 144, 1003, 1987.
19. **Sørenson, T. I. A., Price, R. A., Stunkard, A. J., and Schulsinger, F.,** Genetics of obesity in adult adoptees and their biological siblings, *Br. Med. J.,* 298, 87, 1989.
20. **Stunkard, A. J., Harris, J., Pedersen, N. L., and McClearn, G. E.,** The body mass index of twins who have been reared apart, *N. Engl. J. Med.,* 322, 1483, 1990.
21. **Price, R. A. and Gottesman, I. I.,** Body fat in identical twins reared apart: roles for genes and environment, *Behav. Genet.,* 21, 1, 1991.
22. **Vogler, G. P., Srinivasan, M. R., Stunkard, A. J., Sørenson, T. I. A., and Rao, D. C.,** The significance of genetic and nonshared environmental influences on human obesity: the Danish adoption study, *Am J. Hum. Genet.,* 47(Suppl.), 314, 1990.
23. **Vogler, G. P., Sørenson, T. I. A., Stunkard, A. J., Srinivasan, M. R., and Rao, D. C.,** Genetic and nonshared environmental influences on body mass index in a Danish adoption study, submitted.
24. **Grilo, C. M. and Pogue-Geile, M. F.,** The nature of environmental influences on weight and obesity: a behavior genetic analysis, *Psychol. Bull.,* 110, 520, 1991.

25. **Korkeila, M., Kaprio, J., Rissanen, A., and Koskenvuo, M.,** Effects of gender and age on the heritability of body mass index, *Int. J. Obes.,* 15, 647, 1991.
26. **Price, R. A.,** Increases in prevalence and extent of obesity in post-world war II birth cohorts: implications for genetic analyses, *Behav. Genet.,* 22, 746, 1992.
27. **Bouchard, C., Tremblay, A., Després, J.-P., Nadeau, A., Lupien, P. J., Thériault, G., Dussault, J., Moorjani, S., Pinault, S., and Fournier, G.,** The response to long-term overfeeding in identical twins, *N. Engl. J. Med.,* 322, 1477, 1990.
28. **Malina, R. M. and Bouchard, C.,** Subcutaneous fat distribution during growth, in *Fat Distribution during Growth and Later Health Outcomes,* Alan R. Liss, New York, 1988, 63.
29. **Bouchard, C., Després, J.-P., Mauriège, P., Marcotte, M., Chagnon, M., Dionne, F. T., and Bélanger, A.,** The genes in the constellation of determinants of regional fat distribution, *Int. J. Obes.,* 15, 9, 1991.
30. **Province, M. A. and Rao, D. C.,** Path analysis of family resemblance with temporal trends: applications to height, weight, and quetelet index in northeastern Brazil, *Am. J. Hum. Genet.,* 37, 178, 1985.
31. **Province, M. A. and Rao, D. C.,** Familial aggregation in the presence of temporal trends, *Stat. Med.,* 7, 185, 1988.
32. **Rice, J. P., Cloninger, C. R., and Reich, T.,** Multifactorial inheritance with cultural transmission and assortative mating. I. Description and basic properties of the unitary models, *Am. J. Hum. Genet.,* 30, 618, 1978.
33. **Bayley, N.,** Some increasing parent-child similarities during the growth of children, *J. Educ. Psychol.,* 45, 1, 1954.
34. **Morton, N. E.,** Genetic studies in northeastern Brazil, *Cold Spring Harbor Symp. Quant. Biol.,* 29, 69, 1964.
35. **Cardon, L. R.,** Developmental analysis of the body mass index in the Colorado Adoption Project, *Behav. Genet.,* 21, 563, 1992.
36. **Mueller, W. H.,** Transient environmental changes and age-limited genes as causes of variation in sib-sib and parent-offspring correlations, *Ann. Hum. Biol.,* 5, 395, 1978.
37. **Bouchard, C.,** Transient environmental effects detected in sibling correlations, *Ann. Hum. Biol.,* 7, 89, 1980.
38. **Karlin, S., Williams, P. T., Jensen, S., and Farquhar, J. W.,** Genetic analysis of the Stanford LRC family study data. I. Structural exploratory data analysis of height and weight measurement, *Am. J. Epidemiol.,* 113, 307, 1981.
39. **Zonta, L. A., Jayakar, S. D., Bosisio, M., Galante, A., and Pennetti, V.,** Genetic analysis of human obesity in an Italian sample, *Hum. Hered.,* 37, 129, 1987.
40. **Price, R. A., Ness, R., and Laskarzewski, P.,** Common major gene inheritance of extreme overweight, *Hum. Biol.,* 62, 747, 1990.
41. **Province, M. A., Arnqvist, P., Keller, J., Higgins, M., and Rao, D. C.,** Strong evidence for a major gene for obesity in the large, unselected, total community health study of Tecumseh, *Am. J. Hum. Genet.,* 47(Suppl.), A143, 1990.
42. **Moll, P. P., Burns, T. L., and Lauer, R. M.,** The genetic and environmental sources of body mass index variability: the Muscatine ponderosity family study, *Am. J. Hum. Genet.,* 49, 1243, 1991.
43. **Rice, T., Borecki, I. B., Bouchard, C., and Rao, D. C.,** Segregation analysis of body mass index in an unselected French-Canadian sample: the Québec family study, *Obesity Res.,* 1, 288, 1993.
44. **Lalouel, J. M., Rao, D. C., Morton, N. E., and Elston, R. C.,** A unified model for complex segregation analysis, *Am. J. Hum. Genet.,* 35, 816, 1983.
45. **Borecki, I. B., Rice, T., Bouchard, C., and Rao, D. C.,** Influence of genotype-dependent effects of covariates on the outcome of segregation analysis of the body mass index, *Am. J. Hum. Genet.,* 53, 676, 1993.

46. **Bonney, G. E.,** On the statistical determination of major gene mechanisms in continuous human traits: regressive models, *Am. J. Med. Genet.,* 18, 731, 1984.

47. **Borecki, I. B., Lathrop, G. M., Bonney, G. E., Yaouanq, J., and Rao, D. C.,** Combined segregation and linkage analysis of genetic hemochromatosis using affection status, serum iron, and HLA, *Am. J. Hum. Genet.,* 47, 542, 1990.

48. **Rice, T., Borecki, I. B., Bouchard, C., and Rao, D. C.,** Segregation analysis of fat mass and other body composition measures derived from underwater weighing, *Am. J. Hum. Genet.,* 52, 967, 1993.

49. **Pérusse, L., Tremblay, A., Leblanc, C., Cloninger, C. R., Reich, T., Rice, J., and Bouchard, C.,** Familial resemblance in energy intake: contribution of genetic and environmental factors, *Am. J. Clin. Nutr.,* 47, 629, 1988.

50. **Pérusse, L., Tremblay, A., Leblanc, C., and Bouchard, C.,** Genetic and environmental influences on level of habitual physical activity and exercise participation, *Am. J. Epidemiol.,* 128, 1012, 1989.

Chapter 9

Genetics of Energy Intake and Food Preferences

Louis Pérusse and Claude Bouchard

TABLE OF CONTENTS

I. INTRODUCTION

Advances in molecular biology in the past decade have generated a lot of data confirming the extent of genetic variation in the human genome. The genetic diversity observed between and within populations makes every one of us a genetically unique individual. This concept of genetic individuality is increasingly recognized as an important factor in the etiology of several common diseases since it suggests that not everybody faces the same risk for a particular disease in the population. Considering the importance of nutrition in the development of several chronic diseases like cardiovascular disease, cancer, obesity, diabetes, and osteoporosis, understanding the causes of interindividual differences in energy intake and nutritional requirements is becoming more and more important.

Although it is increasingly recognized that genetic factors play a role in the development and maintenance of obesity, little is known at this time about the nature of the genes involved and how these genes affect the various determinants of body fat. Since variation in energy expenditure and energy intake contributes to interindividual differences in body fat, it is likely that a better understanding of the role of genetic factors in obesity will be obtained by studying the contribution of genetic factors in the two components of the energy balance equation, i.e., energy intake and energy expenditure. This chapter will review the literature about the influence of genes in energy intake and food preferences.

II. FAMILIAL RESEMBLANCE

The presence of familial aggregation in total energy intake and intake of macronutrients (carbohydrates, lipids, and proteins) and micronutrients is a well-documented phenomenon. Thus, dietary habits, total caloric intake, and nutrient intakes have been shown to aggregate in families, with significant resemblance observed among spouses as well as between parents and their children.[1-6] For example, significant familial resemblance has been reported recently for intake of energy and of several nutrients measured in 170 parents (mean age of 33 years) and 91 children (mean age of 4 years) participating in the Framingham Children's Study.[6] Significant correlations were observed among spouses and between parents and their children for most nutrients, with generally higher mother-child than father-child correlations. In order to assess the influence of dietary habits of parents on their child, the authors[6] computed odds ratios for a child's intake of a given

0-8493-4880-3/94/$0.00+$.50

nutrient according to the level of consumption of one or both parents. Results are presented in Table 1. As indicated in this table, children with one parent eating high amounts of total fat, saturated fatty acids, and cholesterol are about two times more likely to consume a diet rich in these nutrients than children whose parents both have low intake of these nutrients (reference group). When nutrient intake is high in both parents, the probability of having a high nutrient intake in children is about three to six times greater. These results suggest that parents may have a profound influence on their children's dietary habits.

In a typical study of familial resemblance in food preferences,[7] ratings of 22 food items were obtained from college students (mean age 19.5) and their parents and mother-child and father-child correlations were computed for each food. The average correlation for all food items was found to be 0.20 in mother-child pairs and 0.04 in father-child pairs. Results of other studies recently reviewed by Cavali-Sforza[8] reveal low to moderate parent-offspring correlations for food preferences, with evidence for a maternal effect as suggested by higher mother-child than father-child correlations in the majority of the studies. These examples illustrate the importance of familial aggregation in energy intake and food preferences. The question arising from these studies is to what extent this familial resemblance could be inherited. This has been addressed in a few studies.

III. HERITABILITY LEVELS

Several twin studies have been undertaken to assess the role of heredity in energy intake and food preferences.[9-15] Most studies have shown greater similarities in dietary intake and food preferences between monozygotic (MZ) twins than between dizygotic (DZ) twins, suggesting that genetic factors may contribute to interindividual differences in dietary habits. However, these findings must be interpreted with caution. For instance, in searching for genetic influences in several biological variables, Heller et al.[15] found that for 12 out of the 13 dietary variables measured using 4-day weighed food diaries the correlations were higher in MZ twins (103 pairs) than in DZ twins (94 pairs). By taking twice the difference between MZ and DZ twin correlations as an estimate of heritability (h^2), they found heritabilities ranging from 3 to 55%, although the genetic variance reached significance only for one variable (intake of complex carbohydrates, $h^2 = 0.55$). They also reported that MZ twins tended to get together and eat together more regularly than DZ twins, suggesting that the greater similarity in energy intake among MZ twin pairs could be partly explained by a greater degree of shared environment. These results illustrate the fact that, depending on the phenotype considered, twin studies may not discriminate well between genetic factors and common environment effects.

Another strategy to assess the role of heredity independently from the possible confounding effects of cultural transmission is to use family data that include information on several types of biological and adopted relatives. This approach has been taken in one

Table 1. **Influence of high nutrient intake in parents on their children's intake**

Parents' intake	Odds ratio on child's intake
Total fat	
One parent	2.8
Both parents	2.8
Saturated fatty acid	
One parent	2.3
Both parents	5.5
Cholesterol	
One parent	1.7
Both parents	6.3

Note: High and low intake groups were defined by the median of the distribution of parents' and children's intakes. Adapted from Reference 6.

study[16] designed to assess the contribution of genetic and environmental factors in total energy intake and macronutrient intake. A total of 1597 individuals from 375 families, which included biological and adopted siblings in addition to MZ and DZ twins, completed a 3-day dietary record from which total energy intake as well as intakes of carbohydrate, lipid, and protein were derived. Significant familial aggregation was found for every energy intake measurement. Familial correlations computed for nine different types of relatives by descent or adoption are presented in Table 2. For all variables the correlations between MZ twins were higher than those between DZ twins, which suggests a genetic basis for the observed familial resemblance. However, a look at the other correlations reveals that individuals sharing the same household environment, whether genetically related or not, were similar in their energy intake, an observation compatible with a weak genetic contribution.

When all these correlations were considered jointly in a model of path analysis, which assumes that the phenotypic variance results from the linear and additive effects of genetic and cultural transmission as well as a residual component that includes nontransmissible environmental factors, it became possible to quantify the fraction of the total phenotypic variance attributable to each component. Results obtained by this strategy using the BETA model of path analysis[16] are summarized in Figure 1. Most of the variation observed for total energy intake (kilojoules per kilogram body weight) and for absolute intakes of carbohydrate, fat, and protein was found to be accounted for by nontransmissible environmental factors (about 70%), while transmissible variance was entirely explained by cultural inheritance (about 30%) with no significant genetic effect (h^2 ranging from 0 to 3%).

The fraction of total energy intake derived from macronutrients was also computed in this study.[16] Results obtained for carbohydrates and fat are presented in Figure 1. When

Table 2. **Familial correlations in various types of relatives for total energy intake and intake of macronutrients**

Type of Relative (*n* pairs)	Total intake (per kg body weight)	Intake in grams		
		Carbohydrate	Fat	Protein
Spouses (339)	0.31	0.37	0.37	0.47
Parent-child (1212)	0.26	0.26	0.27	0.26
Siblings (361)	0.30	0.27	0.23	0.25
Dizygotic twins (60)	0.58	0.45	0.55	0.42
Monozygotic twins (59)	0.69	0.68	0.60	0.65
Uncle (aunt)-nephew (niece) (88)	0.09[a]	0.24	–0.02[a]	0.06[a]
First-degree cousins (95)	0.33	0.23	0.23	0.26
Unrelated sibs (115)	0.21	0.23	0.16[a]	0.25
Foster parent-adopted child (314)	0.29	0.25	0.26	0.33

[a] Nonsignificant correlations. All other correlations, $p < 0.05$.

Adapted from Reference 16.

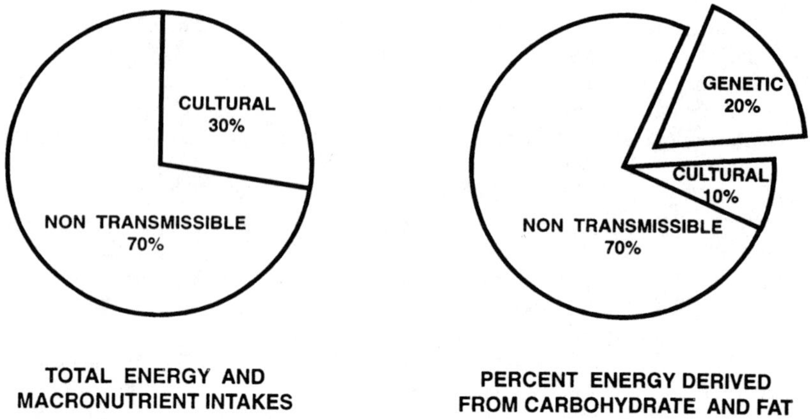

Figure 1. Fraction of the total phenotypic variance in energy and macronutrient intakes (left) and in percentage of energy derived from carbohydrate and fat (right) attributable to nontransmissible, cultural, and genetic factors. (Adapted from Reference 16.)

expressed in percent of total energy intake, intakes of carbohydrate and fat were characterized by a genetic effect of 20%, while cultural transmission and nontransmissible environmental effects explained 10 and 70% of the phenotypic variance, respectively. For percent of energy derived from protein, the genetic effect reached 11% (result not shown).[16] If it is hypothesized that the proportion of macronutrient in the diet reflects preferential choice for certain types of food, these results suggest that food preferences may be partly under genetic control. The existence of possible paternal or maternal effects was also tested in this study, and no evidence was found for any specific paternal or maternal influences in the transmission of the various energy intake components. In summary, the results of this study suggest that energy intake and food preferences are largely influenced by nontransmissible environmental factors and cultural transmission, but that food preferences may be influenced by genetic factors.

The absence of a genetic effect or the very low heritability found for energy intake is not surprising if one considers the large day-to-day variation in energy intake observed for a given individual. Total energy intake and nutrient intakes measured for 7 consecutive days in 329 Hawaiian men of Japanese ancestry[17] are summarized in Table 3. As shown in this table, the within-individual variation in energy intake reached 502 kcal for an average energy intake of 2299 kcal. Considerable within-individual variation was also

Table 3. **Mean and within-individual variability of energy intake and nutrient intakes**

	Mean of 7 days	Within-person SD
Energy intake (kcal)	2299	502
Protein (g)	94	27
Carbohydrates (g)	263	63
Fat (g)	85	29
Alcohol (g)	15	19

Note: Data from 329 Hawaiian men of Japanese ancestry measured for 7 consecutive days.

Adapted from Reference 17.

observed for the protein, carbohydrate, and fat intakes as well as for alcohol intake. These results suggest that energy intake of a given individual may vary considerably during 1 week.

In order to better characterize this within-individual variation in energy intake, Tarasuk and Beaton[18] recently measured energy intake of 13 men (22 to 49 years) and 16 women (20 to 53 years) for 365 consecutive days. Results indicated considerable day-to-day variation in energy intake for a given subject over 1 year. An example of this day-to-day variation for a given subject is illustrated in Figure 2. For this subject, the cubic regression curve accounted for 16% of the variance in energy intake over the year and the average standard deviation of the predicted energy intake values from the fitted regression curve reached 640 kJ. The standard deviations of the predicted intake values were found to range from 322 to 1176 kJ, which illustrates the magnitude of the variation in energy intake over the 1-year period. Despite the apparently random day-to-day variation in energy intake, systematic long-term and weekly patterns of energy intake were detected for all but one subject. On the average, these patterns explained 12.5% (0 to 37%) of an individual's total variance in energy intake across the whole year, but the shape and amplitude of these patterns were found to be specific to each individual. It would be very interesting to determine whether these patterns are also observed for macronutrient intake and test whether they are influenced by genetic factors.

IV. TASTE PREFERENCES

Taste preferences represent a major determinant of food intake and food selection in humans[19] and have already been linked with obesity and weight gain.[20,21] Genetic differences in taste preferences could be partly responsible for the heritability level of about 20% reported above for carbohydrate or lipid food item preference. It has been known for a long time that there are interindividual differences in responses to a variety of taste stimuli (bitterness, sourness, or sweetness). The sensitivity to phenylthiocarbamide (PTC),

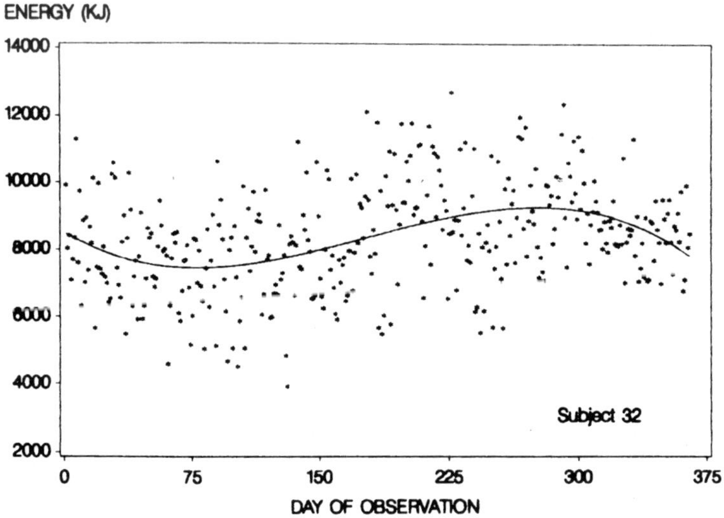

Figure 2. Trend in mean energy intake of one subject over 1 year. The cubic regression curve accounts for 16% of the subject's variance in energy intake over the year. (Adapted from Tarasuk, V. and Beaton, G. H., *Am. J. Clin. Nutr.*, 54, 464, 1991. With permission.)

a bitter substance detected by some individuals (tasters) but not by others (nontasters), has been shown to be inherited as an autosomal recessive trait. Population studies have shown different proportions of tasters and nontasters among populations, with a frequency of nontasters of about 10% among Orientals compared to about 30% among Caucasians.[22] Although taste preference was initially thought to be restricted to bitter substances, there is now evidence that differences in taste perception spread to a variety of other compounds. For instance, it has been shown that tasters are more sensitive to the sweet taste of sucrose and saccharin than nontasters, which suggests that PTC sensitivity could well be a marker of taste preference for several types of food.[22] This hypothesis is in agreement with the results of a recent segregation analysis undertaken in 1152 individuals from 120 families showing that PTC taste status in these families was best explained by a two-locus model, one locus controlling PTC taste and the other a more general taste capacity.[23] Although more studies are needed before a clear link between taste preferences and food preferences can be established, the results available do not exclude the possibility that the genetic effect observed for food preferences results from inherited differences in taste preferences.

V. EATING BEHAVIOR

Despite the recognition that eating behavior may play a role in the development of obesity in humans, very little is known about the role of genes in this behavior. Eating behavior is a broad concept that includes the process of ingestion as well as the attitudes, sensations, experiences, motivations, and physiological processes that accompany ingestion itself.[24] Although various eating patterns are found among obese subjects, a tendency to eat faster (greater amount of food ingested per unit of time) is generally observed among obese adults[24] and children[25] compared to leaner controls. In a study comparing obese and nonobese children, Barkeling et al.[25] also found that obese children did not slow down their eating rate toward the end of the meal as much as normal-weight children and scored lower than the latter for premeal subjective feelings about desire to eat, hunger, and prospective consumption (amount of food they thought they would eat). These observations suggest that the control of appetite may be defective in obese subjects.

No attempts have been made so far to assess the role of heredity in these behaviors. It would be interesting, for example, to know to what extent eating rate is inherited. The distributions of three measures of eating behavior (hunger, disinhibition, and dietary restraint) have been analyzed recently with the aim of finding commingling or mixtures of two or more distributions.[26] Results revealed strong evidence for bimodality since mixtures of two distributions were found to fit the data significantly better than a single distribution. Other studies using path analysis and segregation analysis will be necessary to determine some of the genetic characteristics of eating-behavior phenotypes.

It is generally believed that both genetic and environmental factors influence the mechanisms controlling appetite and satiety.[27] As shown in Table 4, several peptides are known to alter feeding behavior, either by stimulating or inhibiting food intake.[28] It has been suggested that cholecystokinin and neuropeptide Y are two peptides that best fit a series of criteria to qualify as regulators of eating behavior.[29] These peptides, and undoubtedly others, therefore represent potential candidate genes for the study of the impact of genetic variation in food intake and eating behavior. The expression of the neuropeptide Y gene has been shown to be increased in genetically obese animals, an observation which suggests that genes may indeed contribute to the development of disturbed eating behavior and obesity.[30] Moreover, it is also becoming evident that some of the peptides known to stimulate or inhibit food intake are acting specifically on some nutrients such as fat or carbohydrate.[28]

Table 4. **Peptides that influence food intake**

Increase	Decrease
β-Endorphin	Anorectin
Galanin	Caerulein
Growth-hormone-releasing hormone	Cholecystokinin
Growth hormone	Corticotropin-releasing hormone
Insulin	Cyclo His-Pro
Neuropeptide Y	Enterostatin
Peptide YY	Insulin-like growth factor I
Somatostatin (low dose)	Glucagon
	Insulin (CNS)
	Neurotensin
	Neuropeptide K
	Tyrotropin-releasing hormone
	Vasoactive intestinal peptide

Adapted from References 28 and 29.

VI. GENE-NUTRIENT INTERACTION

The literature reviewed thus far indicates a rather moderate role of heredity in energy intake and food preferences. However, it is important to keep in mind that a low heritability level does not mean that genes have nothing to do with nutritional habits. Moreover, one should recall that the interaction between genetics and nutrition may be important in the development of several chronic diseases like coronary heart disease (CHD), hypertension, diabetes, cancer, and obesity, as emphasized by the proceedings of a recent symposium on genetic variation and nutrition.[31] This section will illustrate with a few examples the importance of gene-nutrient interaction in risk factor variation.

The strong epidemiological, clinical, pathological, and experimental evidence linking high blood cholesterol levels to the development of atherosclerosis and CHD has led several countries around the world to the development of consensus documents[32-34] dealing with the necessity to lower the population cholesterol levels by reducing total fat intake, intake of saturated fatty acids, and intake of cholesterol. These dietary recommendations assume *a priori* that all individuals will respond similarly to modifications in their diet. However, it has long been recognized that there are considerable interindividual differences in the response of serum cholesterol to dietary cholesterol.[35] In some individuals (hyporesponders) serum cholesterol level is relatively insensitive to dietary cholesterol, while in others (hyperresponders) the effect appears to be much more important.[36] Although baseline dietary cholesterol was found to be the best predictor of serum cholesterol changes,[35] three lines of evidence suggest that the response could be genetically mediated. First, the same variability in response to dietary cholesterol has also been observed in a variety of animal species, and hypo- and hyperresponsive animal strains have been obtained through selective breeding. Second, baseline serum cholesterol levels have also been found to be correlated with the response in these animal studies. Third, it is known that about 50% of the population variance of serum cholesterol is genetically determined. A fourth line of evidence is now emerging from recent studies on gene effects, as illustrated below.

Measured genetic variation at the apolipoprotein gene loci has been used to study the role of genetic factors in the response to changes in diet. Results of dietary intervention studies conducted on individuals from North Karelia, Finland, revealed that when subjects were switched from their habitual high-fat, low polyunsaturated-to-saturated fatty acid ratio (P/S) diet to a low-fat, high P/S diet for 6 weeks and then switched back to their basal diet, considerable interindividual differences could be observed in the dietary response of serum lipids, lipoproteins, and apolipoproteins. When the results were analyzed taking into account genetic polymorphism of apolipoproteins,[37-40] significant gene-nutrient interactions were found. In the case of apolipoprotein E (apo E) polymorphism, results indicated that subjects homozygous for the E_4 allele exhibited greater reductions in total cholesterol compared to subjects with other genotypes when switched to the low-fat, high P/S diet and greater increases when brought back to the basal diet.[37] Differences in intestinal absorption of cholesterol were also observed between individuals with different apo E genotypes.[41] In addition to the apo E polymorphism, sequence variation detected with the XbaI restriction enzyme on the apo B gene was found to be associated with the response to dietary intervention, subjects carrying the allele associated with the presence of the XbaI cutting site showing greater reductions in total cholesterol, low-density liprotein (LDL) cholesterol, high-density lipoprotein (HDL) cholesterol, and apo B levels.[38] The effects of genetic variation at the apo AII, apo AI-CIII-AIV gene cluster, apo B, apo E, and LDL receptor genes on the response were investigated further on the same cohort.[39] An effect on the response to dietary changes was observed for an MspI RFLP (Restricted Fragment Length Polymorphism) at the apo B gene locus, and it was found to account for 6.3% of the variation in changes of apo AI levels. Results of these studies as well as others were summarized recently.[42] Despite some inconsistencies across studies, it appears that genetic variations at the apo B and apo E gene loci are involved in mediating plasma lipid response to dietary manipulations.

VII. SUMMARY

The results reviewed here reveal the presence of familial resemblance in energy intake and food preferences. Although twin studies suggest that genetic factors contribute to this familial aggregation, nontransmissible environmental factors and cultural transmission account for about 80% of the variation in energy intake and food preferences. Despite low heritability levels, there is increasing evidence that genes are important determinants of individual metabolic response to food intake. This genetic variability among individuals can no longer be ignored and has the potential to put some individuals more at risk than others for developing obesity and other common diseases for which nutrition is a risk factor. Identification of the genes involved in this gene-nutrient interaction as well as a better understanding of the role of genetic factors in taste preferences, eating behavior, and mechanisms of appetite and satiety is likely to increase our knowledge about the genetic basis of obesity.

REFERENCES

1. **Laskarzewski, P., Morrison, J. A., and Khoury, P.,** Parent-child nutrient intake interrelationships in school children ages 6 to 19: the Princeton School District Study, *Am. J. Clin. Nutr.,* 33, 2350, 1980.
2. **Birch, L. L.,** The relationships between children's food preferences and those of their parents, *J. Nutr. Educ.,* 12, 14, 1980.
3. **Lee, J. and Kolonel, L. N.,** Nutrient intakes of husbands and wives: implications for epidemiologic research, *Am. J. Epidemiol.,* 115, 515, 1982.
4. **Kolonel, L. N. and Lee, J.,** Husband-wife correspondence in smoking, drinking, and dietary habits, *Am. J. Clin. Nutr.,* 34, 99, 1981.
5. **Eastwood, M. A., Brydon, W. G., Smith, D. M., and Smith, J. H.,** A study of diet, serum lipids and fecal constituents in spouses, *Am. J. Clin. Nutr.,* 36, 290, 1982.

6. **Oliveria, S. A., Ellison, R. C., Moore, L. L., Gillman, M. W., Garrahie, E. J., and Singer, M.,** Parent-child relationships in nutrient intake: the Framingham Children's Study, *Am. J. Clin. Nutr.,* 56, 593, 1992.
7. **Rozin, P., Fallon, A. E., and Mandell, R.,** Family resemblance in attitudes to foods, *Dev. Psychobiol.,* 20, 309, 1986.
8. **Cavali-Sforza, L. L.,** Cultural transmission and nutrition, in *Genetic Variation and Nutrition,* Simopulos, A. P. and Childs, B., Eds., S. Karger, Basel, 1990, 35.
9. **Greene, L. S., Desor, J. A., and Maller, O.,** Heredity and experience: their relative importance in the development of taste preference in man, *J. Comp. Physiol. Psychol.,* 89, 279, 1975.
10. **Faust, J.,** A twin study of personal preferences, *J. Biosoc. Sci.,* 6, 75, 1976.
11. **Fabsitz, R. R., Garrison, R. J., Feinleib, M., and Hjortland, M.,** A twin analysis of dietary intake: evidence for a need to control for possible environmental influences in MZ and DZ twins, *Behav. Genet.,* 8, 15, 1978.
12. **Wade, J., Milner, J., and Krondl, M.,** Evidence for a physiological regulation of food selection and nutrient intake in twins, *Am. J. Clin. Nutr.,* 34, 143, 1981.
13. **Krondl, M., Coleman, P., Wade, J., and Milner, J.,** A twin study examining the genetic influence on food selection, *Hum. Nutr.,* 37A, 189, 1983.
14. **Rozin, P. and Millman, L.,** Family environment, not heredity accounts for family resemblances in food preferences and attitudes: a twin study, *Appetite,* 8, 125, 1987.
15. **Heller, R. F., O'Connel, D. L., Roberts, D. C. K., Allen, J. R., Knapp, J. C., Steele, P. L., and Silove, D.,** Lifestyle factors in monozygotic and dizygotic twins, *Genet. Epidemiol.,* 5, 311, 1988.
16. **Pérusse, L., Tremblay, A., Leblanc, C., Cloninger, C. R., Reich, T., Rice, J., and Bouchard, C.,** Familial resemblance in energy intake: contribution of genetic and environmental factors, *Am. J. Clin. Nutr.,* 47, 629, 1988.
17. **McGee, D., Rhoads, G., Hankin, J., Yano, K., and Tillotson, J.,** Within-person variability of nutrient intake in a group of Hawaiian men of Japanese ancestry, *Am. J. Clin. Nutr.,* 36, 657, 1982.
18. **Tarasuk, V. and Beaton, G. H.,** The nature and individuality of within-subject variation in energy intake, *Am. J. Clin. Nutr.,* 54, 464, 1991.
19. **Schiffman, S. S. and Warwick, Z. S.,** The biology of taste and food intake, in *The Science of Food Regulation. Food Intake, Taste, Nutrient Partitioning and Energy Expenditure,* Bray, G. A. and Ryan, D. H., Eds., Louisiana State University Press, Baton Rouge, 1992, chap. 2.
20. **Drewnowski, A., Kurth, C. L., and Rahaim, J. E.,** Taste preferences in human obesity: environmental and familial factors, *Am. J. Clin. Nutr.,* 54, 635, 1991.
21. **Drewnowski, A. and Holden-Wiltse, J.,** Taste responses and food preferences in obese women: effects of weight cycling, *Int. J. Obes.,* 16, 639, 1992.
22. **Drewnowski, A.,** Genetics of taste and smell, in *Genetic Variation and Nutrition,* Simopoulos, A. P. and Childs, B., Eds., S. Karger, Basel, 1989, 194.
23. **Olson, J. M., Boehnke, M., Neiswanger, K., Roche, A. F., and Siervogel, R. M.,** Alternative genetic models for the inheritance of the phenylthiocarbamide (PTC) taste deficiency, *Genet. Epidemiol.,* 6, 423, 1989.
24. **Hammer, L. D.,** The development of eating behavior in childhood, *Pediatr. Clin. North Am.,* 39, 379, 1992.
25. **Barkeling, B., Ekman, S., and Rossner, S.,** Eating behavior in obese and normal weight 11-year-old children, *Int. J. Obes.,* 16, 355, 1992.
26. **Allison, D. B., Heshka, S., Gorman, B. S., and Heymsfield, S. B.,** Evidence of commingling in human eating behavior, *Obesity Res.,* 1, 339, 1993.
27. **Blundell, J. E.,** Appetite disturbance and the problems of overweight, *Drugs,* 39(Suppl. 3), 1, 1990.

28. **Bray, G. A.,** The effect of peptides on nutrient intake and the sympathetic nervous system, in *The Science of Food Regulation. Food Intake, Taste, Nutrient Partitioning and Energy Expenditure,* Bray, G. A and Ryan, D. H., Eds., Louisiana State University Press, Baton Rouge, 1992, 257.
29. **Levine, A. S. and Billington, C. J.,** Selected criteria for peptides as regulators of feeding: an overview, in *The Science of Food Regulation. Food Intake, Taste, Nutrient Partitioning and Energy Expenditure,* Bray, G. A. and Ryan, D. H., Eds., Louisiana State University Press, Baton Rouge, 1992, 210.
30. **Leibowitz, S. F.,** Neuropeptide Y and galanin in the central control of food intake and body weight, in *The Science of Food Regulation. Food Intake, Taste, Nutrient Partitioning and Energy Expenditure,* Bray, G. A. and Ryan, D. H., Eds., Louisiana State University Press, Baton Rouge, 1992, 235.
31. **Simopoulos, A. P. and Childs, B., Eds.,** *Genetic Variation and Nutrition,* S. Karger, Basel, 1989.
32. **Anon.,** Consensus Français sur le cholestérol et les dyslipoprotéinémies, *Rev. Prat.,* 39, 971, 1989.
33. **Anon.,** The Canadian Consensus Conference on Cholesterol: final report, *Can. Med. Assoc. J.,* 139(Suppl.), 1, 1988.
34. **Anon.,** The Cholesterol Facts: a summary of the evidence relating dietary fats, serum cholesterol, and coronary heart disease. A joint statement by the American Heart Association and the National Heart, Lung, and Blood Institute, *Circulation,* 81, 1721, 1990.
35. **Hopkins, P. N.,** Effects of dietary cholesterol on serum cholesterol: a meta-analysis and review, *Am. J. Clin. Nutr.,* 55, 1060, 1992.
36. **Beynen, A. C., Katan, M. B., and Van Zutphen, L. F. M.,** Hypo- and hyperresponders: individual differences in the response of serum cholesterol concentration to changes in the diet, *Adv. Lipid Res.,* 22, 115, 1987.
37. **Tikkanen, M. J., Huttunen, J. K., Ehnholm, C., and Pietinen, P.,** Apolipoprotein E4 homozygosity predisposes to serum cholesterol elevation during high fat diet, *Arteriosclerosis,* 10, 285, 1990.
38. **Tikkanen, M. J., Xu, C. F., Hamalainen, T., Talmud, P., Sarna, S., Huttunen, J. K., Pietinen, P., and Humphries, S.,** XbaI polymorphism of the apolipoprotein B gene influences plasma lipid response to diet intervention, *Clin. Genet.,* 37, 327, 1990.
39. **Xu, C. F., Boerwinkle, E., Tikkanen, M. J., Huttunen, J. K., Humphries, S. E., and Talmud, P. J.,** Genetic variation at the apolipoprotein gene loci contribute to response of plasma lipids to dietary changes, *Genet. Epidemiol.,* 7, 261, 1990.
40. **Talmud, P. J., Boerwinkle, E., Xu, C. F., Tikkanen, M. J., Pietinen, P., Huttunen, J. K., and Humphries, S.,** Dietary intake and gene variation influence the response of plasma lipids to dietary intervention, *Genet. Epidemiol.,* 9, 249, 1992.
41. **Kesaniemi, M. A., Ehnholm, C., and Miettinen, T. A.,** Intestinal cholesterol absorption efficiency in man is related to apoprotein E phenotype, *J. Clin. Invest.,* 80, 578, 1987.
42. **Abbey, M.,** The influence of apolipoprotein polymorphism on the response to dietary fat and cholesterol, *Curr. Opinion Lipidol.,* 3, 12, 1992.

Chapter 10

Genetics of Energy Expenditure in Humans

Claude Bouchard, Olivier Dériaz, Louis Pérusse, and Angelo Tremblay

TABLE OF CONTENTS

I. INTRODUCTION

Reduced energy expenditure for a given energy intake level causes positive energy balance and eventually may lead to excess body weight and obesity. Interindividual differences in energy expenditure are among the factors involved in the etiology of obesity. The causes of interindividual differences in energy expenditure are important to consider in the study of the genetic basis of obesity since several studies have reported that most obese subjects do not seem to have higher energy intake than their lean counterparts. Energy expenditure is a complex phenotype that includes various components: basal and resting metabolic rates, thermic effect of food, and energy expenditure of activities, including the energy cost for given activities. Although it is recognized that genetic factors may contribute to the interindividual differences observed in the components of energy expenditure, only a few studies have been reported thus far on this issue.

Two kinds of genetic effects will be considered in this chapter. The first one is the additive genetic effect, or the so-called heritability, and the second one is the genotype-environment interaction effect. The heritability of a given phenotype is the fraction of the phenotypic variance attributable to genetic factors. It is most often assessed from twin or family data obtained on various kinds of relatives by descent or adoption. The genotype-environment interaction effect results from the differential response of genotypes to changes in the environment. For energy expenditure phenotypes, this effect can be estimated using an experimental approach[1] in which the within and between monozygotic (MZ) twin pair responses to standardized positive or negative energy balance conditions are compared.

II. RESTING METABOLIC RATE

A. INDIVIDUAL DIFFERENCES

The common view is that resting metabolic rate (RMR) accounts for about 70% of the daily energy expenditure[2] and is influenced by age and gender.[3] Another prevailing view

0-8493-4880-3/94/$0.00+$.50

is that fat-free mass (FFM) is the single best determinant of RMR variability,[2,4] explaining from about 50 to 80% of the total RMR variance in large samples of heterogeneous individuals. The intraindividual variation in RMR measurements has been estimated to be about 4 to 6%, a value that includes both the normal day-to-day fluctuation in metabolic rate and the technical error associated with the assessment of RMR.[2,5,6]

B. COMMON MISTAKES

RMR is a complex phenotype associated with the metabolic rates of all tissues and organs of the body measured in the basal state after an overnight fast. A contemporary prevailing view fueled by several research papers of the last decade is that body mass and body composition, for any given age and gender class, account for an overwhelming fraction of the RMR variance. In this case, values of 80% and more are commonly quoted. The authors of this review believe that these results apply only when data from a large and very heterogeneous population in terms of body mass are considered — that is, a population with a wide range of body mass, extending typically from 40 to 50 kg to about 90 to 100 kg. When narrow ranges of body mass are considered (e.g., 50 to 60 kg), the relationship becomes much looser. Indeed, the common variance between RMR and body mass and body composition may fall to as low as 20%.

Dériaz et al.[7] discussed this issue in a recent paper. They showed that the relationship between FFM or fat mass (FM) and RMR is a function of the heterogeneity of the population as assessed by the standard deviation of the body composition variable. Their findings are summarized in Figure 1, which has been constructed from the data published in 15 different samples. These observations suggest that body mass and body composition

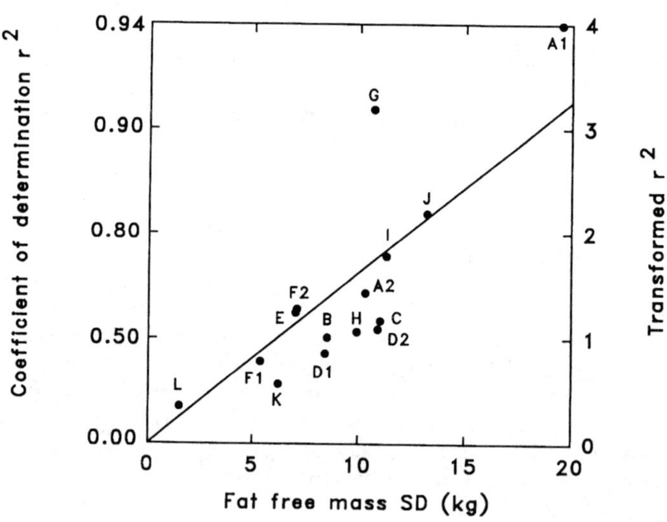

Figure 1. Relationship between the SD of fat-free mass (FFM) and transformed coefficient of determination (r^2) accounted for in resting metabolic rate by FFM from studies reported in the literature. A1 = Christin et al.,[35] white subjects. A2 = Christin et al.,[35] Pima Indian subjects. B = Owen et al.[36] C = Owen et al.[37] D1 = Bernstein et al.,[38] female subjects. D2 = Bernstein et al.,[38] male subjects. E = Jensen et al.[39] F1 = Minghelli et al.,[40] Gambian subjects. F2 = Minghelli et al.,[40] European subjects. G = Astrup et al.[41] H = Heshka et al.[42] I = Ravussin et al.[10] J = Bogardus et al.[9] K = Dériaz et al.,[7] before overfeeding. L = Dériaz et al.,[7] changes induced by overfeeding. The regression through the origin equation is y = 0.163x, r = 0.83, $p < 0.01$. Reproduced from Deriaz et al., *Am. J. Clin. Nutr.*, 56, 840, 1992. With permission.

are not strong determinants of RMR in a given individual. The close relationship reported by many investigators is artificial and is caused by the large heterogeneity of the subjects retained for analysis in these particular studies. From a biological point of view, these high relationships are almost meaningless and have clouded the critical issue of what the true determinants of RMR are.

Another prevailing view is that the skeletal muscle mass is the main determinant of RMR. Most authors who have dealt with the subject matter recognize that FFM is a reasonable indicator of skeletal muscle mass. The same line of reasoning implies that FFM is a valid surrogate marker for the components of RMR that are not caused by variation in skeletal muscle metabolic rate at rest. This is clearly a fallacy. Organ metabolic rates are generally much higher than the skeletal muscle metabolic rate, and they are thought to account for more than 60% of the energy expended at rest. The estimated contributions of kidneys, heart, brain, liver, and skeletal muscle are summarized in Table 1. For instance, the kidneys represent only 0.4% of the body mass, but they may account for about 10% or more of the RMR. In contrast, skeletal muscle represents 43% of body mass, but about 30% of the energy expended at rest results from the skeletal muscle metabolic rate. These observations again suggest that the study of FFM is useful, but not sufficient to explain variation in resting energy expenditure and its regulation.

When RMR is adjusted for FFM, FM, age, and sex, the residual variance remains of considerable importance. For instance, the standard deviation of RMR per kilogram of FFM over 24 h attains about 6 kcal in adults.[3,8] In one study, after adjustment for FFM, FM, age, and gender, the standard deviation of the predicted RMR reached about ±140 kcal per day,[9] which represents about ±10% of the RMR. From a review and meta-analysis of 15 different samples from various studies, the standard deviation of the predicted RMR adjusted for FFM was about 6 W or about 124 kcal/day.[7] Thus, the 95% confidence intervals were about ±250 kcal/day. Thus, the RMR variance unexplained by age, gender, body mass, and body composition remains a phenomenon that undoubtedly has some implications for energy balance. These observations have been instrumental in the development of the hypothesis that familial and genetic factors are perhaps associated with all or a fraction of the unexplained RMR variance.

C. HERITABILITY LEVELS

To test whether this unexplained RMR variance aggregates in families, Bogardus et al.[9] measured RMR and body composition in 130 nondiabetic American Indians (74 men and 56 women), 18 to 39 years of age, from 54 sibships. They found that 83% of the RMR variance was accounted for by FFM, age, and gender. Family membership accounted for

Table 1. **Relative contributions of organ weights to body weight and organ metabolic rates to resting metabolic rate**

	% Total mass	% Resting energy expenditure (range)
Brain	2.0	20–24
Heart	0.4	10–13
Kidneys	0.4	7–20
Liver	2.3	22–27
Skeletal muscle	43.0	22–36

Note: Computed from the data of Holliday,[32] Mottram,[33] and Newsholme and Leech.[34] Values calculated for an adult man (body weight, 70 kg; resting metabolic rate, 7.1 MJ/day).

an additional 11% of the variance in RMR. These results suggest that familial factors independent of FFM, age, and gender contribute to individual differences in RMR. Ravussin et al.[10] also measured total daily (24-h) energy expenditure in 94 siblings (52 males, 42 females) from 36 American Indian families. After adjustment of data for age, gender, and body composition they found significant familial aggregation of 24-h energy expenditure, with an intraclass familial correlation of 0.26. These results suggest that genetic and/or shared familial environmental factors contribute to these interindividual differences in RMR and metabolic rate.

Few attempts have been made to quantify the role of genetic factors in RMR. We have published two studies regarding the heritability of RMR using parent-child and MZ and dizygotic (DZ) twin data.[3,11] Selected results of these two studies are summarized in Table 2. Correlations in MZ twins are always higher than those observed in DZ twins, whether RMR is expressed per kilogram of body weight or FFM. Heritability estimates derived from these results by taking twice the difference between MZ and DZ correlations or twice the parent-offspring correlations suggest that at least 40% of the variance in RMR, after adjustment for age, gender, body mass, and body composition, could be inherited. The heritability of the RMR adjusted for FFM, FM, age, and gender has been further assessed recently in 75 nuclear families of the Quebec Family Study using a path analysis procedure. Results show that about 30% of the variance in RMR adjusted for these concomitants was attributable to genetic inheritance.[12]

A coefficient of heritability of 42% was recently reported for casual metabolic rate measured at rest in 40 pairs of MZ and 40 pairs of DZ male twins (16 to 24 years), but this significant genetic effect was found to be entirely accounted for by body weight.[13] However, when metabolic rate was measured under psychological stress, the authors found evidence for a significant genetic effect, independent of the genetic effect on body weight, accounting for 22% of the variance in the augmented energy expenditure measured during the stress. Metabolic rate was measured during a very short period of time (4 min) and in the late afternoon or evening. Even though the data cannot be considered as valid estimates of RMR, the findings of Hewitt et al.[13] do support the notion of a genotype-dependent response of metabolic rate to environmental stimulus.

III. SUBSTRATE OXIDATION

Although the mechanisms linking high fat consumption to increased body fat stores remain to be elucidated, interindividual differences in substrate oxidation, particularly lipid oxidation, are likely to be involved.[14] The relative proportion of carbohydrate and lipid oxidized can be determined indirectly by measuring the respiratory quotient (RQ) under standardized conditions. Few studies have addressed the role of genetic factors in

Table 2. **A summary of two studies dealing with resting metabolic rate (RMR) in twins and parent-child pairs**

	DZ twins		MZ twins		Parent-child		
	n pairs	r	*n* pairs	r	*n* pairs	r	Ref.
RMR / kg	19	0.21	20	0.45*			11
RMR / kg FFM	19	0.44**	20	0.64**			11
RMR / kg	21	0.38*	37	0.78***	31	0.13	3
RMR / kg FFM	21	0.30	37	0.77***	31	0.21	3
RMR adj. FFM	21	0.38*	37	0.74***	31	0.23	3

Note: * $p < 0.05$, ** $p < 0.01$, *** $p < 0.0001$. DZ = dizygotic; MZ = monozygotic; FFM = fat-free mass; adj. = adjusted.

substrate oxidation. Three lines of evidence suggest that there may be inherited differences in the propensity to oxidize relatively more carbohydrates or lipids. First, twins studies have shown a greater similarity among MZ twins compared to DZ twins in the RQ measured during submaximal exercise, suggesting a role for heredity in substrate oxidation.[3] Second, experimental studies in which MZ twins were submitted to overfeeding or exercise-training suggest a significant within-pair resemblance in the pattern of substrate oxidation following a mixed meal or during submaximal exercise. In a study in which 12 pairs of MZ twins were submitted to a 4.2-MJ (1000-kcal) caloric surplus 6 days a week for a period of 100 days under rigorously controlled conditions of energy intake and activity level,[15] significant within-pair resemblance was found for the changes in RQ at rest and for several hours following a mixed meal.[16] These results suggest that even when energy intake, macronutrient composition of the diet, and physical activity level are standardized for more than 3 months, some individuals oxidize more fat than carbohydrate, and genetic factors appear to play a role in this phenomenon.

In a series of standardized endurance and high-intensity cycle exercise programs performed over the last 10 years in this laboratory with MZ twins, it has been shown that improvements in a given submaximal power output or to maximal exercise were all characterized by a significant within-pair resemblance.[17] For instance, exercise training resulted in a decrease of RQ measured in a relative steady state at a low intensity level, but the changes observed in RQ were not randomly distributed among genotypes. Despite the fact that twins participating in the same exercise program were all subjected to the same training protocol, individuals with the same genotype (within pair) were found to be more similar than unrelated individuals (between pairs) in the changes of RQ, suggesting that the pattern of substrate oxidation changes at low power output levels could be genetically determined.

The third line of evidence comes from the Quebec Family Study. Based on data gathered at rest in a fasted state on about 300 adult subjects from 75 nuclear families, the genetic heritability of the RQ reached about 20%.[12]

IV. THERMIC EFFECT OF FOOD

The thermic effect of food (TEF) is the integrated increase of energy expenditure after food ingestion. TEF is generally divided into an obligatory component, associated with the energy cost of nutrient storage, and a facultative component that has proven to be very difficult to investigate. To our knowledge, only one study has dealt with the heritability of TEF.[3] In that study, energy expenditure was recorded during 4 h after a 1000-kcal carbohydrate meal in 21 pairs of DZ twins and 37 pairs of MZ twins as well as in 31 parent-offspring pairs. Correlations of 0.35, 0.52, and 0.30 in DZ, MZ, and parent-offspring pairs, respectively, were found for TEF. These results suggest a genetic effect of at least 30% and perhaps more for TEF. The biological significance of such a heritability level is highlighted by the fact that the standard deviation of TEF over 4 h in this study reached about 20 kcal, and the 95% confidence intervals were thus ±40 kcal or ±4% of the energy intake.

V. LEVEL OF PHYSICAL ACTIVITY

Studies on the genetic effect of energy expenditure associated with physical activity are also limited. Recently, the level of habitual physical activity was investigated with the Caltrac accelerometer in 100 children 4 to 7 years of age, 99 mothers, and 92 fathers from the Framingham Children's Study.[18] Over the course of 1 year, data were obtained with the mechanical device for about 10 h/day for an average of 9 days in children and 8 days in fathers and mothers. Active fathers (accelerometer counts per hour above the median) or active mothers were more likely to have active offspring than inactive fathers or mothers, with odds ratios of 3.5 and 2.0, respectively. When both parents were active, the children were 5.8 times as likely to be active as children of two inactive parents. These results are compatible with the notion that genetic and/or cultural factors transmitted across generations may predispose a child to be active or inactive. However, other explanations also can be invoked for the familial resemblance in habitual activity level seen in this study.

Studies on the genetic effect for the level of habitual physical activity or the amount of energy expended for daily physical activity as assessed from questionnaires or activity diaries are very limited. Results from a few twin studies have shown that activity level may be partly inherited.[19-23] In these studies, an active person was generally defined as a person always in a hurry or "on the go", one that could qualify as having a "nervous" temperament. Most studies showed that this type of "active temperament" appears to be influenced by heredity. Since spontaneous physical activity or "fidgetting" may account for a substantial fraction of the 24-h energy expenditure measured in a respiratory chamber,[24] these data suggest that inherited differences in activity level as a behavior could have a significant impact on daily energy expenditure.

The influence of heredity on physical activity level has been investigated in a large sample of twins from the Finnish Twin Registry.[25] In this study, leisure-time physical activity was assessed in 1537 MZ and 3057 DZ male twin pairs aged over 18 years. Information on intensity and duration of activity, years of participation in a physical activity, physical activity on the job, and subjective opinion of the subject's own activity level was obtained from questionnaires. These variables were submitted to factor analysis to generate a factor score of physical activity that was used to compute correlations in MZ and DZ twins. Based on these data, the authors reported a heritability level of 62% for age-adjusted physical activity.[25] More recently, Heller et al.[26] reported a significantly higher concordance within MZ twins (94 pairs) than within DZ twins (106 pairs) for exercise participation (participation in vigorous exercise in the past 2 weeks) and estimated the heritability of this phenotype at 39%.

Using data from the 1981 Canada Fitness Survey, the importance of familial resemblance in leisure-time energy expenditure has been studied.[27] A total of 18,073 individuals living in thousands of households across Canada completed a questionnaire on their physical activity habits. Detailed information on frequency, duration, and intensity of activities performed on a daily, weekly, monthly, and yearly basis was obtained and used to determine average daily energy expenditure (in kilojoules per day per kilogram of body weight). Familial correlations of 0.28, 0.12, and 0.21 were obtained in spouses ($n = 1024$ pairs), parent-offspring ($n = 1622$ pairs), and siblings ($n = 1036$), respectively, suggesting a weak contribution of genetic factors in the familial aggregation of leisure-time energy expenditure.[27]

Using data from the Quebec Family Study and the strategy of path analysis, the relative contributions of genetic and nongenetic factors to activity level have been studied.[28] Two different indicators of physical activity, habitual physical activity and exercise participation, were obtained from a 3-day activity record completed by 1610 members of 375 families encompassing 9 types of relatives by descent or adoption. Each day of the activity record was divided into 96 periods of 15 min, and for each 15-min period the individuals had to note, on a scale from 1 to 9, the dominant activity during each period, each score representing a multiple of the RMR. A score of 1 indicated that the individual was at rest, while a score of 9 indicated that the individual was doing an activity with an energy cost equivalent to about 8 times the resting metabolic rate. The scores 1 to 9 were summed over the 96 15-min periods of each day, and the average value for the 3 days was used as the indicator of habitual physical activity. The exercise participation indicator was computed as the average number of periods rated 6, 7, 8, or

9 in each day. These categories were chosen because they corresponded to activities with intensities generally found only in sports or other forms of voluntary exercise. The results obtained are summarized in Figure 2.

Most of the variation in these two indicators of habitual physical activity level was accounted for by nontransmissible environmental factors, with values reaching 71% for habitual physical activity and 88% for exercise participation. The transmission effect across generations was found to be significant, but entirely accounted for by genetic factors for habitual physical activity (with a value of 29%), and by cultural transmission (12%) for exercise participation with no genetic effect. Since habitual physical activity was computed as the sum of all scores (i.e., from 1 to 9) and exercise participation included only the activities rated from 6 to 9, activities rated 1 to 5 were those characterized by a significant genetic effect. These results were interpreted as an indication of inherited differences in the propensity to be spontaneously active.

VI. ENERGY COST OF EXERCISE

The energy cost associated with common body postures or positions (sitting or standing) and with low-intensity activities (walking, climbing stairs, bending, reaching, etc.) repeated several times in the course of a normal day may be an important determinant of the total daily energy expenditure, since there are interindividual differences in oxygen uptake per kilogram of body mass for a given power output. It was hypothesized that these differences could be partly explained by genetic factors. To test this hypothesis, the oxygen uptake required for various submaximal cycle ergometer workloads was measured in 22 pairs of sedentary male DZ twins and 31 pairs of sedentary male MZ twins aged 16 to 29 years.[3] The correlations obtained in DZ and MZ twins are shown in Table 3. The results suggest a significant genetic effect for oxygen uptake per kilogram of body weight at low power output (50, 75, and 100 W), but it became nonsignificant when the energy expenditure reached about 6 times the resting metabolic rate level. In other words, there may well be inherited differences in the energy cost of low-intensity activities even after adjustment for variation in body mass. The significance of this phenomenon for 24-h energy expenditure remains to be investigated and is likely to be of minor significance in comparison to the volume of low-energy-cost spontaneous activities.

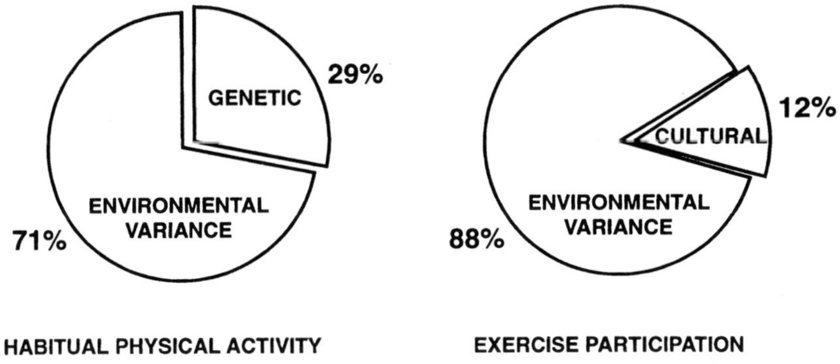

Figure 2. Components of phenotypic variance in habitual physical activity and exercise participation derived from a 3-day activity record. (Drawn from data of Pérusse, L., Tremblay, A., Leblanc, C., and Bouchard, C., *Am. J. Epidemiol.*, 129, 1012, 1989. With permission.)

VII. RESPONSE TO CHANGES IN ENERGY BALANCE

Negative or positive energy balance sustained for a long period influences energy expenditure. The hypothesis that the response of RMR and TEF to changes in energy balance could be genotype dependent was investigated in two different studies with MZ twins. In one study, six pairs of male MZ twins were overfed by 1000 kcal/day for 22 days.[29] Subjects gained body weight and body fat, but there was a nonsignificant 7% increase in RMR. However, interindividual differences in RMR were considerable, but not randomly distributed, as suggested by a significant F ratio for the between-pair over within-pair variances ($F = 4.45$; $p < 0.05$) for RMR expressed in milliliters of O_2 per minute. The intraclass correlation computed to quantify the within-pair resemblance in the response reached 0.63, but it decreased to a nonsignificant level when changes in RMR were adjusted for gains in body mass or FFM.[30] In a more recent report from a long-term overfeeding experiment with identical twins, RMR increased by about 10%.[7] The intrapair resemblance for the changes in RMR brought about by overfeeding in ten pairs of MZ twins was 0.51 ($p< 0.05$). Changes in RMR were not significant, however, when they were adjusted for body mass or FFM increases. During the overfeeding treatment the TEF increased significantly in response to a 1000-kcal mixed meal and the intraclass correlation for TEF changes reached 0.7 ($p < 0.01$).

The same phenomenon was investigated under conditions of negative energy balance generated by exercise. Six other pairs of MZ twins were exercised on a cycle ergometer for the equivalent energy expenditure of 4.2 MJ/day for 22 consecutive days while maintaining a constant energy intake.[31] Although this short-term exercise training program did not produce significant changes in RMR and TEF, there was heterogeneity in the response. Once again, a significant intrapair resemblance was observed for the changes in RMR ($p < 0.05$) and TEF ($p < 0.05$). This whole issue of the role of inherited differences in RMR or TEF when challenged by positive or negative energy balance conditions should be investigated further with protocols of longer duration to induce larger changes that are well beyond the error variance of the metabolic rate measurements. The use of the 24-h room calorimeter to assess resting and sleeping metabolic rates and of the doubly labeled water technique to quantify total energy expenditure would be highly desirable in these future investigations.

VIII. CONCLUSIONS

The studies reviewed here suggest that interindividual differences observed in the various energy expenditure components are partly determined by the genotype. Results of family and twin studies provide evidence for a genetic effect reaching about 30 to 40% of the phenotype variance for RMR adjusted for common determinants such as age, gender, body mass, and body composition. Future studies of the role of genetic variation in RMR should incorporate data on organ metabolic rates as well as on skeletal muscle and fat mass metabolic rates. It appears quite possible that the pattern of relative substrate oxidation is influenced by genetic variation that remains to be characterized. This is an important research avenue, one that certainly would not be in want of

Table 3. **Intraclass correlations for energy cost of submaximal steady state cycle ergometer exercise**

Power output (W)	DZ twins VO_2/kg	MZ twins VO_2/kg
50	0.22	0.67**
75	0.33*	0.72**
100	0.59**	0.82**
125	0.68**	0.79**
150	0.66**	0.75**

Note: * $p < 0.05$; ** $p < 0.001$. DZ = dizygotic; MZ = monozygotic.

Adapted from Bouchard et al.[3]

candidate genes. Genetic transmission is likely important in the familial resemblance observed in habitual physical activity, but the genetic effect appears to influence the propensity toward spontaneous activity rather than exercise participation. The genotype of the individual at undetermined loci also may be a significant determinant of the individual's response to positive or negative energy balance conditions.

REFERENCES

1. **Bouchard, C., Pérusse, L., and Leblanc, C.,** Using MZ twins in experimental research to test for the presence of a genotype-environment interaction effect, *Acta Genet. Med. Gemellol.,* 39, 85, 1990.
2. **Ravussin, E. and Bogardus, C.,** Relationship of genetics, age, and fitness to daily energy expenditure and fuel utilisation, *Am. J. Clin. Nutr.,* 49, 968, 1989.
3. **Bouchard, C., Tremblay, A., Nadeau, A., Després, J. P., Thériault, G., Boulay, M. R., Lortie, G., Leblanc, C., and Fournier, G.,** Genetic effect in resting and exercise metabolic rates, *Metabolism,* 38, 364, 1989.
4. **Miller, A. T., Jr. and Blyth, C. S.,** Lean body mass as a metabolic reference standard, *J. Appl. Physiol.,* 5, 311, 1953.
5. **Bouchard, C.,** Reproducibility of body composition and adipose tissue measurements in humans, in Body Composition Assessment in Youth and Adult. Report of the Sixth Ross Conference on Medical Research, Roche, A. F., Ed., Ross Laboratories, Columbus, OH, 1985, 9.
6. **Henry, C. J. K., Hayter, J., and Rees, D. G.,** The constancy of basal metabolic rate in free-living subjects, *Eur. J. Clin. Nutr.,* 43, 727, 1989.
7. **Dériaz, O., Fournier, G., Tremblay, A., Després, J. P., and Bouchard, C.,** Lean-body-mass composition and resting energy expenditure before and after long-term overfeeding, *Am. J. Clin. Nutr.,* 56, 840, 1992.
8. **Bouchard, C. and Tremblay, A.,** Genetic effects in human energy expenditure components, *Int. J. Obes.,* 14(Suppl. 1), 49, 1990.
9. **Bogardus, C., Lillioja, S., Ravussin, E., Abbott, W., Zawadzki, J. K., Young, A., Knowler, W. C., Jacobowitz, R., and Moll, P. P.,** Familial dependence of the resting metabolic rate, *N. Engl. J. Med.,* 315, 96, 1986.
10. **Ravussin, E., Lillioja, S., Knowler, W. C., Christin, L., Freymond, D., Abbott, G. H., Boyce, V., Howard, B. V., and Bogardus, C.,** Reduced rate of energy expenditure as a risk factor for body weight gain, *N. Engl. J. Med.,* 318, 467, 1988.
11. **Fontaine, E., Savard, R., Tremblay, A., Després, J. P., Poehlman, E. T., and Bouchard, C.,** Resting metabolic rate in monozygotic and dizygotic twins, *Acta Genet. Med. Gemellol.,* 34, 41, 1985.
12. **Dériaz, O., Pérusse, L., Tremblay, A., and Bouchard, C.,** Genetic and environmental effects in resting metabolic rate and respiratory quotient, submitted for publication.
13. **Hewitt, J. K., Stunkard, A. J., Carroll, D., Sims, J., and Turner, J. R.,** A twin study approach towards understanding genetic contributions to body size and metabolic rate, *Acta Genet. Med. Gemellol.,* 40, 133, 1991.
14. **Tremblay, A.,** Human obesity: a defect in lipid oxidation or in thermogenesis?, *Int. J. Obes.,* 16, 953, 1992.
15. **Bouchard, C., Tremblay, A., Després, J. P., Nadeau, A., Lupien, P. J., Thériault, G., Dussault, J., and Moorjani, S.,** The response to long-term overfeeding in identical twins, *N. Engl. J. Med.,* 322, 1477, 1990.
16. **Bouchard, C. and Tremblay, A.,** unpublished results.
17. **Bouchard, C., Dionne, F. T., Simoneau, J. A., and Boulay, M. R.,** Genetics of aerobic and anaerobic performances, *Exercise Sport Sci. Rev.,* 20, 27, 1992.

18. **Moore, L. L., Lombardi, D. A., White, M. J., Campbell, J. L., Oliveria, S. A., and Ellison, S. A.,** Influence of parents' physical activity levels of young children, *J. Pediatr.,* 118, 215, 1991.
19. **Vandenberg, S. G.,** The hereditary abilities study: hereditary components in a psychological test battery, *Am. J. Hum. Genet.,* 14, 220, 1962.
20. **Price, R. A., Vandenberg, S. G., Lyer, H., and Williams, J. S.,** Components of variation in normal personality, *J. Pers. Soc. Psychol.,* 43, 328, 1982.
21. **Loehlin, J. C.,** Heredity, environment and the Thurstone temperament schedule, *Behav. Genet.,* 16, 61, 1986.
22. **Scarr, S.,** Genetic factors in activity motivation, *Child Dev.,* 37, 663, 1966.
23. **Willerman, L.,** Activity level and hyperactivity in twins, *Child Dev.,* 44, 288, 1973.
24. **Ravussin, E., Lillioja, S., Anderson, T. E., Christin, L., and Bogardus, C.,** Determinants of 24-hour energy expenditure in man. Methods and results using a respiratory chamber, *J. Clin. Invest.,* 78, 1568, 1986.
25. **Kaprio, J., Koskenvuo, M., and Sarna, S.,** Cigarette smoking, use of alcohol, and leisure-time physical activity among same-sexed adult male twins, *Prog. Clin. Biol. Res.,* 69, 37, 1981.
26. **Heller, R. F., O'Connel, D. L., Roberts, D. C. K., Allen, J. R., Knapp, J. C., Steele, P. L., and Silove, D.,** Lifestyle factors in monozygotic and dizygotic twins, *Genet. Epidemiol.,* 5, 311, 1988.
27. **Pérusse, L., Leblanc, C., and Bouchard, C.,** Familial resemblance in lifestyle components: results from the Canada Fitness Survey, *Can. J. Public Health,* 79, 201, 1988.
28. **Pérusse, L., Tremblay, A., Leblanc, C., and Bouchard, C.,** Genetic and environmental influences on level of habitual physical activity and exercise participation, *Am. J. Epidemiol.,* 129, 1012, 1989.
29. **Poehlman, E. T., Tremblay, A., Fontaine, E., Després, J. P., Nadeau, A., Dussault, J., and Bouchard, C.,** Genotype dependency of the thermic effect of a meal and associated hormonal changes following short-term overfeeding, *Metabolism,* 35, 30, 1986.
30. **Bouchard, C., Tremblay, A., Després, J. P., Poehlman, E. T., Thériault, G., Nadeau, A., Lupien, P. J., Moorjani, S., and Dussault, J.,** Sensitivity to overfeeding: the Quebec experiment with identical twins, *Prog. Food Nutr. Sci.,* 12, 45, 1988.
31. **Poehlman, E. T., Tremblay, A., Nadeau, A., Dussault, J., Thériault, G., and Bouchard, C.,** Heredity and changes in hormones and metabolic rates with short-term training, *Am. J. Physiol. Endocrinol. Metab.,* 250, E711, 1986.
32. **Holliday, M. A.,** Body composition and energy needs during growth, *Hum. Growth,* Vol. 2, *Postnatal Growth,* 5, 117, 1978.
33. **Mottram, R. F.,** The oxygen consumption of human skeletal muscle in vivo, *J. Physiol.,* 128, 268, 1955.
34. **Newsholme, E. A. and Leech, A. R.,** *Biochemistry for Medical Sciences,* John Wiley & Sons, New York, 1983.
35. **Christin, L., Ravussin, E., Bogardus, C., and Howard, B.,** The effect of propranolol on free fatty acid mobilisation and resting metabolic rate, *Metabolism,* 38, 439, 1989.
36. **Owen, O. E., Kavle, E., Owen, R. S., Polansky, M., Caprio, S., Mozzoli, M. A., Kendrick, Z. V., Bushman, M. C., and Boden, G.,** A reappraisal of caloric requirements in healthy women, *Am. J. Clin. Nutr.,* 44, 1, 1986.
37. **Owen, O. E., Holup, J. L., D'Alessio, D. A., Craig, E. S., Polansky, M., Smalley, K. J., Kavle, E. C., Bushman, M. C., Owen, L. R., Mozzoli, M. A., Kendrick, Z. V., and Boden, G. H.,** A reappraisal of the caloric requirements of men, *Am. J. Clin. Nutr.,* 46, 875, 1987.

38. **Bernstein, R., Thornton, J. C., Yang, M. U., Wang, J., Redmond, A. M., Pierson, R. N., Pi-Sunyer, F. X., and Van Itallie, T. B.,** Prediction of resting metabolic rate in obese patients, *Am. J. Clin. Nutr.,* 37, 595, 1983.
39. **Jensen, M. D., Braun, J. S., Vetter, R. J., and Marsh, H. M.,** Measurement of body potassium with a whole-body counter: relationship between lean body mass and resting energy expenditure, *Mayo Clin. Proc.,* 63, 864, 1988.
40. **Minghelli, G., Schutz, Y., Charbonnier, A., Whitehead, R., and Jéquier, E.,** Twenty-four-hour energy expenditure and basal metabolic rate measured in whole-body indirect calorimeter in Gambian men, *Am. J. Clin. Nutr.,* 51, 563, 1990.
41. **Astrup, A., Thorbeck, G., and Isaksson, B.,** Prediction of 24-h energy expenditure and its components from physical characteristics and body composition in normal humans, *Am. J. Clin. Nutr.,* 52, 777, 1990.
42. **Heshka, S., Yang, M. U., Wang, J., Burt, P., and Pi-Sunyer, F. X.,** Weight loss and change in resting metabolic rate, *Am. J. Clin. Nutr.,* 52, 981, 1990.

Chapter 11

Inherited Susceptibility to Metabolic Complications of Obesity

Roger R. Williams, Paul N. Hopkins, Steven C. Hunt, M. Catherine Schumacher, Barry M. Stults, Lily L. Wu, and Sandra J. Hasstedt

TABLE OF CONTENTS

I. INTRODUCTION

Obesity is strongly associated with multiple metabolic factors that aggregate in families. Many, but not all, obese persons express these metabolic abnormalities. Many, but not all, persons with these metabolic abnormalities are overweight. Among those who are genetically predisposed to metabolic abnormalities, the development of obesity probably increases the likelihood that these abnormalities will be expressed or increases their severity, as illustrated in Figure 1.

Some persons may carry genes that initially cause obesity and subsequently lead to metabolic abnormalities secondary to the long-term effects of obesity. Other persons may carry genes that primarily promote metabolic abnormalities that become more severe if obesity develops. Because many studies have been performed in individuals with both metabolic abnormalities and obesity, it has not been possible to determine whether the primary defect and initial expression first involves obesity or metabolic abnormalities. Cross-sectional data stratified into different ages for given syndromes can help to identify

0-8493-4880-3/94/$0.00+$.50

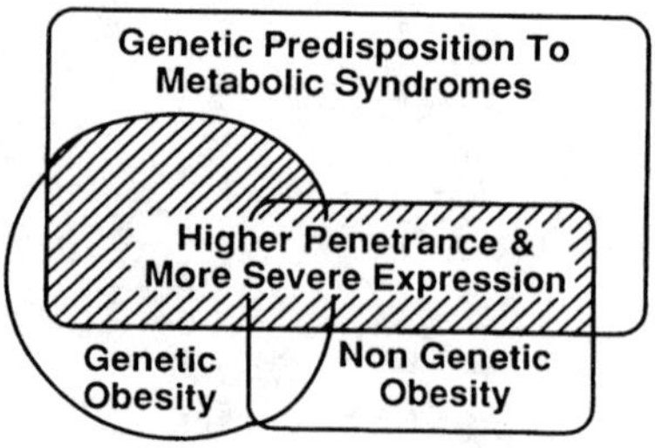

Figure 1. Higher penetrance or more severe expression of metabolic abnormalities (such as hyperinsulinemia, dyslipidemia, and hyperuricemia) are promoted by obesity in genetically susceptible persons.

the earliest expression of abnormalities. Prospective data provide the best answers to this question.

II. THEORIES OF PATHOPHYSIOLOGY

Lipid abnormalities, insulin resistance or hyperinsulinemia, hyperglycemia, hyperuricemia, and frank disorders such as gout, diabetes, and hypertension are all strongly associated with obesity and often with each other. Current theories to explain these coaggregations often invoke an understanding of insulin resistance and/or hyperinsulinemia.

A. INSULIN RESISTANCE IN THE GENERAL POPULATION

Insulin resistance is defined as decreased insulin-mediated rates of whole-body glucose uptake. It can be measured using a combination of the insulin/glucose clamp technique and tracer glucose infusion with indirect calorimetry.[1] The two components of whole-body glucose uptake include glucose oxidation and nonoxidative glucose disposal (glycogen synthesis). Even in healthy persons there is a considerable variation in insulin sensitivity by age and even greater variability between individuals within a given age group. In a study of 124 healthy, normal-weight subjects (ages 19 to 76), mean insulin-mediated glucose disposal decreased by about 40% from the young adults in their mid-20s to older adults in their mid-60s. Within the youngest group of adults, the most insulin-sensitive individual used glucose at a rate four times that of the most insulin-resistant person.

The most common and convenient method to roughly estimate insulin sensitivity is to determine plasma insulin levels in a fasting blood sample or after a standard glucose challenge. In general, insulin sensitivity is inversely related to fasting or stimulated insulin levels. Persons with decreased insulin sensitivity compensate by secreting more insulin to maintain normal glucose levels. In many healthy individuals, increased plasma insulin levels are thought to probably have little or no consequence. However, it is hypothesized that certain genetically predisposed individuals develop serious metabolic abnormalities when insulin resistance and hyperinsulinemia are present.

B. INSULIN RESISTANCE IN OBESITY AND NON-INSULIN-DEPENDENT DIABETES MELLITUS

Insulin clamp studies show that tissue sensitivity to insulin is reduced about 40% in individuals who are 40% over ideal body weight.[1] Both the oxidative and nonoxidative pathways of glucose disposal seem to be involved, and muscle is the primary tissue affected. In most of these obese individuals, impaired insulin action is compensated by higher insulin levels to maintain normal glucose tolerance. With further weight gain or decrease in insulin secretion, incomplete compensation leads initially to impaired glucose tolerance (IGT) and eventually to frank non-insulin-dependent diabetes mellitus (NIDDM).

In the early stages of NIDDM, approximately a two-fold increase in fasting or stimulated plasma insulin level is usually observed when compared to age- and weight-matched controls who do not have NIDDM. Later in the natural history of NIDDM, one can observe a decline in insulin secretion and plasma insulin levels below the average level expected in comparable individuals who do not have NIDDM.[1]

Not all persons with NIDDM are overweight. Those who have normal weight also have insulin resistance and hyperinsulinemia. The magnitude of insulin resistance and hyperinsulinemia observed in normal weight diabetics are approximately the same as those observed in obese nondiabetics. The highest insulin levels and greatest insulin resistance are observed in obese diabetics.

Medical scientists who study insulin resistance stress the fact that insulin resistance and hyperinsulinemia are present for many years in a compensated state with normal glucose tolerance. They hypothesize that many of the metabolic derangements associated with insulin resistance have their onset during this compensated state long before glucose intolerance or frank diabetes would be detected by fasting or stimulated glucose levels. They further hypothesize that since insulin resistance is a characteristic feature of both obesity and NIDDM it may help explain the metabolic consequences often observed in both disorders, including dyslipidemia, hypertension, and atherosclerosis.

C. WEIGHT LOSS AND EXERCISE

In the past it was recognized that weight reduction and physical activity would help reduce the insulin requirement of persons with NIDDM. This observation has now been extended to show that weight reduction and physical exercise also improve insulin sensitivity in persons with less severe hyperinsulinemia. When elevated plasma insulin concentration is reduced by these interventions, blood pressure and triglyceride level also can decline. In one of the most informative studies of obese persons undergoing chronic physical training without weight reduction, it was demonstrated that decreases in blood pressure and triglycerides were observed mainly in obese subjects who had elevated fasting plasma insulin concentrations.[2] Furthermore, the improvement in blood pressure and triglyceride levels correlated closely with the improvement in fasting plasma insulin levels.

D. INSULIN RESISTANCE AND HYPERTENSION

Reaven and Hoffman demonstrated higher fasting and stimulated insulin levels in nonobese hypertensive persons when compared to matched controls without hypertension.[3] Ferrannini and colleagues performed euglycemic insulin-clamp studies on normal-weight young essential hypertensive individuals. They found that insulin-mediated total-body glucose uptake was reduced by 40% in the essential hypertensive group and increasing blood pressure correlated directly with insulin resistance ($r = 0.76$, $p < 0.001$). The insulin resistance was entirely accounted for by a defect in the nonoxidative glucose uptake (glycogen synthesis).[4] Ferrannini et al. further demonstrated with a forearm catheterization technique that muscle is the primary site for the insulin resistance in these patients with essential hypertension.[1]

Reaven gave the label "Syndrome X" for the association of hyperinsulinemia with hypertension in nonobese individuals. Other studies have shown that obese hypertensive individuals also have higher insulin concentrations than nonhypertensive individuals matched for the same level of obesity.[1]

E. SODIUM BALANCE, INSULIN, AND HYPERTENSION

Several investigators have proposed a hypothesis that hyperinsulinemia and/or insulin resistance promote sodium retention, which in turn fosters hypertension. In one of the most informative studies of this hypothesis, Sharma and colleagues[5] identified a group of young normotensives whose blood pressure showed more than a 3 mm change from a high- to low-salt diet. After dividing normotensives into those who were and were not salt sensitive, they investigated the plasma glucose and insulin responses to an oral glucose load on both high- and low-salt diets. They showed significantly higher glucose and insulin levels in the salt-sensitive group on the high-salt diet, but not during the low-salt diet. This would suggest that persons who are genetically susceptible to salt-induced hypertension exhibit insulin resistance and hyperinsulinemia on a high-salt diet that could be ameliorated by salt restriction.

Practical observations regarding sodium balance add credence to the importance of insulin to sodium balance. Studies have consistently shown increased total-body sodium content in hypertensive individuals who are either obese or diabetic. Natriuresis is commonly observed with weight loss, which has an associated decline in plasma insulin levels as well as blood pressure. Conversely, hyperinsulinemia and sodium retention are seen after acute carbohydrate ingestion. A curious phenomena labeled "refeeding edema" has been associated with hyperinsulinemia and sodium retention. The relationship between plasma insulin levels and kidney sodium excretion has been confirmed using euglycemic insulin-clamp studies on healthy young adults. Within 30 to 60 min after a physiological increase in plasma insulin concentration, urinary sodium excretion decreased by as much as 50% of the basal rate.[1] Insulin appears to have an effect on both the proximal and distal parts of the nephron based on observations during micropuncture and microperfusion studies. The changes of insulin causing these effects are within the range of changes observed in obese individuals and considerably less than the insulin levels achieved after the stimulation of a meal.

F. HYPERTENSION AND OTHER METABOLIC FACTORS

Daly and Landsberg have found evidence for insulin-mediated sympathetic stimulation contributing to blood pressure elevation in both obesity and NIDDM.[6] Increased circulating glucose levels seem to suppress sympathetic activity, whereas exogenous insulin administration with sufficient glucose to prevent hypoglycemia stimulates the sympathetic nervous system in humans. Studies also show that hyperinsulinemia is more common among obese individuals with the upper-body fat distribution pattern or with increased intra-abdominal fat accumulation.[6]

Other mechanisms relating insulin to hypertension include stimulation of cation membrane exchange or influences on intracellular cation concentration.[1] It has also been suggested that insulin stimulates growth factors which cause hypertrophy of the vascular wall, narrowing of the resistance vessels, and increased blood pressure (reviewed in Reference 1).

G. INSULIN AND LIPID ABNORMALITIES

A close relationship has been found consistently between hyperinsulinemia and hypertriglyceridemia in several population-based studies in healthy, normal-weight subjects (reviewed in Reference 1). Elevated very-low-density lipoprotein (VLDL) and triglyceride levels are the most striking lipid abnormalities commonly seen in persons with NIDDM and in persons who are obese. Hyperinsulinemia enhances hepatic VLDL synthesis, contributing to the elevated VLDL and triglyceride levels observed. Furthermore, obese individuals have increased plasma concentrations of free fatty acids and glucose, providing extra substrate supply that promotes VLDL formation. Studies have also shown that free fatty acid infusion can result in insulin resistance (reviewed in Reference 7). In patients with elevated triglyceride turnover there is an elevated insulin response to a glucose load. Incubation of cell lines with VLDL results in insulin resistance associated with either a decrease in insulin receptors or post-binding resistance (also reviewed in Reference 7). Thus, there seems to be a potential vicious cycle in which hyperinsulinemia promotes dyslipidemia and dyslipidemia also may promote hyperinsulinemia or insulin resistance.

Low high-density lipoprotein (HDL) levels are also characteristic, although not quite as prominent as high triglyceride and VLDL levels, in persons with NIDDM, obesity, and hyperinsulinemia. An inverse relationship of HDL concentration with both triglyceride and insulin levels has been demonstrated in numerous studies (reviewed in Reference 1). In some studies it appears to be due to an enhanced rate of apoprotein (apo) A1/HDL degradation even beyond an also enhanced rate of apo A1/HDL synthesis.

H. CORONARY HEART DISEASE AND INSULIN-RELATED RISK FACTORS

It is well known that coronary heart disease (CHD) risk is higher in individuals with low HDL cholesterol, with hypertension, and also with insulin resistance.[8] Studies have shown consistently that, while presence of NIDDM is a risk factor for CHD, duration of diabetes is not a quantitative risk factor for CHD. It is hypothesized that a long period of insulin resistance, hyperinsulinemia, and subtle or even overt metabolic abnormalities such as dyslipidemia and hypertension precede the frank onset of hyperglycemia and diabetes by many years. Thus, it could be that atherogenesis has been developing long before the diagnosis of NIDDM. A similar pathophysiological diathesis toward atherosclerosis is thought to exist among individuals with insulin resistance due to obesity or other factors even if they never develop glucose intolerance or diabetes.

III. FAMILIAL METABOLIC SYNDROMES

Table 1 presents a summary of familial syndromes with a constellation of metabolic abnormalities relating to the pathophysiological mechanisms discussed above. This table summarizes overlapping metabolic abnormalities in each of these different syndromes and indicates the type of studies supporting familial aggregation or genetic determination.

A. NON-INSULIN-DEPENDENT DIABETES MELLITUS (NIDDM)

NIDDM occurs in about 2 to 5% of the general adult population of the U.S. NIDDM is highly concordant among identical twins (reviewed in References 1 and 8), and even the age of onset is very similar in co-twin pairs. In offspring of two diabetic parents, NIDDM occurs in approximately 70 to 90%. In first-degree relatives the incidence is about 40%.[1] The frequency of lipid abnormalities and hypertension in diabetics approaches 50%. Most persons with NIDDM are also overweight, although, as described above, NIDDM can occur in individuals who are not obese. If genetic factors lead to serious obesity, NIDDM would be an expected complication. In persons with a genetic predisposition to NIDDM (i.e., through inherited tendency toward insulin resistance) the concurrent development of obesity would certainly increase the liability of diabetes and perhaps produce an earlier age of onset or more severe expression. Weight reduction, exercise, dietary carbohydrate regulation, and oral medications to improve insulin sensitivity can all help reduce hyperinsulinemia, normalize glucose levels, and improve lipid abnormalities.

B. IMPAIRED GLUCOSE TOLERANCE

Depending on the specific definition used, IGT is as common as or more common than NIDDM. Metabolic abnormalities and long-term atherosclerotic complications are similar. The associations with obesity and the response to exercise, weight reduction, and dietary carbohydrate regulation also parallel observations for NIDDM.

C. PRE-NON-INSULIN-DEPENDENT DIABETES MELLITUS

Prospective studies of individuals who later developed NIDDM showed that baseline predictors included central obesity, lipid abnormalities, hypertension, and, most prominently, increased triglyceride levels.[9,10] This suggests that hypertriglyceridemia may be one of the most sensitive and most conveniently measured indicators of underlying insulin resistance.

Table 1. **Multiple metabolic syndromes and obesity**

Condition or Syndromes	HBP	High TGL	Low HDL	High LDL	High Apo B	High VLDL	Obesity	Early CHD	High insulin		High glucose		Genetic/ Familial
									Fast	Post	Fast	Post	
1. Pre-HBP/BBP	++++	+++	++	0	?	?	+++	?	+	?	0	0	FT
2. FDH	+++	++++	+++	+	+++	+++	+	+++	++	+++	0	+	FT
3. FCHL	++	+++	++	++	+++	+++	+	+++	?	?	0	+	FL
4. Syndrome X	+++	+++	++	0	?	?	0	?	+	+++	0	0	?
5. Pre-NIDDM	+	+++	++	0	?	?	+++	?	+++	+++	++	+++	S
6. IGT	+	++	+	+	?	?	++	++	++	++++	+	+++	FT
7. NIDDM	+++	++++	+++	++	?	++	+++	+++	V	V	++	++++	FT
8. Gout/high uric acid	++	++++	++	+	?	++	+++	+	?	?	++	+++	FS
9. Dense LDL	+	++++	++	0	++	++	+	++	?	?	?	?	TSL
10. Hetz LPL def.	+	++++	++++	0	+	++++	0	?	0	?	0	?	M

Note: Approximate degree of association is indicated from weakly (+) to strongly (++++) positive, unknown (?), not associated (0), or variable (V). HBP/BBP = high or borderline blood pressure; TGL = triglycerides; HDL = high-density lipoprotein; LDL = low-density lipoprotein; Apo B = apoprotein B; VLDL = very-low-density lipoprotein; CHD = coronary heart disease; FDH = familial dyslipidemic hypertension; FCHL = familial combined hyperlipidemia; IGT = impaired glucose tolerance; NIDDM = non-insulin-dependant diabetes mellitus. Genetic/familial abbreviations: F = familial aggregation; T = twin, MZ > DZ; S = segregating major gene; L = genetic linkage; M = mutation found; C = familial correlation. Pre-HBP and Pre-NIDDM are profiles in persons who later developed hypertension or NIDDM, respectively. Hetz LPL def. = heterozygous lipoprotein lipase deficiency (see text).

A substantial major gene effect has been suggested[11] for hyperinsulinemia among first-degree relatives of persons with NIDDM (thus suggesting that these are prediabetic individuals). Maximum likelihood segregation analysis among normoglycemic relatives of index cases with NIDDM revealed a recessive trait. Affected homozygotes (6% of the general population) had fasting insulin levels three times higher than persons with the other genotypes. Persons with this genotype were somewhat more obese (body mass index of 29.0 vs. 26.4 kg/m^2) and had dyslipidemia more often than persons with the other genotype (triglycerides above the 90th percentile in 36% and HDL cholesterol levels below the 10th percentile in 57% compared to persons with other genotypes, respectively, at 17% and 30%). Hypertension was present in 40% of these homozygotes for hyperinsulinemia, compared to only 18% of age-matched persons with the other genotypes in the same family.[11]

D. GOUT AND INCREASED URIC ACID

While the exact mechanisms are not known, the frequency and coaggregation of these multiple metabolic abnormalities with gout and hyperuricemia are striking. Among individuals with gout 80% have abnormal triglyceride levels, and among persons with hypertriglyceridemia approximately 70% have hyperuricemia (defined as 2 SD above the mean level for specific age and sex categories).[13] Familial aggregation of gout and hyperuricemia has been well documented, and segregation analysis also suggests strong genetic determination.[13] While not all persons who have gout or hyperuricemia are overweight, obesity is a well-known strong correlate of gout and hyperuricemia. In prospective studies, increased plasma uric acid is also a predictor of future development of both hypertension and coronary artery disease.[1,14]

E. FAMILIAL COMBINED HYPERLIPIDEMIA

Approximately 1 to 2% of the general population is estimated to have familial combined hyperlipidemia (FCHL), defined as the occurrence of elevated triglyceride and total cholesterol level above the 90th percentile in two or more first-degree relatives. Other standardized definitions require higher percentiles or elevations in measured low-density lipoprotein (LDL) and VLDL cholesterol levels. The specific genetic mechanism for this condition has not been defined, although strong familial aggregation and suggested dominant transmission have been mentioned in textbooks regarding this disorder. As a clinical syndrome with probable genetic heterogeneity, FCHL is one of the most common causes of early familial coronary disease, being present in approximately 30% of families with early familial CHD.[15] A strong association of FCHL with obesity and NIDDM has been reported.[16] Studies also indicate that persons with FCHL are prone to develop hypertension and hyperinsulinemia.[7] At least one linkage study suggests a possible major gene contributor to at least a subset of persons with FCHL.[17]

F. SYNDROME X

This term, coined by Reaven for nonobese hypertensives who tend to have hyperinsulinemia,[3] has also been studied perspectively by Haffner and colleagues.[18] Fasting insulin at baseline was related to the occurrence of hypertension, decreased HDL cholesterol, increased triglycerides, and NIDDM 8 years later. Hyperinsulinemia was not related to LDL or total cholesterol. Even after adjusting for obesity and body fat distribution, fasting insulin at baseline was a strong predictor of future abnormalities in HDL and triglycerides.

G. FAMILIAL DYSLIPIDEMIC HYPERTENSION

Population-based pairs of siblings with hypertension diagnosed before age 55 are also found to have strong significant coaggregation of lipid abnormalities, most prominently hypertriglyceridemia and low HDL cholesterol.[19] Familial dyslipidemic hypertension (FDH) was found to be present in approximately 12% of patients with essential hypertension and in 1 to 2% of persons in the general population. Approximately one third of these individuals met classic criteria for FCHL. The studies showed that 90th percentile obesity was present three times more often than expected in the general population. Most, but not all, individuals with FDH have some degree of obesity. Hyperinsulinemia, central obesity, elevated levels of apolipoprotein B, and higher percentage of dense LDL subfractions also have been observed among persons with FDH.[7]

Dyslipidemic hypertension was also studied using the same criteria among the 1028 middle-aged white male twin participants in the NHLBI (National Heart, Lung, and Blood Institute) twin study. Concordance for dyslipidemic hypertension was three times greater among MZ than DZ twins.[20] The frequency of FDH among hypertensives and among the general population was similar in the NHLBI study as in the Utah study.[19,20] In a 16-year follow-up from the time of diagnosis of FDH, the NHLBI twin study showed that dyslipidemia and hypertension produced a coronary mortality rate four times higher than either dyslipidemia alone or hypertension alone. Thus, dyslipidemic hypertension seems to produce an especially severe propensity toward early coronary disease. Among 18 MZ twin pairs who were discordant (i.e., one had dyslipidemic hypertension and one did not), the dyslipidemic hypertensive twin was always heavier than the unaffected co-twin. Thus, NHLBI twin study results indicate that dyslipidemic hypertension is strongly influenced by genetic factors, but nongenetic obesity is an important factor related to the expression of this clinically important syndrome.[20]

H. PREHYPERTENSION OR BORDERLINE BLOOD PRESSURE

Prospective studies in Utah and San Antonio were able to identify baseline factors in individuals who developed hypertension 8 years later.[14,21] Baseline blood pressure and triglyceride levels were strong predictors, as were obesity, unfavorable body fat distribution, and 2-h poststimulation levels of insulin and glucose. After adjusting for obesity in multivariate analyses, triglyceride, blood pressure, and HDL cholesterol remain significant predictors of hypertension. As previously mentioned, the Utah study also showed uric acid to be a strong predictor. Blood pressures in general and borderline or slightly elevated blood pressures also correlate strongly in families and are highly concordant among MZ twins more than DZ twins, suggesting a strong genetic component for the determination of a prehypertensive status.

I. HETEROZYGOUS LIPOPROTEIN LIPASE DEFICIENCY

The possibility of a single mutation predisposing to dyslipidemia and hypertension is suggested from a large Utah pedigree studied by Wilson and colleagues.[22] Starting with a proband homozygous for a mutation of the lipoprotein lipase (LPL) locus that resulted in nonfunctional enzyme, 126 members were screened using hybridization of DNA with allele-specific probes; 29 heterozygous carriers of the mutant allele were detected. Based on studies in adipose tissue, LPL activity in such single gene carriers was found to be reduced to approximately 50% of normal. Carriers over age 40 showed a significant increase in hypertriglyceridemia (58% above the 95th age/gender-specific percentile), low HDL cholesterol (58% below the 5th percentile), and hypertension (68%). While these gene carriers had significantly increased rates of dyslipidemia and hypertension, they did not have an increased frequency of obesity or hyperinsulinemia compared to noncarriers of the same age and gender. However, persons who carried this mutant LPL allele and did not have lipid abnormalities were significantly thinner and had lower fasting plasma insulin levels than those who had expressed the lipid abnormalities. Finally, persons under age 40 who carried this mutant allele did not have any significant differences in lipid abnormalities or other manifestations. This is a practical example of how genes can operate in the "real world". A single copy of this gene has no effect in younger people; in older people it has a strong effect, but is significantly influenced by other factors such as obesity and hyperinsulinemia.

J. DENSE LOW-DENSITY LIPOPROTEIN SUBFRACTIONS

Subclasses of LDL can be detected using gradient gel electrophoresis of plasma. Patients with the predominantly dense LDL subclass have been shown to have approximately a three-fold increased risk of myocardial infarction independent of age, sex, and relative weight. Plasma levels of HDL cholesterol and triglyceride are very strong predictors of dense LDL pattern. Since this dense LDL subclass is often found in persons with high triglyceride and low HDL levels, it is often found in persons with FCHL or FDH.[7] There appears to be substantial genetic determination based on twin studies in Utah,[28] segregation analysis,[23] and genetic linkage.[24] Additional unpublished data in Utah[28] suggest that exercise training can significantly improve the profile for LDL subfractions. Because of the strong influence of obesity on triglycerides and HDL, it is likely a significant factor influencing LDL subfractions.

IV. AN INTEGRATED VIEW

Table 1 shows considerable similarities for the characteristics of each of these syndromes. It is unlikely that each of them represents a separate and discrete condition. It seems more likely that each of them represents a different way of looking at some of the same pathophysiological mechanisms resulting from some of the same underlying genetic and environmental factors. All of them probably result from the combined effects of four or five specific genetic and environmental factors. Many of them probably have two or three of these specific causal factors in common.

Five different types of causal factors can contribute to such syndromes. In the first category of causal factors, *single major gene* effects are responsible for the predominant determination of a given trait. Major gene effects are striking, but uncommon. One example is LPL deficiency, discussed above as a predominant cause of high triglyceride and low HDL levels in heterozygous carriers.[22] Another example would be heterozygous familial hypercholesterolemia, which causes twice-normal LDL cholesterol levels and very early coronary disease in males and females.[24] Another example is glucocorticoid-remediable aldosteronism, a single gene leading to early serious hypertension with strokes in the mid-40s.[25] In each of these disorders a single gene has a predominant effect which is modulated to some degree by other factors such as age and obesity, but the predominant expression is attributable to a single gene in heterozygous carriers.

As a second genetic category, *multiple discrete susceptibility genes* cause predispositions that are strongly dependent on other factors for expression. Examples would include urinary kallikrein excretion, which shows strong major gene effects and seems to offer a liability for hypertension, but not predominant determination.[26] Low potassium intake is an important environmental cofactor for renal kallikrein. Another recently determined gene from molecular studies is the angiotensinogen locus, which seems to promote moderately severe blood pressure elevation in about 5% of persons with hypertension.[27] Again, by itself this gene probably does not cause hypertension.[27] Many common disorders probably require two or three of these common genetic mechanisms to produce a strong genetic predisposition. Thus, hypertension or lipid abnormalities that are common usually reflect the combined effects of one or two of these multiple discrete genes in addition to other factors such as age and environment.

As a third category, *blended polygenic effects* are thought to be common determinants for all major quantitative cardiovascular risk factors such as cholesterol, weight, and blood pressure. No single gene can be identified with significant individual contributions (in contrast to single major genes or multiple discrete genes discussed above). On the other hand, polygenes are thought to account for about 50% of the variability of many of these risk factors and act in a quantitative blended fashion such that a high level from one parent and a low level from another parent generally result in an average in-between level in most of the children. For many persons considered "abnormal" in medical screening studies, some cutoff point in the continuous distribution is chosen. Persons above that point with abnormalities are often simply in the upper tail of the polygenic distribution.

As a fourth category, *environmental factors* are often shared among family members, including such prominent risk factors as dietary intake, physical activity, and cigarette smoking. It is sometimes difficult to distinguish polygenic effects from shared environmental effects since both of them tend to have a sort of blending effect. It is interesting to note that shared environmental effects can be transmitted more completely in families than some genetic effects. For example, smoking avoidance may be shared by all members of the sibship and all of their offspring, whereas major genes are shared by only 50% of siblings and offspring.

The fifth category has been studied by many epidemiologists. *Individual environmental factors* are unique to a given individual, not shared with other members of their family, and are obviously important in determining individual risk.

Each of the above five types of genetic and environmental factors can be considered as different classes or types of building blocks. Within each of these groups there are multiple factors contributing to a given condition such as hypertension, obesity, or lipid abnormalities. The somewhat complicated but still definable combination of these factors can lead to the observed risk in any given individual.

Once this model has been visualized, the role of obesity in susceptibility to metabolic complications can be considered. A few severe syndromes (some persons with morbid obesity) may be determined by major genes yet to be defined. Some families are observed in which multiple siblings have morbid obesity and yet other siblings are unaffected, suggesting major gene effects.

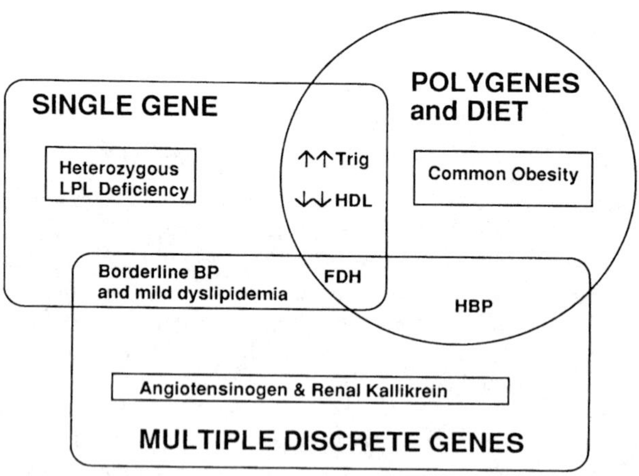

Figure 2. Hypothetical model based on developing research results. Polygenes and dietary factors that lead to ordinary obesity also promote hypertension (HBP) in persons with multiple discrete susceptibility genes (angiotensinogen and renal kallikrein). A single major gene (lipoprotein lipase deficiency) predisposes to dyslipidemia, which is severe in obese persons (very high triglycerides, very low high-density lipoprotein). Familial dyslipidemic hypertension (FDH) could develop in persons with all three tendencies.

More often obesity is likely attributable to multiple discrete genes or blended polygenes. A strong role for genetics in the determination of obesity is based on other studies already reviewed in this volume. In many individuals, shared environmental factors and individual environmental factors such as exercise and diet can also affect the level of obesity.

In any given individual who has a genetic susceptibility to hypertension, lipid abnormalities, or diabetes, a single major gene would have a high probability of promoting expression, multiple discrete genes may have a moderate probability of promoting expression, and blended polygenes or shared environmental factors promoting obesity would certainly have an effect, but perhaps would be less prominent.

It seems likely that some of the conditions in Table 1 may be reflecting underlying major gene effects. Such seems to be the case for subsets of persons with diabetes, gout, and certain lipid abnormalities. Many of the less striking but more common metabolic abnormalities, such as in impaired glucose intolerance, common lipid abnormalities, moderate hypertension, or ordinary hyperuricemia, probably involve multiple discrete genes, with either genetic or nongenetic obesity playing an important role in determining the degree of expression. The hypothetical model in Figure 2 illustrates how these causal factors may overlap to produce dyslipidemia and hypertension.

What practical use can result from an understanding of these possible models? Presently a detailed medical family history helps detect a strong familial predisposition to disorders such as hypertension, lipid abnormalities, or CHD. The same detailed family history also can help identify strong family tendencies toward obesity and related metabolic abnormalities. Since most of these abnormalities have a strong increase in expression with age, it seems important to identify risks through family history analysis while some family members are still young so that certain preventive interventions (such as modification of diet and exercise) could help prevent or delay these complications.

Over the next decade it is very likely that molecular biology will provide practical tools for the early diagnosis of persons with genetic susceptibility to these metabolic complications related to obesity. If gene testing was used to identify young children who had a high probability of developing severe dyslipidemia, hypertension, or atherosclerosis at a later stage, and if it was known that obesity played an important role in these families, one could invest in targeted interventions for these high-risk persons to help avoid these complications. Nonetheless, the real world is a complicated place, and it is likely that even the most sophisticated diagnostic tools will not solve all of our problems. Even if all of the pathophysiological mechanisms were understood, and even if certain mechanisms such as weight reduction and dietary restriction would help produce the desired prevention, clinicians and behavioral scientists would face the challenging task of learning how to be effective in modifying human behavior.

REFERENCES

1. **DeFronzo, R. A. and Ferrannini, E.,** Insulin resistance: a multifaceted syndrome responsible for NIDDM, obesity, hypertension, dyslipidemia, and atherosclerotic cardiovascular disease, *Diabetes Care,* 14, 173, 1991.
2. **Krotkiewski, M., Mandroukas, K., Sjostrom, L., Sullivan, L., Wetterqvist, H., and Bjorntorp, P.,** Effects of long-term physical training on body fat, metabolism, and blood pressure in obesity, *Metabolism,* 28, 650, 1979.
3. **Reaven, G. M. and Hoffman, B. B.,** A role for insulin in the aetiology and course of hypertension, *Lancet,* 2, 435, 1987.
4. **Ferrannini, E., Buzzigoli, G., Bonadonna, R., Giorico, M.A., Oleggini, M., Graziadei, L., Pedrinelli, R., Brandi, L., and Bevilacqua, S.,** Insulin resistance in essential hypertension, *N. Engl. J. Med.,* 317, 350, 1987.

5. **Sharma, A. M., Ruland, K., Spies, K. P., and Distler, A.,** Salt sensitivity in young normotensive subjects is associated with a hyperinsulinemic response to oral glucose, *J. Hypertension,* 9, 329, 1991.
6. **Daly, P. A. and Landsberg, L.,** Hypertension in obesity and NIDDM — role of insulin and sympathetic nervous system, *Diabetes Care,* 14, 240, 1991.
7. **Hunt, S. C., Wu, L. L., Hopkins, P. N., Stults, B. M., Kuida, H., Ramirez, M. E., Lalouel, J. M., and Williams, R. R.,** Apolipoprotein, low density lipoprotein subfraction, and insulin associations with familial combined hyperlipidemia: study of Utah patients with familial dyslipidemic hypertension, *Arteriosclerosis,* 9, 335, 1989.
8. **Williams, R. R., Schumacher, M. C., Hunt, S. C., Wu, L. L., Hopkins, P. N., and Kuida, H.,** The genetics of hypertension, coronary atherosclerosis, and non insulin dependent diabetes mellitus (NIDDM): heterogeneity and covariation, in *Genes and Gene Products in the Development of Diabetes Mellitus: Basic and Clinical Aspects,* Nerup, J., Mandrup-Poulsen, T., and Hokfelt, B., Eds., Excerpta Medica, Amsterdam, 1989, 387.
9. **Schumacher, M. C., Hunt, S. C., Stephenson, S. H., Wu, L. L., and Williams, R. R.,** Risk factors for cardiovascular disease predict the development of diabetes among Utah families, *Epidemiology,* 3, 459, 1992.
10. **Haffner, S. M., Stern, M. P., Hazuda, H. P., Mitchell, B. M., and Patterson, J. K.,** Cardiovascular risk factors in confirmed prediabetic individuals, *JAMA,* 263, 2893, 1990.
11. **Schumacher, M. C., Hasstedt, S. J., Hunt, S. C., Williams, R. R., and Elbein, S. C.,** Major gene effect for insulin levels in familial NIDDM pedigrees, *Diabetes,* 41, 416, 1992.
12. **Schumacher, M. C., Hunt, S. C., Maxwell, T. M., Williams, R. R., Wu, L. L., and Elbein, S. C.,** Dyslipidemias among normoglycemic members of familial NIDDM pedigrees, *Diabetes Care,* 15, 1285, 1992.
13. **Palella, T. D. and Fox, I. H.,** Hyperuricemia and gout, in *The Metabolic Basis of Inherited Disease,* 6th ed., Scriver, C. R., Beaudet, A. L., Sly, W. S., and Valle, D., Eds., McGraw Hill, New York, 1989, 965.
14. **Hunt, S. C., Stephenson, S. H., Hopkins, P. N., and Williams, R. R.,** Predictors of an increased risk of future hypertension in Utah: a screening analysis, *Hypertension,* 17, 969, 1991.
15. **Williams, R. R., Hopkins, P. N., Hunt, S. C., Wu, L. L., Hasstedt, S. J., Lalouel, J. M., Ash, K. O., Stults, B. M., and Kuida, H.,** Population-based frequency of dyslipidemia syndromes in coronary-prone families in Utah, *Arch. Intern. Med.,* 150, 582, 1990.
16. **Iverius, P. H. and Brunzell, J. D.,** Obesity and common genetic metabolic disorders, *Ann. Intern. Med.,* 103, 1050, 1985.
17. **Wojciechowski, A. P., Farrall, M., Cullen, P., and Wilson, T. M.,** Familial combined hyperlipidemia linked to the apolipoprotein AI-CII-AIV gene cluster on chromosome 11q23–q24, *Nature,* 349, 161, 1991.
18. **Haffner, S. M., Valdez, R. A., Hazuda, H. P., Mitchell, B. D., Morales, P. A., and Stern, M. P.,** Prospective analysis of the insulin resistance syndrome (Syndrome X), *Diabetes,* 41, 715, 1992.
19. **Williams, R. R., Hunt, S. C., Hopkins, P. N., Stults, B. M., Wu, L. L., Hasstedt, S. J., Barlow, G. K., Stephenson, S. H., Lalouel, J. M., and Kuida, H.,** Familial dyslipidemic hypertension: evidence from 58 Utah families for a syndrome present in approximately 12% of patients with essential hypertension, *JAMA,* 259, 3579, 1988.
20. **Selby, J. V., Newman, B., Quiroga, J., Christian, J. C., Austin, M. A., and Fabsitz, M. A.,** Concordance for dyslipidemic hypertension in male twins, *JAMA,* 265, 2079, 1991.

21. **Haffner, S. M., Ferrannini, E., Hazuda, H. P., and Stern, M. P.,** Clustering of cardiovascular risk factors in confirmed prehypertensive individuals, *Hypertension,* 20, 38, 1992.
22. **Wilson, D. E., Emi, M., Iverius, P. H., Hata, A., Wu, L. L., Hillas, E., Williams, R. R., and Lalouel, J. M.,** Phenotypic expression of heterozygous lipoprotein lipase deficiency in the extended pedigree of a proband homozygous for a missense mutation, *J. Clin. Invest.,* 86, 735, 1990 (74 references).
23. **Austin, M. A., King, M. C., Vranizan, K. M., and Krauss, R. M.,** Atherogenic lipoprotein phenotype: a proposed genetic marker for coronary heart disease risk, *Circulation,* 82, 495, 1990.
24. **Nishina, P. M., Johnson, J. P., Naggert, J. K., and Krauss, R. M.,** Linkage of atherogenic lipoprotein phenotype to the low density lipoprotein receptor locus on the short arm of chromosome 19, *Proc. Natl. Acad. Sci. U.S.A.,* 89, 708, 1992.
25. **Lifton, R. P., Dluhy, R. G., Powers, M., Rich, G. M., Cook, S., Ulick, S., and Lalouel, J. M.,** A chimeric 11-beta-hydroxylase/aldosterone synthetase gene causes glucocorticoid-remediable aldosteronism and human hypertension, *Nature,* 365, 262, 1992.
26. **Berry, T. D., Hasstedt, S. J., Hunt, S. C., Wu, L. L., Smith, J. B., Ash, K. O., Kuida, H., and Williams, R. R.,** A gene for high urinary kallikrein may protect against hypertension in Utah kindreds, *Hypertension,* 13, 3, 1989.
27. **Jeunemaitre, X., Soubrier, F., Kotelevtsev, Y. V., Lifton, R. P., Williams, C. S., Charru, A., Hunt, S. C., Hopkins, P. N., Williams, R. R., Lalouel, J. M., and Corvol, P.,** Molecular basis of human hypertension: role of angiotensinogen, *Cell,* 71, 169, 1992.
28. **Williams, R. R.,** unpublished data, 1990.

Chapter 12

Animal Models of Genetic Obesity: Peripheral Tissue Changes

Patricia R. Johnson and Francine Gregoire

TABLE OF CONTENTS

I. INTRODUCTION

Animals that deposit excessive amounts of body fat and become obese as a result of inheritance of single Mendelian genes for obesity have been known since 1905, when Cuenot first described the yellow obese mouse.[1] Since that time several other mouse and rat strains that carry obesity genes have been identified and described (see Table 1), and a number of major reviews of these genetically obese rodent models have been written.[2-5] In all of the obese rodents described thus far, the obesity is accompanied by a variety of other pathologies, including hyperinsulinemia, hyperglycemia, non-insulin-dependent diabetes (NIDDM), insulin resistance, hypertension, hyperlipemias, altered thermogenesis, impairments in cardiovascular function, and impairments in reproductive function. These various pathologies vary in degree and kind among the obese rodents and in general are considered to be secondary accompaniments to the obesity. Since these same pathologies are also present in many cases of human obesity, the various obese rodents have been utilized widely as models of human obesity with its associated pathologies. Although several of the genes that produce these obese phenotypes have been localized to a specific chromosome (see Table 1), in no case has the gene been cloned, nor has its specific protein product, or site of action, been identified. Several laboratories are currently engaged in efforts to clone the *ob* and *db* mouse genes, and both have been mapped,[6,7] as has the *fa* gene in the rat.[8] When one of the obesity genes is finally available to study, it should prove highly instructive to decipher the pathway(s) by which a single Mendelian gene leads to the multiple metabolic and behavioral changes that are seen in obesity,

0-8493-4880-3/94/$0.00+$.50

Table 1. **Summary of single gene mutations producing obesity in rodents**

Species	Strain	Genotype	Phenotype	Chromosome location	Ref
Mouse	C3BL/6J	*ob/ob*	Obese; hyperglycemic	6	73
	C3BL/KsJ	*ob/ob*	Obese; severely diabetic	6	73
	C3BL/KsJ	*db/db*	Obese; severely diabetic	4	126
	C3BL/6J	*db/db*	Obese; hyperglycemic	4	73
	Yellow	A^{y}/a	Obese	2	1
	Viable yellow	A^{vy}/a	Obese, slow development; mild hyperinsulinemia; normoglycemic	2	130
	HRS/J-fat	*fat/fat*	Obese; hyperinsulinemic; normoglycemic	8	127
	C57BL/6J-Hbb	*tub/tub*	Obese, slow development; hyperinsulinemic; normoglycemic	7	127
Rat	Zucker	*fa/fa*	Obese; hyperinsulinemic; normoglycemic	5	128
	Zucker/DRT	*fa/fa*	Obese; diabetic	5	76
	WDF	*fa/fa*	Obese; diabetic	5	129
	SHR/N-cp	*cp/cp*	Obese; hypertensive		75
	LA/N-cp	*cp/cp*	Obese; normotensive		75
	JCR:LA/N-cp	*cp/cp*	Obese; atherosclerotic/myocardial lesions in males		131

including the interactions that occur between the single gene and the genetic background on which it is expressed.

Given the immensity of the literature that exists on animal models of genetic obesity, the task of reviewing requires that limitations be set on the material to be addressed. Two significant hypotheses have been advanced over the years as to the initial site of the lesion(s) produced by mutant genes that lead to the obesity syndrome. One presents the view that the first changes occur in the central nervous system and the other that the periphery is the site of primary action of mutant genes leading to obesity. Substantial evidence and arguments support each of these hypotheses. The role of the central nervous system has been thoroughly reviewed;[2] thus, this chapter shall focus on the most recent findings relating to the type of changes that have been reported for peripheral tissue (white adipose tissue, brown adipose tissue, skeletal muscle, and pancreas) metabolism and gene expression in obese compared to lean rodent models.

II. WHITE ADIPOSE TISSUE

White adipose tissue is the site of lipid storage by the organism, and it is the tissue that can expand to an extraordinary extent during the course of the development of obesity. The expansion occurs by the processes of proliferation of new adipocytes (i.e., hyperplasia) and enlargement of adipocytes (i.e., hypertrophy). The animal models of genetic obesity, for the most part, exhibit both adipocyte hyperplasia and hypertrophy.

A. GLUCOSE TRANSPORTER EXPRESSION

In most animal models of genetic obesity, whether or not associated with NIDDM, insulin-resistant glucose utilization is observed *in vivo* in peripheral tissues, primarily skeletal muscle and adipose tissue. There are several steps at which the insulin resistance can be manifested, including transport, phosphorylation, and metabolism. In adipose cells, glucose transport is mediated through the action of two different glucose transporters, GLUT1 and GLUT4. GLUT1 is much less abundant than GLUT4 and is considered to be primarily a constitutive glucose transporter that contributes little, if any, to the effects of insulin[9] on glucose transport, whereas GLUT4 is primarily responsible for glucose uptake in response to insulin.[10] Several recent studies have addressed the potential role of GLUT4 in the pathogenesis of insulin-resistant glucose uptake in different models of genetically obese rodents as well as in obese humans.[11-18] Until now, published data appear equivocal since increased[15,18] or decreased[13,19] glucose transport activity may be found associated with increased,[15,18] unchanged,[11,13,17] or decreased[11,13,14,18] levels of GLUT4 protein and mRNA. Intrinsic differences between the different models used, in terms of heterogeneity or degree of obesity, level of hyperinsulinemia and degree of insulin resistance, and presence or absence of hyperglycemia, may be implicated, at least in part, in the generation of these divergent results. On the other hand, normalization with respect to expression of results appears to be a critical issue, since altered metabolic states such as obesity and diabetes have been shown to profoundly affect total cellular RNA and protein content.[9,18]

In the Zucker rat, the early stages of obesity are correlated in adipose tissue with an insulin-hyperresponsive glucose uptake that can be attributed, at least in part, to changes in the abundance of GLUT4.[20] Adipocytes isolated from young Zucker rats display an enhanced glucose utilization rate which is associated with increased expression of GLUT4 mRNA and protein.[15,16,18] This overexpression is observed even before the emergence of hyperinsulinemia, indicating that the genotype may be a major regulatory factor of GLUT4 expression in adipose tissue.[15] By contrast, in 20-week-old obese Zucker rats, despite the persistent increase in insulin-stimulated glucose uptake rate, GLUT4 protein, but not mRNA, is decreased.[18] This finding suggests that the translocation or intrinsic activity of GLUT4 may be altered at this age.[20] On the other hand, both basal glucose uptake and GLUT1 mRNA, as well as protein, are significantly increased in 20-week-old obese Zucker rats, suggesting that GLUT1 may contribute to insulin-stimulated glucose transport in adipose cells from these obese rats.[18,20] The discrepancy between GLUT4 mRNA and protein levels indicates that the transcription of the GLUT4 gene may not be proportional to the steady-state level of the protein,[17,18,21] thus suggesting that posttranscriptional mechanisms may be involved in controlling GLUT4 levels.

A clear decrease in levels of GLUT4 protein in adipose tissue of nondiabetic human subjects also has been reported,[14] whereas others show no significant alterations in GLUT4 expression in obese mildly diabetic Zucker rats (ZDF/drt)[11] and obese nondiabetic human subjects.[13] In general, in obese rodents as well as in obese human subjects, the presence of NIDDM seems to induce a more profound down-regulation in GLUT4 mRNA and protein levels.[11,13,14,18] In severely diabetic ZDF/drt rats and in yellow obese mice *(A^y/a)*, the alterations seen in GLUT4 protein levels appear not to be associated with obesity per se, but are secondary to the severely diabetic state, suggesting that glucose itself may be an important contributing regulator of glucose transporter protein levels.[11] By contrast, GLUT4 mRNA and protein levels are found to be unaltered in adipose tissue of *db/db* mice, suggesting that in this particular model the insulin resistance seen is not related to a pretranslational change in GLUT4 expression, but may be related to changes in signal transduction, translocation, or functional activity of the protein.[17] To summarize these data, it is safe to say that no clear picture has emerged as to a contribution of glucose transporter activity in adipose tissue that is consistent across strains of obese and obese/diabetic animal models and humans. Thus, it appears unlikely that the alterations that do occur in glucose transporter expression in these genetically obese animals are in any way primary to the underlying genetic defect.

B. ADIPSIN AND TUMOR NECROSIS FACTOR-α

Adipsin is a differentiation-dependent serine protease which is an abundant secreted protein of fat tissue. Adipsin mRNA is expressed in white and brown adipose tissues and, to a lesser extent, in sciatic nerve.[22] A high level of adipsin gene expression is also seen in human adipose tissue.[23] Adipsin mRNA and circulating protein are greatly reduced in several rodent models of genetic obesity, usually after the emergence of hyperinsulinemia.[24-29] The dramatic down-regulation of adipsin seen in genetic obesity suggests a possible link between adipsin and adipose tissue metabolism or systemic energy balance.[25] Adipsin has complement factor D activity and catalyzes the first and rate-limiting step in the alternative pathway of complement activation.[24] Adipocytes were also recently reported to synthesize two other essential components of the alternative pathway (factors C3 and B) and locally activate the proximal portion of this pathway, in the absence of infectious agents and without triggering the terminal lytic part of the pathway.[30] Furthermore, this pathway appears to be dysregulated in several models of obesity, since adipose tissue from *ob/ob* mice is deficient in this localized activation of the alternative pathway.[30] These results, which indicate that constitutive complement activation occurs in adipose tissue, but is impaired in the obese state, suggest a previously unsuspected role for adipose tissue in immune system biology. More recently, tumor necrosis factor-alpha (TNF-α) mRNA expression has been reported in adipose tissue of genetically obese rodents, including *ob/ob*, *tub/tub*, and *db/db* mice and the Zucker *fa/fa* rat.[31] The endogenous expression of TNF-α mRNA, evident only in adipose tissue and spleen, was elevated only in adipose tissue from these obese rodents when they were compared with their lean littermates. TNF-α protein was also elevated locally and systemically. When local protein production was examined, a significant amount of TNF-α secretion was observed, obese adipose tissue secreting twice as much TNF-α as did lean adipose tissue. The amount of TNF-α in the circulation is low but significantly elevated in obese animals. Chronic treatment of cultured murine 3T3-F442A adipocytes with very low doses (2 ng/ml) of TNF-α leads to specific down-regulation of GLUT4 mRNA; other genes that are expressed in a differentiation-dependent manner, such as lipoprotein lipase (LPL), aP2 (adipocyte P_2, a fatty acid binding protein), glycerol-3-phosphate dehydrogenase (GPDH), and adipsin, are unaffected. These data suggest that TNF-α could be a mediator of abnormal gene expression in obesity-diabetes syndromes and that it may affect glucose homeostasis.[31] In the Zucker *fa/fa* rat, neutralization of TNF-α by injection of a recombinant soluble TNF-α receptor-immunoglobulin G chimeric protein leads to a significant increase in the peripheral uptake of glucose in response to insulin, suggesting that TNF-α is involved in obesity-linked insulin resistance.[31] These intriguing findings may provide additional clues as to the role of cytokines in the regulation of adipose tissue and energy metabolism in states of altered energy balance, such as obesity, NIDDM, and cachexia.

C. LIPOPROTEIN LIPASE AND OTHER LIPOGENIC ENZYMES

Elevated LPL activity in adipose tissue is a well-known feature in genetically obese rodents[32-35] and in obese humans.[36,37] The mechanisms by which LPL is increased in fat cells of obese Zucker rats have been investigated; the data provide new insights concerning the regulation of LPL activity.[35] As expected, LPL activity is elevated in obese adipose tissue when expressed either on a per cell basis or per unit fat cell surface area to account for the difference in fat cell size between lean and obese adipose deposits. In the presence of heparin, obese-derived cells secrete more LPL than do lean-derived cells. Absolute rates of LPL synthesis per fat cell are increased in obese when compared with lean rats, accounting for the increase in LPL activity per cell. LPL mRNA expressed per cell is also increased. However, the relative rate of LPL synthesis (percent of total protein synthesis) and the levels of LPL mRNA as percent of total RNA are similar in fat cells from lean and obese rats, leading to the conclusion that the increase in LPL activity in the adipose tissue of genetically obese Zucker rats is not due to a specific abnormality in LPL gene expression or synthesis, but rather to a generalized increase in protein synthetic activity.[35] Several investigators have suggested that posttranscriptional and/or posttranslational mechanisms contribute to the increased LPL activity seen in obesity. In obese weight-reduced Zucker rats, although the changes in mRNA contribute to the changes seen in LPL enzyme activity, they do not entirely account for the magnitude of the change.[37] Moreover, the presence of specific cell surface binding sites for LPL on freshly isolated lean- and obese-derived rat fat cells has been demonstrated.[35] Obese-derived fat cells show an increased capacity for LPL binding on a per cell basis which is also slightly increased when the data are expressed per unit cell surface area. In addition, the ability of fat cells from obese Zucker rats to degrade LPL is directly proportional to their increased binding capacity.[35] Since a certain proportion of cell surface LPL is likely to leave that area and travel to its site of action on the luminal surface of endothelial cells, the variation in the number of LPL molecules bound and degraded by enlarged adipocytes may be an important posttranslational mechanism that controls rates of LPL secretion to its extracellular site of action.[35] The increase seen in LPL activity in obese Zucker rats is also reported to be one of the earliest manifestations of the *fa* gene, occurring before elevation in plasma insulin.[32,38] Greenwood proposed that, in obese rats, abnormalities in adipose tissue LPL might play a central role in an abnormal partitioning of fuel toward storage in adipose tissue relative to muscle.[39,40] Recent data obtained on weight-reduced obese Zucker rats provide support for the "LPL hypothesis". After weight reduction of both lean and obese Zucker rats as well as lean Sprague-Dawley rats, LPL activity is increased in adipose tissue, but decreased in cardiac muscle. These data show that sustained weight reduction results in coordinate changes in tissue-specific LPL, favoring delivery of lipoprotein triglyceride fatty acids to adipose tissue relative to cardiac muscle and the restoration of energy stores.[37]

In addition to LPL, the increased fat storage capacity seen in obese Zucker rats is also known to be affected by tissue-specific increases in the activities, mRNA levels, and gene transcription of a number of other lipid storage-related enzymes in adipose tissue (see Table 2).[33,41-46] The overexpression of glyceraldehyde-3-phosphate dehydrogenase (GAPDH), fatty acid synthetase (FAS), and malic enzyme (ME) seen in adipose tissue of preobese pups appears to be related to increased transcriptional activity,[33,44] suggesting the existence of a common trans-acting factor(s) that could be under direct or indirect control of the *fa* gene, and that triggers enhanced expression of these genes in adipose tissue of genetically obese rats.[33] After weaning, a dramatic increase in enzyme activities, mRNA levels, and gene transcription takes place (Table 2). Since frank hyperinsulinemia has already developed by this time in obese rats,[41,47] this phenomenon is most likely the reflection of the amplifying effect of hyperinsulinemia on expression of these genes. This effect of insulin is mainly obvious for activity, mRNA levels, and gene transcription of GPDH, since differences between lean and obese Zucker rats in these parameters become apparent only after weaning.[33]

D. G PROTEINS AND LIPOLYSIS

Alterations in adipocyte catecholamine-stimulated lipolysis have been noted in several models of genetic obesity, including *ob/ob* and *db/db* mice and the Zucker *fa/fa* rat.[48-51] Adipocytes of *ob/ob* mice and obese Zucker rats display an impaired adenylate cyclase

Table 2. **Levels of enzyme activity, mRNA, and gene transcription in obese Zucker rats before (A) and after (B) weaning**

Enzyme	Activity	mRNA	Gene transcription	Ref.
	A. Before weaning (normoinsulinemia)			
LPL	+	+	nd	32,33
GAPDH	+	+	+	33
FAS	+	+	+	43,44
ME	+	+	+	33
ACC	+	+	nd	43
GPDH	0	0	0	33
	B. After weaning (hyperinsulinemia)			
LPL	++	+	nd	33,35,37,45
GAPDH	++	++	++	33
FAS	++	++	++	43,44
ME	++	++	++	33
ACC	++	++	nd	43
GPDH	++	++	++	33
ACS	++	++	nd	43,45
PC	++	nd	nd	46

Note: 0, no increase in obese vs. lean; +, slight but significant increase; ++, marked increase; nd, not determined. LPL, lipoprotein lipase; GAPDH, glyceraldehyde-3-phosphate dehydrogenase; FAS, fatty acid synthetase; ME, malic enzyme; ACC, acetyl-CoA carboxylase; GPDH, glycerol-3-phosphate dehydrogenase; ACS, acetyl CoA synthetase; PC, pyruvate carboxylase.

activity in response to adrenergic stimuli,[48,49,51,52] that appears to be related to a defect at the level of the G-protein signaling system, since alterations in G protein status are found in these two models of genetic obesity. In the *ob/ob* mouse, both the stimulatory (through G_s) and the inhibitory (through G_i) regulation of adenylate cyclase are altered; this is correlated with a significant decrease in the levels of specific isoforms of the **a** subunits of G_s (42- and 45/46-kDa isoforms) and $G_{i\,a1}$ (41-kDa isoform), whereas no differences are detected in the levels of the **b** subunits.[48,50,51,54] In adipocytes from the obese Zucker rat, the levels of $G_{s\,a}$ as well as $G_{i\,a}$ are also markedly reduced when compared to membrane preparations from lean rats.[49,51] By contrast, in the *db/db* obese mutant, the abnormal kinetics of adenylate cyclase cannot be explained by a defect in the G protein system since similar proportions of the various isoforms of G_s and G_i are present in adipocytes of the *db/db* mouse compared to its lean control.[50,51] Since a deficiency in β adrenergic receptors is detected in adipocytes of the *db* mutant, the resistance of adenylate cyclase to catecholamines seen in adipose tissue of *db/db* mice could be explained by this deficit rather than by a lower abundance of the **a** subunit of G_s and G_i.[50,51] Further studies of the G-protein signaling system in obese rodent models are certainly warranted by these provocative findings.

III. SKELETAL MUSCLE

Insulin resistance is a characteristic feature of obesity and NIDDM. Although various defects in insulin action have been described in muscle and other organs from insulin-resistant rodents, as well as humans, the molecular mechanisms causing insulin resistance remain unclear. *In vivo,* skeletal muscle is the primary site of glucose disposal and, thus, the most important site for expression of insulin resistance.

A. GLUCOSE TRANSPORTER EXPRESSION

The insulin-resistant stage observed in obese-derived skeletal muscle is characterized by an impaired insulin-stimulated glucose uptake. Since the insulin-sensitive glucose transporter GLUT4 is also present in muscle, as well as adipose tissue,[55] potential defects in GLUT4 expression have been suggested to explain the markedly reduced glucose transport activity. A slight, but significant, reduction in GLUT4 protein levels (down to about 20 to 25%) has been reported for obese ZDF/drt rats and yellow *(A^{vy}/a)* mice,[11] as well as for morbidly obese human subjects with or without NIDDM.[56] However, most of the current studies have found no evidence for an impaired expression (mRNA and protein) of the major insulin-responsive glucose transporter in skeletal muscles derived from genetically obese rodents, including *ob/ob* and *db/db* mice and Zucker and Wistar diabetic fatty (WDF) rats, as well as in muscles from obese humans, in the presence or absence of NIDDM.[12,15,17,57-65] In the Zucker *fa/fa* rat, as indicated above, no change in muscle GLUT4 expression is observed, but alteration in translocation of this transporter is reported.[63] In the human studies, since the same muscles have been analyzed (vastus lateralis and/or rectus abdominis), the divergent results obtained in different studies are usually attributed to the heterogeneity of the obesity syndrome and/or to the large variation in muscle GLUT4 protein seen in normal subjects.[56,57,61] In obese rodents, various muscles displaying differences in fiber types are often used (gastrocnemius vs. soleus and/or quadriceps), suggesting that the variations reported in GLUT4 protein levels may be due, at least in part, to potential differences in glucose transporter expression in different fiber types.[11,61,62] Taken together with the results on adipose tissue, these studies clearly do establish the existence of a tissue-specific regulation of GLUT4 expression, so that transporter expression in insulin-resistant states, is much more affected in adipose cells than in muscle.[20,61] These studies also suggest that the changes in insulin-stimulated glucose transport seen in obese-derived muscle may be primarily due to alterations in the subcellular distribution or function of glucose transporters rather than to alterations in their level of expression.[17,20,61] Given that skeletal muscle is considered quantitatively more significant than adipose tissue in accounting for total-body insulin resistance, studies to date leave us with little in the way of consensus concerning how glucose transporter activity contributes to overall insulin resistance.

B. INSULIN RECEPTORS AND POSTRECEPTOR EVENTS

In obese-derived muscles, alterations in insulin action have been attributed to defects in insulin binding, to autophosphorylation of insulin receptor tyrosine kinase, and/or to insulin receptor tyrosine kinase activity. In most rodent models of obesity the decrease in insulin action is associated with a decrease in insulin binding, but autophosphorylation of the insulin receptor has been reported to be decreased or unchanged. In *ob/ob* mice the decrease seen in insulin action in muscle is associated with a decrease in receptor number, but the activity of the receptor tyrosine kinase against exogenous substrates, when corrected per insulin binding, appears to be normal.[66] The major defects in this model seem, therefore, to be a decrease in the number of insulin receptors and alterations at the postreceptor level. A significant reduction (~50%) in tyrosyl phosphorylation of a protein termed insulin receptor substrate-1 (IRS-1), or pp185, is indeed observed after insulin stimulation in *ob/ob* mouse muscle.[67] *In vitro,* the decrease in the phosphorylation of this cytoplasmic protein, which is known to be a direct substrate of the insulin receptor, is associated with defective insulin signaling.[67] This finding suggests that alterations in phosphorylation of IRS-1 may be a major factor in the insulin resistance of *ob/ob* mice. In *db/db* mice, insulin binding activity as well as tyrosine kinase activity expressed per insulin binding do not differ between obese and lean preparations,[66] demonstrating differences in insulin receptor regulation between the *ob/ob* and *db/db* models. Striking differences are also observed between the Zucker and WDF *fa/fa* rats, two congenic strains carrying the *fa* gene on different backgrounds.[68] Obese Zucker and obese WDF rats exhibit marked down-regulation of the insulin receptor, insulin receptor number being significantly lower in obese WDF compared to obese Zucker rats. In addition, only obese WDF rats display a decrease in tyrosine kinase activity per receptor compared to their lean controls and to obese Zucker rats.[69] In humans, all hyperinsulinemic obese subjects with or without NIDDM have a reduced number of insulin receptors in skeletal muscles.[70] The ability of insulin receptor tyrosine kinase to phosphorylate external substrates is also reduced.[70-72] In summary, a more consistent picture emerges with respect to insulin receptor dysregulation in animal models of obesity than is the case with respect to glucose transporters.

IV. PANCREAS

Among the candidates for a peripheral mechanism responsible for the onset of obesity is the endocrine pancreas, which displays abnormalities in most animal models of obesity, all of which are hyperinsulinemic and some frankly diabetic. Pancreatic function has been studied extensively, primarily in obese rodents.

A. HYPERINSULINEMIA

The fact that all genetically obese rodents are characterized by hyperinsulinemia[2,4] has led to the suggestion that insulin may play a primary role in the development and expression of obesity. Genetically obese rodents can also exhibit some degree of hyperglycemia, as seen in murine *(ob/ob* and *db/db)*[73] and rat (WDF *fa/fa,* SHR/N-cp [spontaneously hypertensive], ZDF-drt)[74-76] models, leading to the development of diabetes. Hyperinsulinemia is also characteristic of nongenetic models of obesity, e.g., the ventromedial hypothalamic-lesioned (VMH) obese rat and monkey,[2] spontaneously obese Rhesus monkeys,[77] and obese humans.[78] Although hyperinsulinemia is a well established feature of genetic as well as nongenetic obesity, its underlying mechanisms are still not totally understood. Both hypertrophy and hyperplasia of β-cells characterize pancreatic islets in obese rodents.[73] These factors *per se,* or hyperstimulation of these cells by a variety of secretogogues, both neural and hormonal, must be responsible for the major hypersecretion of insulin observed in obese rodents. It is also possible that impaired suppression of β-cell insulin secretion by inhibitory factors could contribute to the hypersecretion.

B. INSULIN SECRETION

A number of investigators have proposed that in the obese Zucker rat excessive parasympathetic activity via the vagus nerve mediates hypersecretion of insulin,[79-81] as it does for the VMH-lesioned rat.[82] This stimulation of vagal drive to pancreatic β-cells may be centrally mediated, at least in part, by glucocorticoids.[80] In *ob/ob* mice, a tonic elevation in vagal activity and/or an exaggerated muscarinic receptor sensitivity contribute to the persistent hyperinsulinemia seen in this model.[83] However, in a recent study no evidence was found for increased parasympathetic activity in obese-derived *ob/ob* islets, although even normal parasympathetic nervous system activity in the pancreas would contribute to hyperinsulinemia since the glucose hyperresponsiveness of *ob/ob* islets increases the islet response to acetylcholine.[84] This finding suggests that the major alteration in *ob/ob* mouse islets is in glucose sensitivity and responsiveness, which subsequently increase *ob/ob* islet susceptibility to neural regulation of insulin secretion.[84]

Alterations in the ionic permeability of the β-cell membrane also has been suggested as a cause of the hypersecretion of insulin in obese *ob/ob* mice.[85-87] However, although the presence in *ob/ob* mouse of a defective ATP-sensitive K^+ channel has been questioned repeatedly,[87-92] Fournier et al.[93] have recently concluded that the hypersecretory response of obese mouse β-cells is not related to an altered behavior of their ATP-sensitive potassium channels.

Galanin, a neuropeptide which has been proposed as a sympathetic neurotransmitter in the endocrine pancreas,[94] also has been suggested to be involved in development of hyperinsulinemia.[95] The pancreatic content of this 29-amino-acid peptide, which is known to inhibit insulin release both *in vivo* and *in vitro,*[94,96] has been reported to be decreased in the pancreas of obese *ob/ob* mice.[95]

The importance of insulin is underlined by the fact that this hormone plays a role in the stimulation of lipid deposition in adipose tissue, in the regulation of food intake, in sympathic neural activity, and in the overall regulation of body weight.[2] In obese *db/db* mice as well as in obese Zucker *fa/fa* rats, changes in insulin gene expression and pancreatic insulin content occur with the development of hyperinsulinemia. A fourfold elevation in plasma insulin and in pancreatic proinsulin mRNA is found in 5-week-old *db/db* mice. These levels decrease as the animals age and become increasingly glucose intolerant.[97,98] In obese Zucker rats, the preproinsulin mRNA (ppImRNA) levels and pancreatic content at 5 and 14 weeks of age are significantly higher than those of lean littermates.[99] On the contrary, WDF *fa/fa* rats at 5 and 14 weeks of age were found to have no differences in ppImRNA levels or in insulin content when compared to lean animals.[99,100] These results indicate that insulin genes are subject to differing regulation in these two animal models of obesity, resulting in the development of frank diabetes in WDF *fa/fa* rats, but not in Zucker *fa/fa* rats.[99] Pancreatic preproinsulin mRNA and plasma insulin increase to a greater extent with age in obese Zucker rats than in lean ones, suggesting that increased fat deposition is associated with enhanced insulin gene expression in these animals. Although insulin appears to play a role in the expression of the obese phenotype, it has been shown that hyperinsulinemia itself is not a necessary condition for the development of obesity in the Zucker *fa/fa* rat.[101]

Abnormalities in the insulin secretory pattern also have been reported for several obese nondiabetic as well as obese diabetic models. The most common alteration is a paradoxically high insulin secretion at low glucose levels that is observed in most rodent models of obesity, including obese *ob/ob* mice,[84,85] obese Zucker rats,[102] and obese nondiabetic LA/N-cp and obese diabetic SHR/N-cp rats.[103] This insulin secretory response to low glucose suggests a sensitization to glucose which is somehow related to the abnormal function of the (still unidentified) *fa* and *cp* mutant gene products.[103] In obese diabetic SHR/N-cp rats, an impaired response of insulin secretion to high glucose is also observed. This alteration is absent in obese LA/N-cp rats as well as in prediabetic obese SHR rats, suggesting that hyperglycemia is required for expression of the defect.[103] A decrease in the glucose sensitivity of pancreatic β-cells was also reported for obese Zucker rats fed a diabetogenic diet, the progressive development of hyperglycemia induced by the diet leading to an impaired β-cell sensitivity to glucose.[104]

The normal insulin secretory response to hyperglycemia is dependent on glucose uptake into β-cells, mediated through the action of the glucose transporter GLUT2.[105,106] In *db/db* mice, as well as in the Zucker substrain ZDF/drt, which is diabetic as well as obese, impaired glucose-stimulated insulin secretion is associated with down-regulation of the normal β-cell glucose transporter, GLUT2. GLUT2 protein and/or GLUT2 mRNA levels were lower than the levels detected in lean controls.[105-108] Unger suggests that this down-regulation in GLUT2 expression may be the cause of diabetic hyperglycemia.[106,108] However, since the decrease in GLUT2 expression appears to be reversible when islets are placed in nondiabetic conditions,[105] this hypothesis may not be substantiated. In addition, this laboratory has obtained results in the WDF strain showing no decrease in GLUT2 mRNA in pancreas of frankly diabetic obese male rats.[109] The reasons for these discrepancies between species and strains remain to be established, but at this point it appears unlikely that impaired regulation of insulin secretion associated with obesity and NIDDM can be explained solely by differences in GLUT2 expression.

C. GLUCAGON

Among the pancreatic secretions, glucagon is an important regulator of hepatic glucose production and has been thought to be involved in obesity-related abnormalities of glucose tolerance. Glucagon levels in obesity remain controversial since normal, elevated, and decreased levels have all been reported under various conditions. Higher glucagon levels have been reported in obese humans, especially in subjects with fatty liver and hypertriglyceridemia,[110] but also in persons displaying abdominal obesity.[111]

D. PANCREATIC POLYPEPTIDE AND SOMATOSTATIN

Pancreatic polypeptide (PP) levels have also been reported to be normal, elevated, and depressed in obese subjects, but the majority of the data obtained in humans reveal normal values for PP and somatostatin.[111] Somatostatin is a potent inhibitor of pancreatic insulin release, and a potential role for somatostatin in the pathogenesis of hyperinsulinemia has been suggested.[112] In *ob/ob* mice, lower than normal concentrations were reported for both the pancreas and the stomach.[113] By contrast, in obese Zucker and obese SHR/N-cp rats, pancreatic levels of somatostatin were significantly higher than those seen in lean littermates. Gastric somatostatin levels were reduced, but only in obese Zucker rats.[112]

E. AMYLIN

The pancreatic levels of islet amyloid polypeptide (IAPP), or amylin, are also perturbed in obese rodents. IAPP is a 37-amino-acid peptide produced by the β-cell and cosecreted with insulin. Its release appears to be regulated by glucose and other insulin secretagogues. IAPP has been suggested to have a role in the development of NIDDM as well as to be involved in peripheral insulin resistance.[114] In obese Zucker rats, as well as in the

VMH-lesioned rat, concentrations of IAPP in islets were found to be elevated when compared to lean or sham-operated controls, and in both models obese-derived isolated islets secreted larger amounts of IAPP than did lean-derived islets. These findings indicate that both overproduction and hypersecretion of IAPP occur in animals with obesity and hyperinsulinemia.[115,116]

In summary, it is well established that severe abnormalities occur in the regulation of pancreatic endocrine function in obese animal models. In most ways the problems reported reflect the pathologies seen in humans with NIDDM; thus, a number of these rodent strains remain excellent candidates for studies designed to tease apart the complex interactions of obesity and non-insulin-dependent diabetes.

V. BROWN ADIPOSE TISSUE

Brown adipose tissue (BAT) is the principal site of nonshivering thermogenesis in many mammals, and in some species it also plays an important role in the regulation of energy balance.[117] In many models of obesity the capacity for facultative thermogenesis is decreased. In the newborn Zucker *fa/fa* rat, BAT is thermogenically quiescent, with a low level of expression of thermogenin message (UCP mRNA). Like *ob/ob* and *db/db* mice, the newborn *fa/fa* rat is extremely cold intolerant and displays a decreased capacity of thyroxine (T4) to 5,3′-triiodothyronine (T3) conversion in BAT.[117,118] This decreased capacity for T3 production is one of the earliest known changes detectable in Zucker *fa/fa* pups, confirming that BAT is the earliest known site of *fa/fa* genotype expression.[118] However, in contrast to *ob/ob* and *db/db* mice, *fa/fa* pups respond normally to cold stress by increasing BAT thyroxine 5′-deiodinase activity to the same extent as their lean counterparts.[118] After weaning, the capacity for T4 to T3 conversion is restored in BAT, but is dramatically reduced in liver, the concentration of serum free T3 remaining lower in obese than in lean Zucker rats.[118] In the adult *fa/fa* rat, diet-induced activation of BAT thermogenesis fails to occur. BAT is usually in a quiescent and atrophied state, with a progressive reduction in UCP mRNA level and mitochondria UCP concentration and a low sympathetic nervous system activity.[117] A reduced level of mitochondrial GTP binding is detectable, even in BAT of rats that are only heterozygous for the *fa* gene. Sympathetic nervous system activity in BAT of *ob/ob* as well as *db/db* mice is also low, resulting in atrophy of BAT, with a low level of GTP binding and of UCP in the mitochondria and a reduced capacity to respond to noradrenaline or to acute cold exposure by an increase in thermogenesis.[117] The yellow mouse *(A^{vy}/a)* also displays reduced GTP binding and has reduced sympathic nervous system activity, but BAT in yellow obese mice is of normal size (protein and DNA) and appears to be maintained in a reasonably functional state since thermogenesis is increased by both cold exposure and injection of noradrenaline.[117] In corpulent rat models, marked differences in BAT thermogenic capacity exist between the obese nondiabetic LA/N-cp and the obese diabetic SHR/N-cp rats.[119] In SHR rats, a decrease in total BAT protein content and total tissue cytochrome oxidase as well as a decrease in insulin stimulation of glucose transport and a decreased responsiveness and sensitivity to norepinephrine are observed. All of these parameters are normal in the obese nondiabetic LA/N-cp rat, suggesting that the mechanism leading to obesity in these two strains is different.[120] Insulin-stimulated glucose utilization is also markedly decreased in BAT of obese Zucker rats.[121] This decrease in the effect of insulin could not be attributed to the alteration of GLUT4 expression since a similar level of expression for GLUT4 mRNA, as well as GLUT4 protein, was detected in BAT from lean and obese Zucker rats.[121] In most models of genetic obesity there is an apparent association between insulin resistance in BAT and defective thermogenesis. In *db/db* and *ob/ob* mice as well as in Zucker *fa/fa* rats there is an early and selective development of insulin resistance in BAT, before it appears in other tissues.[117,122,123] This may contribute to the atrophied state of BAT that is seen in these models. Insulin resistance does not appear to affect the basal activity of the thermogenic mitochondrial proton conductance pathway, but studies on *ob/ob* mice suggest that it does impair the acute cold-induced activation of the pathway. Insulin resistance in BAT also may lead to a decreased mitochondriogenesis, as suggested for *ob/ob* mice[124] and SHR/N-cp rats,[119] and to a decrease in induction of uncoupling protein on cold exposure,[124,125] which results in a reduced thermogenic capacity. This series of events could, therefore, contribute to the development of obesity.

VI. FUTURE DIRECTIONS

To date, none of the studies of gene products that have been considered as potential candidates for one of the obese mutant genes in rodent models have led to direct identification of the primary lesion(s) produced by the mutant gene. To date, none of the mutant genes have been cloned and sequenced; thus, their protein products remain unknown. The fact that there are so many specific abnormalities of metabolic regulation and gene expression occurring in obese rodent models has led our laboratory to propose that the lesion(s) produced by obese mutant genes is likely to be a regulatory defect that is subsequently expressed in various ways in different tissues — i.e., a pleotropic effect. Further studies designed to look at regulatory pathways in early stages of development of obesity appear to be a fruitful approach, as well as continued efforts to clone and sequence the mutant genes.

REFERENCES

1. **Cuenot, G.,** Pure strains and their combination in the mouse, *Arch. Zool. Exp. Genet.,* 122, 123, 1905
2. **Bray, G. A., York, D. A., and Fisler, J. S.,** Experimental obesity: a homeostatic failure due to defective nutrient stimulation of the sympathetic nervous system, *Vitam. Horm. N.Y.,* 45, 1, 1989.
3. **Argiles, J. M.,** The obese Zucker rat: a choice for fat metabolism. Twenty years of research on the insights of the Zucker mutation, *Prog. Lipid Res.,* 28, 53, 1989.
4. **Johnson, P. R., Greenwood, M. R. C., Horwitz, B. A., and Stern, J. S.,** Animal models of obesity: genetic aspects, in *Annual Review of Nutrition,* Annual Reviews, Palo Alto, CA, 1991, 325.
5. **Magrum, L. J., Horwitz, B. A., and Stern, J. S.,** Animal models of obesity: diet, inactivity and genetics, in Proc. 1992 Vahoney Symp., Kritchevsky, D. and Bonfield, C., Eds., in press.
6. **Bahary, N., Leibel, R. L., Joseph, L., and Friedman, J. M.,** Molecular mapping of the mouse *db* mutation, *Proc. Natl. Acad. Sci. U.S.A.,* 87, 8642, 1990.
7. **Friedman, J. M., Leibel, R. L., Siegel, D. S., Walsh, J., and Bahary, N.,** Molecular mapping of the mouse *ob* mutation, *Genomics,* 11, 1054, 1991.
8. **Truett, E. E., Bahary, N., Friedman, J. M., and Leibel, R. L.,** Rat obesity gene fatty *(fa)* maps to chromosome 5: evidence for homology with the mouse gene diabetes *(db), Proc. Natl. Acad. Sci. U.S.A.,* 88, 7806, 1991.
9. **Kahn, B. B. and Flier, J.,** Regulation of glucose transporter gene expression in vitro and in vivo, *Diabetes Care,* 13, 548, 1990.
10. **Charron, M. J., Brosius, F. C., Alper, S. L., and Lodish, H. F.,** A novel glucose transporter protein expressed predominately in insulin-responsive tissues, *Proc. Natl. Acad. Sci. U.S.A.,* 86, 2535, 1989.

11. **Slieker, L. J., Sundell, K. L., Heath, W. F., Osborne, H. E., Bue, J., Manetta, J., and Sportman, J. R.,** Glucose transporter levels in tissue of spontaneously diabetic Zucker fa/fa rat (ZDF/drt) and viable yellow mouse (A^{vy}/a), *Diabetes,* 41, 187, 1992.
12. **Yamamoto, T., Fukumoto, H., Koh, G., Yano H., Yasuda, K., Masuda, K., Ikeda, H., Imura, H., and Seino, Y.,** Liver and muscle-fat type glucose transporter gene expression in obese and diabetic rats, *Biochem. Biophys. Res. Commun.,* 175, 995, 1991.
13. **Sinha, M. K., Raineri-Maldonado, C., Buchanan, C., Pories, W., Carter-Su, C., Pilch, P. F., and Caro, J.,** Adipose tissue glucose transporters in NIDDM. Decreased levels of muscle/fat isoform, *Diabetes,* 40, 472, 1991.
14. **Garvey, W. T., Maianu, L., Hueckstead, T. P., Birnbaum, M. J., Molina, J. M., and Ciaraldi, T. P.,** Pretranslational suppression of a glucose transporter protein causes insulin resistance in adipocytes from patients with non-insulin-dependent diabetes mellitus and obesity, *J. Clin. Invest.,* 87, 1072, 1991.
15. **Hainault, I., Guerre-Millo, M., Guichard, C., and Lavau, M.,** Differential regulation of adipose tissue glucose transporters in genetic obesity (fatty rat). Selective increase in the adipose tissue/muscle glucose transporter (GLUT4) expression, *J. Clin. Invest.,* 87, 1127, 1991.
16. **Guerre-Millo, M., Lavau, M., Horne, J. S., and Wardzala, L. J.,** Proposed mechanism for increased insulin-mediated glucose transport in adipose cells from young rats. Large intracellular pool of glucose transporters, *J. Biol. Chem.,* 260, 2197, 1985.
17. **Koranyi, L., James, D., Mueckler, M., and Permutt, M. A.,** Glucose transporter levels in spontaneously obese (db/db) insulin-resistant mice, *J. Clin. Invest.,* 85, 962, 1990.
18. **Pedersen, O., Kahn, C. R., and Kahn, B. B.,** Divergent regulation of the GLUT1 and GLUT4 glucose transporters in isolated adipocytes from Zucker rats, *J. Clin. Invest.,* 89, 1964, 1992.
19. **Baly, D. L., Zarnowski, M. J., Carswell, N., and Michaelis, O. E.,** Insulin resistant transport activity in adipose cells from the SHR/N-corpulent rat, *J. Nutr.,* 119, 628, 1989.
20. **Kahn, B. B. and Pedersen, O.,** Tissue-specific regulation of glucose transporters in different forms of obesity, *Proc. Soc. Exp. Biol. Med.,* 200, 214, 1992.
21. **Kahn, B. B., Cushman, S. W., and Flier, J. S.,** Regulation of glucose transporter-specific mRNA levels in rat adipose cells with fasting and refeeding, *J. Clin. Invest.,* 83, 199, 1989.
22. **Cook, K. S., Min, H.-Y., Johnson, D., Chaplinsky, R. J., Flier, J. S., Hunt, C. R., and Spiegelman, B. M.,** Adipsin: a circulating serine protease homolog secreted by adipose tissue and sciatic nerve, *Science,* 237, 402, 1987.
23. **White, T. R., Damm, D., Hancock, N., Rosen, B. S., Lowell, B. B., Usher, P., Flier, J. S., and Spiegelman, B. M.,** Human adipsin is identical to complement factor D and is expressed at high levels in adipose tissue, *J. Biol. Chem.,* 267, 9210, 1992.
24. **Rosen, B., Cook, K. S., Yaglom, J., Groves, D. L., Volanakis, J. E., Damm, D., White, T., and Spiegelman, B. M.,** Adipsin and complement factor D activity: an immuno-related defect in obesity, *Science,* 244, 1483, 1989.
25. **Rosen, B., Cook, K. S., Yaglom, J., Groves, D. L., Volanakis, J. E., Damm, D., White, T., and Spiegelman, B. M.,** Adipsin and the alternative pathway of complement in the regulation of energy balance, in *Obesity: Towards a Molecular Approach,* Spiegelman, B. M. and Ricquier, E., Eds., Alan R. Liss, New York, 1990, 273.
26. **Flier, J. S., Lowell, B., Napolitano, A., Usher, P., Rosen, B., Cook, K., and Spiegelman, B.,** Adipsin: regulation and dysregulation in obesity and other metabolic states, *Recent Prog. Horm. Res.,* 45, 567, 1989.

27. **Dugail, I., Quignard-Boulange, A., Le Liepvre, X., and Lavau, M.,** Impairment of adipsin expression is secondary to the onset of obesity in db/db mice, *J. Biol. Chem.,* 265, 1831, 1990.
28. **Johnson, P. R., Spiegelman, B. M., Rosen, B., Turkenkopf, I., Ree, H., and Greenwood, M. R. C.,** Reduced adipsin mRNA and circulating adipsin protein are modulated by adrenal steroids in obese Zucker rats, *Am. J. Physiol.,* 259, R184, 1990.
29. **Shillabeer, G., Hornford, J., Forden, J. M., Wong, N. C. W., Russel, J. C., and Lau, D. C. W.,** Fatty acid synthase and adipsin mRNA levels in obese and lean JCR:LA-cp rats: effect of diet, *J. Lipid Res.,* 33, 31, 1992.
30. **Choy, L. N., Rosen, B. S., and Spiegelman, B. M.,** An endogenous pathway of complement from adipose cells, *J. Biol. Chem.,* 267, 12736, 1992.
31. **Hotamisligil, G. S., Shargill, N. S., and Spiegelman, B. M.,** Adipose expression of tumor necrosis factor-a: direct role in obesity-linked insulin resistance, *Science,* 259, 87, 1993.
32. **Gruen, R., Hietanen, E., and Greenwood, M. R. C.,** Increased adipose tissue lipoprotein lipase activity during the development of the genetically obese rat (fa/fa), *Metab. Clin. Exp.,* 27, 1955, 1978.
33. **Dugail, I., Quignard-Boulange, A., Le Liepvre, X., Ardouin, B., and Lavau, M.,** Gene expression of lipid storage-related enzymes in adipose tissue of the genetically obese Zucker rat, *Biochem. J.,* 281, 607, 1992.
34. **Lemmonier, D., de Gasquet, P., Mackay, S., Planche, E., Alexiu, A., Rosselin, G., and Loiseau, A.,** Different levels of food restriction have opposite effects on adipocyte cellularity and lipoprotein-lipase activity in obese rats, *Diabete Metab.,* 15, 394, 1989.
35. **Fried, S. K, Turkenkopf, I. J., Goldberg, I. J., Doolittle, M. H., Kirchgessner, T. G., Schotz, M. C., Johnson, P. R., and Greenwood, M. R. C.,** Mechanisms of increased lipoprotein lipase in fat cells of obese Zucker rats, *Am. J. Physiol.,* 261, E653, 1991.
36. **Ong, J. M. and Kern, P. A.,** Effect of feeding and obesity on lipoprotein lipase activity, immunoreactive protein, and messenger RNA levels in human adipose tissue, *J. Clin. Invest.,* 84, 305, 1989.
37. **Bessesen, D. H., Robertson, A. D., and Eckel, R. H.,** Weight reduction increases adipose but decreases cardiac LPL in reduced-obese-Zucker rats, *Am. J. Physiol.,* 261, E246, 1991.
38. **Boulange, A., Planche, E., and de Gasquet, P.,** Onset of genetic obesity in the absence of hyperphagia during the first week of life in the Zucker rat (fa/fa), *J. Lipid Res.,* 20, 857,1979.
39. **Greenwood, M. R. C.,** Enzymatic alterations in the obese: long or short-term regulatory errors?, *Int. J. Obes.,* 8, 561, 1984.
40. **Greenwood, M. R. C.,** The relationship of enzyme activity to feeding behavior in rats: lipoprotein lipase as the metabolic gatekeeper, *Int. J. Obes.,* 9, 67, 1985.
41. **Bazin, R. and Lavau, M.,** Development of hepatic and adipose tissue lipogenic enzymes and insulinemia during suckling and weaning on to a high-fat diet in Zucker rats, *J. Lipid Res.,* 23, 839, 1982.
42. **Dugail, I., Quignard-Boulange, A., Brigant, L., Etienne, J., Noe, L., and Lavau, M.,** Increased lipoprotein lipase content in the adipose tissue of suckling and weaning obese Zucker rats, *Biochem. J.,* 249, 45, 1988.
43. **Penicaud, L., Ferre, P., Assimacoupoulos-Jeannet, F., Perdereau, D., Leturque, A., Jeanrenaud, B., Picon, L., and Girard, J.,** Increased gene expression of lipogenic enzymes and glucose transporter in white adipose tissue of suckling and weaned obese Zucker rats, *Biochem. J.,* 279, 303, 1991.

44. **Guichard, C., Dugail, I., Le Liepvre, X., and Lavau, M.,** Genetic regulation of fatty acid synthetase expression in adipose tissue: overtranscription of the gene in genetically obese rats, *J. Lipid Res.,* 33, 679, 1992.
45. **Shimomura, I., Tokunaga, K., Jiao, S., Funahashi, T., Keno, Y., Kobatake, T., Kotani, K., Suzuki, H., Yamamoto, T., Tarui, S., and Matsuzawa, Y.,** Marked enhancement of acyl-CoA synthetase activity and mRNA, parallel to lipoprotein lipase mRNA, in adipose tissues of Zucker obese rats (fa/fa), *Biochim. Biophys. Acta,* 1124, 112, 1992.
46. **Lynch, C. J., McCall, K. M., Billingsley, M. L., Bohlen, L. M., Hreniuk, S. P., Martin, L. F., Witters, L. A., and Vannucci, S. J.,** Pyruvate carboxylase in genetic obesity, *Am. J. Physiol.,* 262, E608, 1992.
47. **Turkenkopf, I. J., Johnson, P. R., and Greenwood, M. R. C.,** Development of pancreatic and plasma insulin in prenatal and suckling Zucker rats, *Am. J. Physiol.,* 242, E220, 1982.
48. **Begin-Heick, N.,** Absence of inhibitory effect of guanine nucleotides on adenylate cyclase activity in white adipocyte membranes of the ob/ob mouse. Effect of the ob gene, *J. Biol. Chem.,* 260, 6187, 1985.
49. **Strassheim, D., Palmer, T., Milligan, G., and Houslay, M. D.,** Alterations in G-protein expression and the hormonal regulation of adenylate cyclase in the adipocytes of obese (fa/fa) Zucker rats, *Biochem. J.,* 276, 197, 1991.
50. **Begin-Heick, N.,** a-Subunits of G(s) and G(i) in adipocyte plasma membranes of genetically diabetic (db db) mice, *Am. J. Physiol.,* 263, C121, 1992.
51. **Begin-Heick, N. and McFarlane-Anderson, N.,** G-Proteins in obesity, in *G-Proteins — Signal Transduction and Disease,* Milligan, G. and Wakelam, M., Eds., Academic Press, New York, 1992, 129.
52. **Naim, M., Katz, Y., Brand, J. G., and Kare, M. R.,** Nonreceptor-mediated responses of adenylate cyclase in membranes from liver, muscle, and white and brown adipose tissue of obese (fa/fa) and lean (Fa/) Zucker rats, *Proc. Soc. Exp. Biol. Med.,* 195, 369, 1990.
53. **Strassheim, D., Palmer, T., and Houslay, M. D.,** Genetically acquired diabetes: adipocyte guanine nucleotide regulatory protein expression and adenylate cyclase regulation, *Biochim. Biophys. Acta,* 1096, 121, 1991.
54. **Begin-Heick, N.,** Quantification of the a and b subunits of the transducing elements (G_s and G_i) of adenylate cyclase in adipocyte membranes from lean and obese (ob/ob) mice, *Biochem. J.,* 268, 83, 1990.
55. **James, D. E., Brown, R., Navarro, J., and Pilch, P. F.,** Insulin regulatable tissues express a unique insulin-sensitive glucose transport protein, *Nature,* 333, 183, 1988.
56. **Dohm, G. L., Elton, C. W., Friedman, J. E., Pilch, P. F., Pories, W. J., Atkinson, S. M., Jr., and Caro, J. F.,** Decreased expression of glucose transporter in muscle from insulin-resistant patients, *Am. J. Physiol.,* 260, E459, 1991.
57. **Pedersen, O., Bak, J. F., Andersen, P. H., Lund, S., Moller, D. E., Flier, J. S., and Kahn B. B.,** Evidence against altered expression of GLUT1 or GLUT4 in skeletal muscle of patients with obesity or NIDDM, *Diabetes,* 39, 865, 1990.
58. **Handberg, A., Vaag, A., Damsbo, P., Beck-Nielsen, H., and Vinten, J.,** Expression of insulin regulatable glucose transporters in skeletal muscle from type 2 (non-insulin-dependent) diabetic patients, *Diabetologia,* 33, 625, 1990.
59. **Friedman, J. E., Sherman, W. M., Reed, M. J., Elton, C. W., Dohm, G. L.,** Exercise training increases glucose transporter protein GLUT4 in skeletal muscle of obese Zucker (fa/fa) rats, *FEBS Lett.,* 268, 13, 1990.

60. **Friedman, J. E., Dohm, G. L., Leggett-Frazier, N., Elton, C. W., Tapscott, E. B., Pories, W. P., and Caro, J.,** Restoration of insulin responsiveness in skeletal muscle of morbidly obese patients after weight loss. Effect on muscle glucose transport and glucose transporter GLUT4, *J. Clin. Invest.,* 89, 701, 1992.
61. **Garvey, T. W., Maianu, L., Hancock, J. A., Golichowski, A. M., and Baron, A.,** Gene expression of GLUT4 in skeletal muscle from insulin-resistant patients with obesity, IGT, GDM, and NIDDM, *Diabetes,* 41, 465, 1992.
62. **Brozinick, J. T., Etgen, G. J., Yaspelkis, B. B., and Ivy, J. L.,** Contraction-activated glucose uptake is normal in insulin-resistant muscle in the obese Zucker rat, *J. Appl. Physiol.,* 73, 382, 1992.
63. **King, P. A., Horton, E. D., Hirshman, M. F., and Horton, E. S.,** Insulin resistance in obese Zucker (fa/fa) skeletal muscle is associated with a failure of glucose transporter translocation, *J. Clin. Invest.,* 90, 1568, 1992.
64. **Seino, Y., Yamamoto, T., and Koh, G.,** Insulin and glucose transporter gene expression in obesity and diabetes, *Proc. Soc. Exp. Biol. Med.,* 200, 210, 1992.
65. **Zarjeski, N., Doyle, P., and Jeanrenaud, B.,** Muscle insulin resistance may not be a primary etiological factor in the genetically obese fa/fa rat, *Endocrinology,* 130, 1564, 1992.
66. **Vicario, P., Brady, E. J., Slater, E. E., and Saperstein, R.,** Insulin receptor tyrosine kinase activity is unaltered in ob/ob and db/db mouse skeletal muscle membranes, *Life Sci.,* 41, 1233, 1987.
67. **Saad, M. J., Araki, E., Miralpeix, M., Rothenberg, P. L., White, M. F., and Kahn, C. R.,** Regulation of insulin receptor substrate-1 in liver and muscle of animal models of insulin resistance, *J. Clin. Invest.,* 90, 1839, 1992.
68. **Kava, R., Peterson, R. G., West, D. B., and Greenwood, M. R. C.,** Wistar diabetic fatty rat, *ILAR News,* 32, 9, 1990.
69. **Greene, S. F., Johnson, P. R., Eiffert, K. C., Greenwood, M. R. C., and Stern, J. S.,** unpublished data.
70. **Beck-Nielsen, H.,** Insulin resistance in skeletal muscles of patients with diabetes mellitus, *Diabetes Metab. Rev.,* 5, 487, 1989.
71. **Caro, J. F., Dohm, L. G., Pories, W. J., and Sinha, M. K.,** Cellular alteration in liver, skeletal muscle, and adipose tissue responsible for insulin resistance in obesity and type II diabetes, *Diabetes Metab. Rev.,* 5, 665, 1989.
72. **Arner, P., Pollare, T., Lithell, H., and Livingston, J. N.,** Defective insulin receptor kinase in human skeletal muscle in obesity and type 2 (non-insulin-dependent) diabetes mellitus, *Diabetologia,* 30, 437, 1987.
73. **Coleman, D. L.,** Obese and diabetes: two mutant genes causing diabetes-obesity syndromes in mice, *Diabetologia,* 14, 141, 1978.
74. **Ikeda, H., Shino, A., Matsuo, T., Iwatsuka, H., and Suzuoki, Z.,** A new genetically obese-hyperglycemic rat (Wistar fatty), *Diabetes,* 30, 1045, 1981.
75. **Hansen, C. T.,** Two new congenic strains for nutrition and obesity research, *Fed. Proc.,* 42, 537, 1983.
76. **Clark, J. B., Palmer, C. J., and Shaw, W. N.,** The diabetic Zucker fatty rat, *Proc. Soc. Exp. Biol. Med.,* 173, 68, 1983.
77. **Hansen, B. C. and Bodkin, N. L.,** B-Cell hyperresponsiveness: earliest events in development of diabetes in monkeys, *Am. J. Physiol.,* 259, R612, 1990.
78. **Elahi, D., Nagulesparan, M., Herscopf, R. J., Muller, D. C., Tobin, J. D., Blix, P. M., Rubenstein, A. I. L., Unger, R. H., and Andres, R.,** Feedback inhibition of the insulin secretion by insulin. Relation to the hyperinsulinemia of obesity, *N. Engl. J. Med.,* 306, 1196, 1982.

79. **Rohner-Jeanrenaud, F., Hochstrasser, A. C., and Jeanrenaud, B.,** Hyperinsulinemia of preobese and obese fa/fa rats is partly vagus nerve mediated, *Am. J. Physiol.,* 244, E317, 1983.
80. **Stubbs, M. and York, D.,** Central glucocorticoid regulation of parasympathic drive to pancreatic B-cells in the obese fa/fa rat, *Int. J. Obes.,* 15, 547, 1991.
81. **Lee, H. C., Curry, D. L., and Stern, J. S.,** Direct effect of CNS on insulin hypersecretion in obese Zucker rats: involvement of vagus nerve, *Am. J. Physiol.,* 256, E439, 1989.
82. **Campfield, L. A., Smith, F. J., and LeMagnen, J.,** Altered endocrine pancreatic function following vagotomy: possible behavioral and metabolic bases for assessing completeness of vagotomy, *J. Auton. Nerv. Syst.,* 9, 283, 1983.
83. **Fukudo, S., Virnelli, S., Kuhn, C. M., Cochrane, C., Feinglos, M. N., and Surwit, R. S.,** Muscarinic stimulation and antagonism and glucoregulation in nondiabetic and obese hyperglycemic mice, *Diabetes,* 38, 1433, 1989.
84. **Tassava, T. M., Okuda, T., and Romsos, D. R.,** Insulin secretion from ob/ob mouse pancreatic islets: effects of neurotransmitters, *Am. J. Physiol.,* 262, E338, 1992.
85. **Black, M. A., Heick, H. M., and Begin-Heick, N.,** Abnormal regulation of insulin secretion in the genetically obese (ob/ob) mice, *Biochem. J.,* 238, 863, 1986.
86. **Black, M. A., Fournier, L., Heick, H. M., and Begin-Heick, N.,** Different insulin-secretory responses to calcium-channel blockers in islets of lean and obese (ob/ob) mice, *Biochem. J.,* 249, 401, 1988.
87. **Black, M. A., Heick, H. M., and Begin-Heick, N.,** Abnormal regulation of cAMP accumulation in pancreatic islets of obese mice, *Am. J. Physiol.,* 255, E833, 1988.
88. **Rosario, L.,** Differential effects of the K^+ channel blockers apamin and quinine on glucose-induced electrical activity in pancreatic b-cells from a strain of ob/ob (obese) mice, *FEBS Lett.,* 188, 302, 1985.
89. **Rosario, L., Atwater, I., and Rojas, E.,** Membrane potential measurements in islets of Langerhans from ob/ob obese mice suggest an alteration in [$Ca2^+$]-activated K^+ permeability, *Q. J. Exp. Physiol.,* 70, 137, 1985.
90. **Scott, A. M., Dawson, C. M., and Goncalves, A. A.,** Comparison of glucose-induced changes in electrical activity, insulin release, lactate output and potassium permeability between normal and ob/ob mouse islets: effects of cooling, *J. Endocrinology,* 107, 265, 1985.
91. **Fournier, L., Heick, H. M. C., and Begin-Heick, N.,** The influence of K^+-induced membrane depolarization on insulin secretion in islets of lean and obese (ob/ob) mice, *Biochem. Cell Biol.,* 68, 243, 1990.
92. **Kukuljan, M., Yi Li, M., and Atwater, I.,** Characterization of potassium channels in pancreatic b cells from ob/ob mice, *FEBS Lett.,* 266, 105,1990.
93. **Fournier, L., Begin-Heick, N., Whitfield, J. F., and Schwartz, J.-L.,** Comparison of the properties of the ATP-sensitive K+ channels of pancreatic b-cells of lean and obese (ob/ob) C57BL/6J mice, *J. Membr. Biol.,* 129, 267, 1992.
94. **Dunning, B. E., Ahren, B., Veith, R. C., Bottcher, G., Sundler, F., and Taborsky, G. J.,** Galanin: a novel pancreatic neuropeptide, *Am. J. Physiol.,* 255, E785, 1986.
95. **Dunning, B. E. and Ahren, B.,** Reduced pancreatic content of the inhibitory neurotransmitter galanin in genetically obese, hyperinsulinemic mice, *Pancreas,* 7, 233, 1992.
96. **Ahren, B., Arkhammar, P., Berggren, P. O., and Nilsson, T.,** Galanin inhibits glucose-stimulated insulin release by a mechanism involving hyperpolarization and lowering of cytoplasmic free Ca^{2+} concentration, *Biochem. Biophys. Res. Commun.,* 140, 1059, 1986.

97. **Orland, M. J., Chyn, R., and Permutt, M. A.,** Modulation of proinsulin mRNA after partial pancreatectomy in rats: relationship to glucose homeostasis, *J. Clin. Invest.,* 75, 2047, 1985.
98. **Orland, M. J. and Permutt, M. A.,** Quantitative analysis of pancreatic proinsulin mRNA in genetically diabetic (db/db) mice, *Diabetes,* 36, 341, 1987.
99. **Koh, G., Seino, Y., Usami, M., Ikeda, H., Yamamoto, T., Tsuda, K., Taminato, T., and Imura, H.,** Importance of impaired insulin-gene expression in occurrence of diabetes in obese rats, *Diabetes,* 39, 1050, 1990.
100. **Seino, Y., Yamamoto, T., and Koh, G.,** Insulin and glucose transporter gene expression in obesity and diabetes, *Proc. Soc. Exp. Biol. Med.,* 200, 210, 1992.
101. **Chan, C. P. and Stern, J. S.,** Adipose lipoprotein lipase in insulin-treated diabetic lean and obese Zucker rats, *Am. J. Physiol.,* 242, E445, 1982.
102. **Curry, D. L. and Stern, J. S.,** Dynamics of insulin hypersecretion by obese Zucker rats, *Metabolism,* 34, 791, 1985.
103. **Recant, L., Voyles, N. R., Timmers, K. I., Bathena, S. J., Solomon, D., Wilkins, S., and Michaelis, O. E.,** Comparison of insulin secretory patterns in obese nondiabetic LA/N-cp and obese diabetic SHR/N-cp rats, *Diabetes,* 38, 691, 1989.
104. **Furnsinn, M., Komjati, M., Madsen, O. D., Schneider, B., and Waldhausel, N.,** Lifelong sequential changes in glucose tolerance and insulin secretion in genetically obese Zucker rats fafa fed a diabetogenic diet, *Endocrinology,* 128, 1093, 1992.
105. **Thorens, B., Wu, Y.-J., Leahy, J. L., and Weir, G. C.,** The loss of GLUT2 expression by glucose-unresponsive b cells of db/db mice is reversible and is induced by the diabetic environment, *J. Clin. Invest.,* 90, 77, 1992.
106. **Unger, R. H.,** Diabetic hyperglycemia: link to impaired glucose transport in pancreatic b cells, *Science,* 251, 1200, 1991.
107. **Johnson, J. H., Ogawa, A., Chen, L., Orci, L., Newgard, C. B., Alam, T., and Unger, R. H.,** Underexpression of beta cell high Km glucose transporter in non-insulin-dependent diabetes, *Science,* 250, 546, 1990.
108. **Orci, L., Johnson, J. H., and Unger, R. H.,** Evidence that down-regulation of beta cell glucose transporters in non-insulin-dependent diabetes may be the cause of hyperglycemia, *Proc. Natl. Acad. Sci. U.S.A.,* 87, 9953, 1990.
109. **Albright, A., Gregoire, F., Greene, S., Gaudette, K., Greenwood, M. R. C., and Johnson, P. R.,** unpublished data.
110. **Starke, A., Erhardt, G., Berger, M., and Zimmerman, H.,** Elevated pancreatic glucagon in obesity, *Diabetes,* 33, 277, 1984.
111. **Van Gaal, L., Vanderkam, S., Duysburgh, I., and De Leeuw, I.,** Endocrine abnormalities related to total and regional fat mass accumulation, *Acta Clin. Belg.,* 47, 37, 1992.
112. **Voyles, N. R., Bhathena, S. J., Kennedy, B., Wilkins, S. D., Michaelis, O. E., Zalenski, C. M., Timmers, J. I., and Recant, L.,** Tissue somatostatin levels in three models of genetic obesity in rats, *Proc. Soc. Exp. Biol. Med.,* 185, 49, 1987.
113. **Patel, C. Y., Orci, L., and Bankier, A.,** Decreased pancreatic somatostatin (SRIF) concentration in spontaneously diabetic mice, *Endocrinology,* 99, 1415, 1976.
114. **Koranyi, L., Tanizawa, Y., Penicaud, L., Natef, N., Girard, J., and Permutt, M. A.,** Developmental regulation of amylin and insulin-gene expression in lean (Fa/Fa) and obese (fa/fa) Zucker rats, *Diabetes,* 41, 685, 1992.
115. **Tokuyama, Y., Kanatsuka, A., Ohsawa, H., Yamaguchi, T., Makino, H., Yoshida, S., Nagase, H., and Inoue, S.,** Hypersecretion of IAPP from the islets of VMH-lesioned rats and obese Zucker rats, *Endocrinology,* 128, 2739, 1991.
116. **Tokuyama, Y., Kanatsuka, A., Ohsawa, H., Yamaguchi, T., Makino, H., Yoshida, S., Nagase, H., and Inoue, S.,** Hypersecretion of IAPP from the islets of VMH-lesioned rats and obese Zucker rats, *Diabetes Res. Clin. Pract.,* 15, 23, 1992.

117. **Himms-Hagen, J.,** Brown adipose tissue thermogenesis and obesity, *Prog. Lipid Res.,* 28, 67, 1989.
118. **Marie, V., Dupuy, F., and Bazin, R.,** Decreased T4-to-T3 conversion in brown adipose tissue of Zucker fa/fa pups before the onset of obesity, *Am. J. Physiol.,* 263, E115, 1992.
119. **Marette, A., Deshaie, Y., Collet, A. J., Tulp, O., and Bukowiecki, L. J.,** Major thermogenic defect associated with insulin resistance in brown adipose tissue of obese diabetic SHR/N-cp rats, *Am. J. Physiol.,* 261, E204, 1991.
120. **Marette, A., Tulp, O., and Bukowiecki, L. J.,** Mechanism linking insulin resistance to defective thermogenesis in brown adipose tissue of obese diabetic SHR/N-cp rats, *Int. J. Obesity,* 15, 823, 1991.
121. **Assimacoupoulos-Jeannet, F., Greco-Perotto, R., Terrataz, J., Meier, M. K., and Jeanrenaud, B.,** Effect of a b-adrenergic agonist on glucose transport and insulin-responsive glucose transporters (GLUT4) in brown adipose tissue of control and obese fa/fa rats, *Pflugers Arch.,* 421, 52, 1992.
122. **Mercer, S. W. and Trayhurn, P.,** Developmental changes in fatty acid synthesis in interscapular brown adipose tissue of lean and genetically obese (ob/ob) mice, *Biochem. J.,* 212, 393, 1983.
123. **Trayhurn, P. and Wusteman, M. C.,** Lipogenesis in genetically diabetic (db/db) mice: developmental changes in brown adipose tissue, white adipose tissue and the liver, *Biochim. Biophys. Acta,* 1047, 168, 1990.
124. **Milner, R. E. and Trayhurn, P.,** Cold induced changes in uncoupling protein and GDP binding sites in brown fat of ob/ob mice, *Am. J. Physiol.,* 257, R292, 1989.
125. **Mercer, S. W. and Trayhurn, P.,** Effects of ciglitazone on insulin resistance and thermogenic responsiveness to acute cold in brown adipose tissue of genetically obese (ob/ob) mice, *FEBS Lett.,* 195, 12, 1986.
126. **Coleman, D. L. and Hummel, K. P.,** Studies with the mutation, diabetes, in the mouse, *Diabetologia,* 3, 238, 1967.
127. **Coleman, D. L. and Eicher, E. M.,** Fat (fat) and tubby (tub): two autosomal recessive mutations causing obesity syndromes in the mouse, *J. Hered.,* 81, 424, 1990.
128. **Zucker, L. M. and Zucker, T. F.,** Fatty, a new mutation in the rat, *J. Hered.,* 52, 275, 1961.
129. **Ikeda, H., Shino, A., Matsuo, T., Iwatsuka, H., and Suzuoki, Z.,** A new genetically obese-hyperglycemic rat (Wistar fatty), *Diabetes,* 30, 1045, 1981.
130. **Danforth, C. H.,** Hereditary adiposity in mice, *J. Hered.,* 18, 153, 1927.
131. **Russell, J. C. and Amy, R. M.,** Early atherosclerotic lesions in a susceptible rat model, *Atherosclerosis,* 60, 119, 1986.

Chapter 13

Identification of Genes Underlying Polygenic Obesity in Animal Models

Craig H. Warden and Janis S. Fisler

TABLE OF CONTENTS

0-8493-4880-3/94/$0.00+$.50

I. INTRODUCTION

While it has been difficult to directly identify the genes underlying obesity in humans, animal models clearly have important advantages for both genetic and biochemical studies. A new era in the analysis of obesity has begun with the recent development of methods for genetic analysis of polygenic traits in virtually any animal model. Although the recognition of genetic loci contributing to obesity in animal models is not intrinsically significant, the identification of obesity loci in animals will pinpoint "candidate loci" that can be tested in humans. It also may be possible to use "positional cloning" in animal models to clone genes underlying obesity. Perhaps most importantly, these studies will provide insights into mechanisms leading to obesity.

II. THE CONTRIBUTION OF POLYGENES TO OBESITY

A number of rodent models of obesity due to autosomal dominant or recessive inheritance of single genes have been described.[1-3] Studies of polygenic obesity in rodents are fewer[1-3] and the underlying genes not nearly so well defined. Several inbred (New Zealand Obese [NZO], KK) and hybrid (C3H × I (F1) and *Mus spretus* × C57BL/6J) mouse models of polygenic obesity, as well as a potentially useful model of polygenic obesity in rats (Osborne-Mendel × S 5B/Pl), will be described in this chapter.

Evidence for Mendelian inheritance in human obesity has been provided by studies of families, twins, and adoptees. It has long been recognized that obesity runs in families: most obese individuals have at least one parent who is obese, and the risk of obesity in first-degree relatives is estimated to be double that of the general population.[4] More definitive evidence for the role of genetics in human obesity is provided by studies of monozygotic and dizygotic twins. The body mass index of monozygotic twins is more likely to be similar than that of dizygotic twins; additionally, in twins who have been reared apart, genetic influences on body mass index are substantial (60 to 75% of variance), whereas childhood environment has little or no influence.[5] Long-term overfeeding of monozygotic twins results in weight gains of between 4.3 and 13.3 kg, with the response being about three times more variable between twin pairs than within twin pairs.[6] Some studies have concluded that the heritability of the body mass index is quite low (about 5%), but is much higher for fat mass and regional fat distribution (25 to 30%).[6,7] Studies of human subjects cannot, however, determine the number of genes involved in a trait. Therefore, it is not possible to state whether human obesity is polygenic or is perhaps monogenic with reduced penetrance modified by a second gene. For a more complete description of the genetics of human obesity see Chapters 4 to 8 in this volume.

III. GENERAL APPROACHES TO COMPLEX DISEASES

A. PHENOTYPE DOWN

The two basic approaches to identifying the genes underlying complex diseases such as obesity can be called "phenotype down" and "genotype up" (Figure 1).

In the phenotype down approach, the products of the genes underlying disease are isolated directly and protein sequences, antibodies, or function of those products are then used to isolate the underlying genes. Success with this approach usually requires that the results of the genetic variation are large, that tissues or cells expressing the altered gene product are accessible, and that some clues about the type of variation can be deduced.[8] While numerous phenotypic and biochemical differences have been identified between lean and obese animals and humans, none of these differences has been shown conclu-

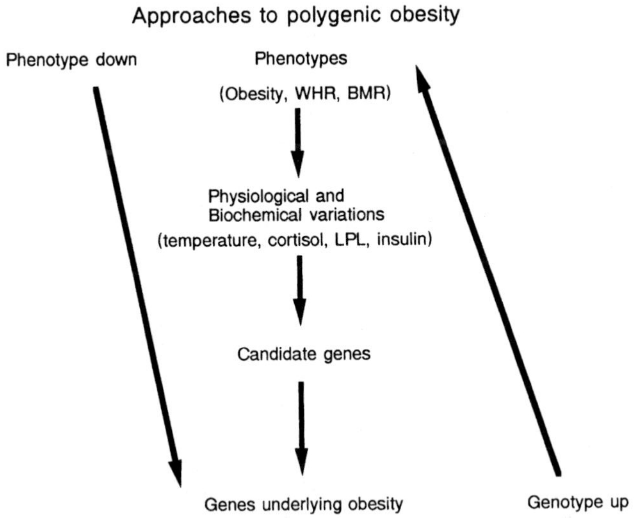

Figure 1. Outline of the phenotype down and genotype up methods used to identify the genes underlying inherited metabolic diseases. WHR, waist/hip ratio; BMR, basal metabolic rate; LPL, lipoprotein lipase.

sively to cause any form of obesity.[9-12] The candidate gene approach is a phenotype down technique in which a candidate protein is identified and its gene is tested for genetic association with obesity phenotypes. For example, the biochemical approach has identified serum insulin and adipose tissue lipoprotein lipase (LPL) activity as candidates to cause obesity. These candidate genes have been tested for linkage or association with obesity in humans, but to date there is no consensus on the role of either LPL or insulin in obesity.

While the biochemical and candidate gene approaches have proved relatively useful in studies of the genetic control of cholesterol metabolism,[13-15] they have not been as useful in the study of obesity. A problem with these approaches is that they require more understanding of the underlying molecular mechanisms than is currently available for obesity.

B. GENOTYPE UP

The genotype up approach is the second major approach to identify genes underlying obesity (Figure 1). In this method one identifies genetic polymorphisms that segregate (correlate or associate) with obesity. Positional cloning has been a powerful genotype up approach for identification and characterization of genes for monogenic disorders in which no biochemical or candidate gene can be identified. Positional cloning involves (1) the identification of genetic markers linked to a disease gene by testing for cosegregation of the disease phenotype with genetic markers covering the genome, (2) cloning regions of the genome surrounding those genetic markers linked to the disease, and (3) testing whether genes present in the cloned regions have properties consistent with the disease gene, such as alterations in expression in affected individuals. A strength of the positional cloning approach is that it is not dependent on an understanding of the disease. The last several years have seen the successful cloning of several genes causing human disease by the positional genetics methodology, including those for familial adenomatous polyposis[16,17] and cystic fibrosis.[18-20] Given the current difficulty in locating consensus candidate genes, genotype up or positional cloning of genes is very likely to be important in pinpointing the genes underlying obesity.

IV. ANIMAL MODELS ARE PARTICULARLY POWERFUL IN THE ANALYSIS OF COMPLEX DISEASES

Unfortunately, traditional positional cloning approaches are difficult to use in human studies of complex polygenic traits such as obesity. First, it is difficult or impossible to identify the responsible genetic loci since multiple independently segregating loci (unlinked genes on separate chromosomes) may contribute to obesity. This problem is exacerbated by the problem of genetic heterogeneity (in which the same disorder is caused in different individuals by different genetic defects) and by environmental influences such as diet. Classical examples of genetic heterogeneity include disruption of a biochemical pathway at any of its steps, and disruption of a gene or of the transcription factors responsible for the expression of that gene. These problems greatly complicate the identification of the responsible gene by chromosome walking and jumping from a linked genetic marker to the disease gene. In the case of monogenic disorders the walk from a linked marker to the gene underlying the disease is guided by the frequency of genetic recombination: as one nears the gene responsible for the trait, the recombination frequency must decrease to zero. However, it is difficult to determine how far a marker is from the responsible gene in the case of polygenic disorders because recombination frequency calculations are greatly complicated by the independent inheritance of other unlinked loci affecting the phenotype. For instance, suppose that two loci, A and B, are linked to obesity and to each other in an animal model system. Further suppose that another unlinked gene also causes obesity in this animal model. Ideally one would determine whether A or B is closer to the obesity gene by determining which gene has less recombination with obesity in a cross. However, this will be impossible in a multifactorial model since any one individual also may inherit alleles of the other gene(s) that cause obesity. It is sometimes possible to identify genes for complex traits in large families that have such a large effect that the defect segregates as a monogenic disorder. An example is the identification of a locus for maturity onset diabetes of the young (MODY) in a large family that is linked to adenosine deaminase on chromosome 20.[21]

Virtually all of these problems can be eliminated by the use of animal models to study polygenic multifactorial traits (Table 1). Control is the major advantage of animal studies — control of heterogeneity, breeding, and physiological and biochemical studies and control of germ-line transmission in transgenics and targeted mutations for hypothesis testing. These advantages make it possible to pursue approaches to directly identify genes underlying polygenic obesity in animal models, to use positional cloning to identify the specific genes responsible, and to test hypotheses about causes and treatments of obesity in animal models.

V. METHODS TO IDENTIFY LOCI UNDERLYING COMPLEX TRAITS IN ANIMAL MODELS

This chapter concentrates on genotype up methods for the identification of loci underlying obesity and its risk factors by surveying the entire genome of experimental animal models. Recently, a technique for mapping Mendelian factors underlying quantitative traits, in virtually any animal model, using genetic linkage maps has been described.[22,23] The quantitative trait locus (QTL) method requires no knowledge of, or assumptions concerning, the biological nature of the characteristics or defects being tracked. This technique has been applied to the mapping of Mendelian factors that underlie continuous variables in tomatoes[24] and, more recently, the technique has been used to identify genes

Table 1. **Advantages of using animal models in the study of polygenic traits**

Problem	Advantages of animal models
Heterogeneity	Minimize heterogeneity; inbred animals can be kept in uniform environments on identical diets
Breeding	Can design genetic crosses as desired
Physiological studies	Can use surgery, diets, environment, and sacrifices as needed for hypothesis testing and biochemical studies
Variations	Availability of a wide variety of phenotypes in different inbred strains permits study of numerous traits
Hypothesis testing	Ability to make transgenics and targeted mutations permits hypotheses tests about roles of specific genes in complex diseases
Therapies	Can use both spontaneous and artificially produced animal models to test new therapies

for obesity in the mouse[25] and hypertension in the rat.[23,26] The QTL method can identify chromosomal regions regulating a trait in any animal model system for which two key resources are available — inbred strains and a complete linkage map of the genome.[22,23]

The methods to identify quantitative trait loci can be divided into four steps, which are illustrated for a hypothetical example (Figure 2): (1) two different inbred strains are first crossed to produce F2 or backcross progeny, (2) all of the progeny are individually genotyped for markers that are spread throughout the genome, (3) phenotypes are assayed for all of the progeny, and (4) statistical associations of markers and phenotypes are performed to identify loci underlying the traits. For quantitative traits these associations can reveal quantitative trait loci (QTLs), while for yes/no traits the associations can be revealed by a chi-square analysis. Each of these points is discussed in more detail below.

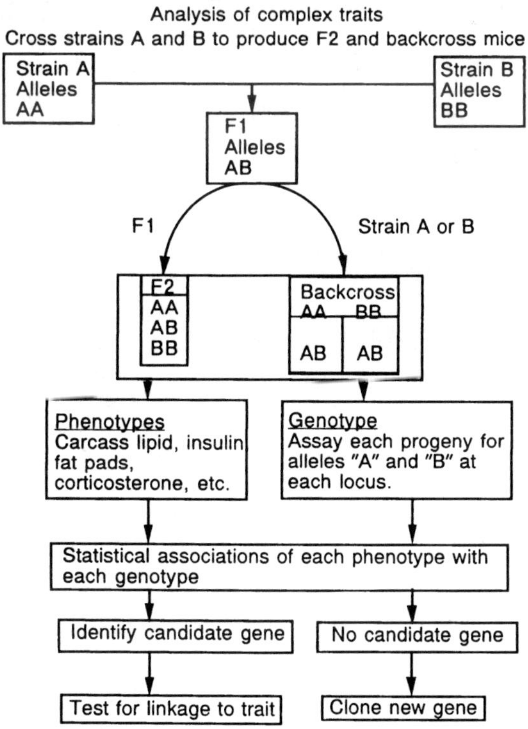

Figure 2. Outline of the methods to analyze complex traits in animal models. Strain A (genotype AA) is crossed with strain B (genotype BB) to produce F1 animals with genotype AB. F1 animals are crossed with each other to produce F2 animals with genotype AA, AB, or BB or with one of the parental strains to produce backcrosses with genotype AA,AB or BB,AB, depending on the parental strains used for the backcross. Phenotypes, genotypes, and quantitative trait loci are assayed as described in the text.

A. GENETIC CROSSES OF STRAINS DIFFERING IN POLYGENIC TRAITS

There are three major considerations in setting up crosses. First, the parental strains used should be inbred. Inbred strains, produced by 20 or more generations of brother × sister mating, provide the basic resource for analysis of monogenic and polygenic traits. The genes passed on by any one animal of an inbred strain will be identical to those of any other animal of that strain; thus, animals from an inbred strain provide an invariant gene pool that can be used for all subsequent experiments.

Second, identification of polymorphisms is simplified by the use of strains which are evolutionarily divergent. For example, in studies with mice it is possible to construct crosses between different species which are only interfertile in the laboratory. Restriction fragment length polymorphisms (RFLPs) can be identified easily for genetic markers in interspecific crosses. On the other hand, many of the markers presently being developed, such as microsatellite elements, are highly polymorphic among closely related strains of *Mus domesticus.*[27] The use of widely divergent strains also may be a disadvantage since a greater number of loci may contribute to the phenotypic differences between the parental strains and, thus, complicate QTL analysis.

Third, identification of individual QTLs with relatively large phenotypic effects may be difficult when the means of the parental strains differ by less than 2 SD for the trait under consideration. As discussed later, this would complicate the cloning of genes underlying QTLs. On the other hand, different strains coincidentally may have similar phenotypes while exhibiting substantial genetic differences. In crosses involving such parental strains, the phenotypes of the progeny are expected to span a much wider range of values than the parents. One such instance of this phenomenon, the obesity of *M. spretus* × C57BL/6J mice, is discussed below.

B. PHENOTYPING

The methods used for phenotyping will depend on the trait of interest. The most specific measure available should be used. For example, percent of carcass weight as fat is a better measure of obesity than body weight or body mass index. Particular care should be taken to minimize the error of the assay since nongenetic variation will reduce the power of the method. QTL mapping can be applied to any continuously variable trait which can be measured, such as carcass lipid, plasma insulin or glucose levels, oxygen consumption, or weight gain induced by a high-fat diet.

C. GENOTYPING

Genotyping means to identify which of the two parental strains has contributed alleles to a specific locus in each F2 or backcross animal (Figure 2). The two most common methods for genotyping are polymerase chain reaction (PCR) assay of simple sequence repeats (SSRs) and RFLPs of complementary DNA (cDNA) or genomic clones. The most common SSR consists of a variable number of (CA)n repeats, is present at approximately 100,000 copies per genome, and is so polymorphic that any two inbred mouse or rat strains will, on average, be polymorphic at 50% of existing SSR loci.[23,28] Genotyping with SSR primers is faster and cheaper than with RFLPs, in part because reactions can be performed in 96-well PCR plates and in part because more than 1500 mouse and 200 rat SSR primer pairs are available at low cost from Research Genetics (Birmingham, AL). Genotyping by RFLPs requires that one acquire and prepare cDNA or genomic clones, prepare Southern blots, and probe the blots. Genotyping by RFLPs remains useful when one needs to test a specific candidate gene for linkage to a trait.

D. STATISTICAL TESTS OF ASSOCIATION

1. Surveys of the Genome for Loci Underlying Quantitative Traits

Many of the correlates and risk factors of obesity can be considered as quantitative diseases since many of its associated markers, such as carcass lipid, waist-hip ratio, basal metabolic rate, and blood triglycerides, insulin, and glucose, are quantitative. Although complete surveys of the genome for loci underlying quantitative traits are not a new concept, the method has become feasible only recently due to the development of both numerous highly polymorphic genetic markers that span the genome and mathematical methods for data analysis.

A linear regression of phenotype on genotype, such as an analysis of variance, is the classical method for identifying whether the difference between the means of the different genotypes is significantly different from zero at loci that might underlie complex traits. If A and B denote inbred strains and we assume a backcross with A as the recurrent parent, then there would be two possible genotypes in the backcross, AA and AB. In an F2 intercross there would be three genotypes: AA, AB, and BB (see Figure 2). Finding a significant phenotypic difference between animals with different genotypes suggests that the locus, or one to which it is tightly linked, controls a measurably detectable difference in the phenotype. This approach is limited by both the number and spacing of the individual loci genotyped, since linear regression can be used only to detect linkage to each genotyped locus. The major difficulty is that one cannot distinguish a small, close QTL from a large but distant one. This technique has been improved by implementing several modifications.[22]

2. Quantitative Trait Locus Mapping with Mapmaker

The ability to analyze phenotype and genotype information for QTLs in model systems is combined in the Mapmaker[29] and Mapmaker/QTL programs.[22] The QTL analysis requires the construction of genetic linkage maps of ordered markers which can be constructed from primary data using the Mapmaker program.[29] This program is interactive and relatively easy to use; the linkage maps constructed can be used directly by the Mapmaker/QTL program. Mapmaker/QTL uses genetic linkage maps along with quantitative phenotype data to locate QTLs by an efficient interval mapping method that calculates log-of-the-odds (LOD) scores for each quantitative trait at 1- to 2-centimorgan (cM) intervals between each marker.[23] This gives Mapmaker/QTL the ability to detect QTLs in between linked markers. LOD scores provide a measure of the significance of linkage of trait and genotype. A LOD score of 3.0 or greater is a statistically significant evidence of linkage. While Mapmaker/QTL is an easy-to-use interactive program, it nevertheless should be used with some care. For instance, since the program uses a missing data algorithm to estimate the genotypes between markers, in some cases the estimated genotypes may give false positive LOD score results. Thus, the Mapmaker/QTL program cannot be used to prove the existence of a QTL between two linked markers, but rather guides one in the selection of additional markers to genotype in a cross at the sites of putative QTLs.

VI. EXAMPLES OF THE MAPPING OF LOCI DETERMINING POLYGENIC TRAITS

A. THE *MUS SPRETUS* × C57BL/6J (BSB) MODEL OF OBESITY

A new model of polygenic obesity has arisen by crossing two interfertile species of mice (*M. spretus* × C57BL/6J; see Section VII.A). Chow-fed backcross progeny (BSB mice) range from very lean to massively obese (up to 95 g body weight in older mice). Obesity in this model is associated with hyperinsulinemia, insulin resistance, and hypertriglyceridemia as is commonly seen in obese humans.[30] Using QTL mapping with RFLP and microsatellite maps, two genetic loci which are coincident for plasma cholesterol and obesity were identified.[25] Statistical analysis revealed that distal mouse chromosome 7 exhibited significant linkage both to plasma total cholesterol (LOD score 5.8) and to carcass lipid (LOD score 3.8).[25] This locus accounts for 17% of the variance in plasma cholesterol in males and 5% in females. The same locus explains 8% of the variance in carcass lipid. Located approximately 10 cM proximal to this locus on chromosome 7 is the recessive mutation *tubby* which results in obesity in mice. A locus identified on chromosome 6 also shows significant linkage to plasma total cholesterol (LOD score 5.6), accounting for 8% of the variance in total cholesterol, and to a subcutaneous fat pad (LOD score 2.8), accounting for 16% of the variance in the femoral fat pad, but shows no linkage to carcass lipid.[25] The chromosome 6 locus is approximately 4 cM from the *obese* gene. It is therefore possible that variations of the *tubby* and *obese* mutations are involved in these traits in BSB mice. If so, it would imply that variants of these genes could be involved in multigenic obesity and, thus, could be involved in human obesity.

B. IDENTIFICATION OF GENES FOR ESSENTIAL HYPERTENSION

Blood pressure is influenced by multiple genetic loci, and efforts to identify these loci in human subjects have been largely unsuccessful. In contrast, recent genetic studies with rat models of spontaneous and salt-induced hypertension have yielded several genetic loci that contribute to blood pressure. Using QTL mapping, a gene having a major effect on sodium-loaded blood pressure, accounting for approximately 20% of the variance, was placed on rat chromosome 10.[23,26] The locus was found to be closely linked to the rat gene encoding angiotensin-converting enzyme (ACE), the enzyme responsible for converting angiotensin I into angiotensin II and inactivating bradykinin; thus, the gene encoding ACE was identified as a candidate gene. A locus on rat chromosome 18 affecting baseline blood pressure and, more weakly, sodium-loaded blood pressure was also identified.

The candidate gene approach also has been used successfully with the Dahl salt hypertension sensitive (S) and resistant (R) rat strains, which differ at multiple loci affecting blood pressure, to indicate that the renin gene may contribute to the difference in blood pressure.[31] The investigators showed that a polymorphism of the renin gene segregated with blood pressure in an F2 population from a cross between S and R animals. Subsequently, a renin gene polymorphism also was found to correlate with blood pressure in an F2 cross derived from the parental rat strains SHR (hypertensive) and Lewis (normal).[32] The importance of renin gene expression in the control of blood pressure has been confirmed recently using transgenic rats[33] and mice.[34]

VII. ANIMAL MODELS OF POLYGENIC OBESITY

There are several rodent models of polygenic obesity. In the mouse these include the inbred NZO and Japanese KK mice and the hybrid Wellesley and *M. spretus* × C57BL/6J backcross mice. There are fewer models of polygenic obesity in rats, but a potentially useful model is the Osborne-Mendel × S 5B/PI rat cross.

A. MOUSE MODELS

1. Advantages of the Mouse for Genetic Studies

Mice are the model of choice for genetic studies, primarily due to the existence of hundreds of inbred strains, but also due to the availability of other powerful genetic tools, such as a genetic map which currently includes over 3000 mapped loci (GBASE, 1993, The Jackson Laboratory, Bar Harbor, ME), making it second only to the human map in completeness. Moreover, the homology relationships between mouse and human chromosomes have been well defined.[35] It is frequently possible to identify the chromosomal location of a gene in humans by mapping it in mice.

2. Mouse Models of Polygenic Obesity

Models of polygenic obesity in the mouse have been reviewed previously.[1-3] The NZO mouse and the Japanese KK mouse are inbred strains which spontaneously develop obesity. Spontaneous obesity is also observed in hybrid models such as the Wellesley mouse (C3H × I (F1) hybrid) and the BSB mouse (*M. spretus* × C57BL/6J backcross). Dietary fat readily induces obesity in the Japanese KK mouse[36] and in the C3H and A strains,[37] but not in C57BL/6J and I strains.[37] Recently, West and associates reported a survey of nine inbred mouse strains.[38] Six strains had a significant increase in carcass lipid in response to a high-fat and high-sucrose diet, whereas three strains did not. Most sensitive to dietary-induced obesity were AKR/J, C57L/J, and A/J strains, whereas SJL/J, I/STN, and SWR/J mice were resistant to the diet.[38] Unfortunately, a survey of sensitivity to spontaneous obesity has not been done in a large series of inbred strains. Therefore, the best choices for the study of spontaneous obesity models are not readily apparent.

Although the precise mode of inheritance is not understood in any of these models, the obesity is generally thought to be polygenic.[39,40] The obesity and diabetes in the Japanese KK mouse may result from a dominant gene with incomplete penetrance and a modifier gene.[41]

a. *New Zealand Obese (NZO) Mouse*

The inbred NZO mouse was selectively bred for obesity.[39] This mouse can become massively obese, with weight in adult males ranging from 45 to 89 g (up to 75% body fat). The fat is primarily stored in the abdomen.[42] NZO mice are hyperinsulinemic, but, depending on age and sex, are not severely hyperglycemic. A recent study employing a hyperinsulinemic clamp has shown hepatic glucose overproduction, brown fat and skeletal muscle insulin resistance, and impaired first-phase insulin secretion in the NZO mouse.[43] The NZO mouse is also sensitive to a high-fat diet, which converts the obesity in this mouse from a primarily hypertrophic obesity to a hypertrophic-hyperplastic obesity.[44] For a more detailed review of the metabolic characteristics of the NZO mouse see Reference 2.

The NZC strain, developed from the same progenitor mice as the NZO strain, has normal weight and has been used as a control for the NZO strain. The NZC mouse, however, develops congenital cystic kidneys and ovarian tumors[45] and, thus, may not be a suitable control strain. C57BL/6J mice also have been used as a control strain in metabolic studies with the NZO mouse. With the advent of microsatellite genotyping, either of these control strains should have sufficient genetic diversity from NZO mice and provide appropriate crosses for genetic studies. The advantage of the NZC strain as a control is that it should differ from the NZO strain by relatively few genes.

b. *Japanese KK Mouse*

The Japanese KK mouse also was bred for large body size.[46] The obesity in this strain is moderate and tends to diminish in older mice. During the period of weight gain, Japanese KK mice are hyperphagic and develop hyperinsulinemia and a moderately impaired glucose tolerance which can be prevented by dietary restriction. For a more detailed review of the metabolic characteristics of the Japanese KK mouse see Reference 2.

c. *C3H × I (F1) (Wellesley) Mouse*

The Wellesley mouse is the F1 hybrid resulting from a cross between strains C3H and I.[47] It develops moderate spontaneous obesity, with a maximum weight of about 50 g after 3 to 4 months of age. The mice are hyperinsulinemic and moderately hyperglycemic. These abnormalities are intensified by a diet containing 11% fat by weight and can be prevented by diet restriction.[48] F2 mice, resulting from an F1 × F1 cross, would have the range of genotypes and phenotypes necessary for QTL mapping (see Figure 2).

d. *Mus spretus × C57BL/6J Backcross (BSB) Mouse*

A new mouse model of polygenic obesity, involving progeny of a cross between *M. spretus* and C57BL/6J *(M. musculus)*,[30] has been identified.[30] A particular advantage of the *M. musculus* × *M. spretus* cross is that these mice are widely diverged (at least 3 million years), making the identification of DNA polymorphisms between strains relatively straightforward. Although these progenitor strains are interfertile, the F1 males are sterile. Therefore, genetic analysis requires that F1 females be backcrossed to either parental strain. It is in the progeny of the F1 females backcrossed to the C57BL/6J males that the variation in obesity has been found. The backcross progeny are either genotype BB or SB at any locus.

Young C57BL/6J mice and F1 hybrids (*M. spretus* × C57BL/6J) have about 13% body fat, whereas young *M. spretus* are very lean. Obesity is first observed in the backcross mice, where body fat varies from less than 1% to greater than 50% of wet carcass weight. The simplest model for this observation is that obesity results from the interactions of two genes and that one locus must be homozygous for C57BL/6J alleles (BB) while the other locus is heterozygous (SB), since this is the only combination of two genes which is unique to backcross mice. It is possible that there are actually three or more genes involved in this obesity, with two or more genes for either homozygous BB or heterozygous SB type of loci. Thus, backcross obesity may be an example of a heterozygous epistasis interaction between two or more genes. This is a mechanism which might be of considerable importance in outbred populations such as humans, where both heterozygosity and homozygosity are common. It has been demonstrated experimentally that obesity genes help animals survive prolonged fasts; that is, there may be evolutionary selection favoring mice heterozygous for obesity genes.[49]

B. RAT MODELS

The larger size of rats makes them more useful than mice for measurements of many traits, but this same increased size makes rats much more expensive to breed and maintain. Although the current genetic map of rats includes over 400 loci which have been mapped to 20 of the 22 rat chromosomes,[23,50] this is approximately an order of magnitude fewer markers than on the mouse (GBASE, 1993) and human genetic maps (Genome Data Base, a Howard Hughes Medical Institute project in collaboration with The Johns Hopkins University School of Medicine). However, the last practical barrier to QTL mapping in rats has been removed with the advent of rat SSR markers.[23,51]

One model of polygenic obesity in rats has been studied extensively. Schemmel and colleagues,[52] in a survey of seven strains of rats, showed that feeding rats a diet containing 60% of its calories as fat produced the greatest increase in body fat in Osborne-Mendel rats, an intermediate increase in body fat in animals of most other strains, and only a very small weight gain in rats of the S 5B/Pl strain. From this, a useful model for the study of dietary-fat-induced obesity has been developed.[53] By using inbred Osborne-Mendel and S 5B/Pl rats in the crosses, as outlined in Figure 2, and genotyping and measuring response of body fatness to dietary fat in the F2 progeny, the standard QTL mapping technique could be applied to this model.

VIII. FROM QUANTITATIVE TRAIT LOCUS TO GENE

A. QUANTITATIVE TRAIT LOCI PROVIDE INSIGHTS INTO THE CAUSES OF COMPLEX DISEASES

Identification of a QTL is only one of the results of mapping quantitative loci modulating obesity. For instance, one can search for correlations among QTLs for dissimilar traits, thereby providing new data on the molecular, genetic, and biochemical mechanisms of obesity. An example of this is the finding of a locus on chromosome 7 coincident for obesity and plasma cholesterol in BSB mice (see Section VI.A).[25] In addition, one of the potentially most powerful features of QTL mapping is its ability to decompose traits into their separate parts. As an example, QTL mapping will help in the identification of biochemical sexual dimorphisms, since loci that underlie complex diseases and which are unique to one sex can be identified more easily through the study of individual loci than by the study of whole-body trait values.

B. CLONING OF GENES UNDERLYING POLYGENIC OBESITY

While identification of QTLs is a first step toward understanding obesity, a full understanding of obesity will require the use of positional cloning to identify those genes that underlie obesity. While a full discussion of positional cloning is beyond the scope of this chapter, it includes the following steps: (1) breeding of QTL congenic animals, (2) fine mapping of the phenotype, (3) identifying candidate genes in the area of the QTL, and (4) proving that a single candidate gene is the QTL gene. These are discussed in turn below.

1. Breeding QTL Congenics

The method for breeding of QTL congenics is summarized in Figure 3. As a hypothetical example, suppose that there are two QTLs for percent carcass lipid in a polygenic animal model with five chromosomes (Figure 3). Refined mapping and positional cloning can be accomplished only in a genetic cross in which strains A and B differ by a single gene. This is because correlation of a trait with a gene cannot be done precisely if two unlinked QTLs affect the trait. Thus, after identification of QTLs in a multifactorial model, it will be

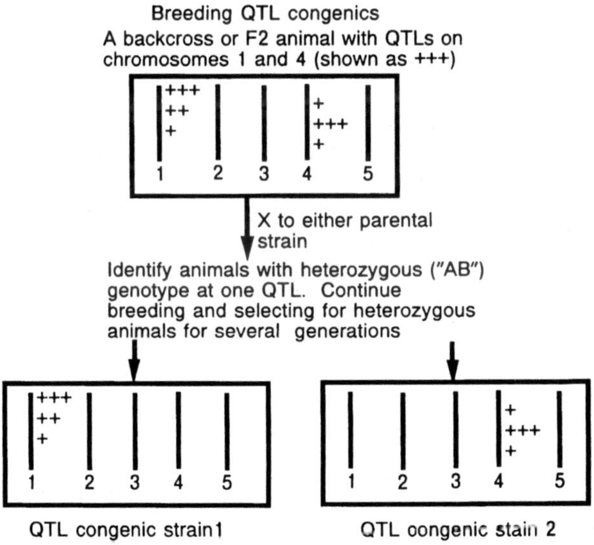

Figure 3. Breeding of quantitative trait locus (QTL) congenics. The breeding of QTL congenics can be illustrated by a hypothetical model system with five chromosomes and QTLs for a trait on chromosomes 1 and 4. Pluses indicate log-of-the-odds (LOD) score and position for a QTL. The first step of breeding QTL congenics would be to identify a backcross or F2 animal that has the genotype of AB at the chromosome 1 and 4 QTLs. The second step is to cross this animal with one of the parental strains. Progeny would be genotyped at the chromosome 1 and 4 QTLs, and heterozygous animals would be identified. These animals would be used for an additional cycle of breeding, and progeny heterozygous at each QTL would be identified. These cycles would be repeated for 2 to 20 rounds. The QTL congenic strains would each have a single QTL that modulates the relevant trait. These QTL congenics would be used for fine mapping as described in the text.

necessary to derive new strains that differ from one of the parental strains by a single QTL (QTL congenics). This can be accomplished by several cycles of breeding and selection for the AB genotype at the QTL at each round of breeding. For example, suppose that a backcross mouse is bred to either parental strain, and the progeny are assayed for the AB genotype at each QTL (Figure 3). Progeny with AB genotypes at only one QTL could then be picked for a second round of breeding to the same parental strain. The cycle could be repeated several times until a new strain had been produced that contained the AB genotype at only one QTL and was otherwise identical to the parental strain used for the cross. These QTL congenics could then be crossed to the parental strain one more time and several hundred progeny collected for fine mapping of the trait, since differences of phenotype would now be due to the segregation of a single gene. This final cross is essentially identical to the crosses being used to clone genes causing single-gene obesity, such as *db.*[54]

2. Fine Mapping

Fine mapping is necessary because there are approximately 3×10^9 base pairs (bp) in the mammalian genome. Since the total recombinational length of the mouse genome is 1600 cM, there are approximately 2×10^6 bp per centimorgan in the mouse. It has been estimated that there are 100,000 expressed genes in mammals; therefore, on average there will be 30,000 bp per gene, or 50 genes per centimorgan in the mouse. If one has mapped a gene to a specific location ± 1 cM, there will be approximately 100 expressed genes in that region which must be examined for their role in the QTL. Thus, it is clear that positional cloning requires resolution of less than 1 cM.

3. Identification of Candidate Quantitative Trait Locus Genes

This topic is very broad and includes the generation of many specific probes in the region of the QTL and testing of these probes for linkage to the trait by linkage mapping[55] in the cross of the QTL congenic with the parental strain. Ideally one could identify a gene as underlying the QTL by showing that there is no recombination between this gene and the QTL. However, this will not be practical because a resolution of 1 cM requires a cross of at least 100 animals and there are approximately 50 genes per centimorgan. Thus, identification of the one gene underlying obesity entirely by linkage mapping would require a resolution of 0.02 cM and a cross of at least 5000 animals. This is clearly impractical. The work involved in breeding and genotyping a cross of QTL congenics will still lead to a pool of at least 50 to 100 genes that are candidates for the QTL gene. Other important parts of this step include the identification of cDNA clones that may code for the QTL gene.

4. Proving that a Single Gene Underlies the Quantitative Trait Locus

Since there may be many candidate cDNA clones that could underlie the QTL, it will be necessary to prove that one of them underlies obesity. This step will be difficult. It will require that one examine alleles of the genes in mice that differ for the trait, examine tissue expression of the genes, and perhaps construct transgenics and targeted mutations to prove finally that one single gene underlies obesity in this QTL congenic.

C. HOMOLOGY TO HUMANS

While no animal model is perfect, a growing number of animal models exist in which mutations of the same genes in animals and humans lead to homologous diseases (Table 2). Ancestral mammalian chromosomes have been shuffled in identifiable segments during evolution. Thus, the same genes are in the same order in mouse and human chromosomal segments. The average length of conserved chromosomal segments between mice and humans has been calculated as 10 to 20 cM.[56] The basic approach to using

Table 2. **Mouse models of human disease**

Gene or locus	Animal model	Human disease	Phenotype	Ref.
CFTR	Targeted mouse	Cystic fibrosis	Failure to thrive, defective chloride transport, many others	57,58
Glucocerebrosidase	Knock-out mouse	Gaucher's disease	Lipid accumulation in macrophages and early death	59
Histocompatibility locus	Nonobese diabetic (NOD) mouse	IDDM	Insulin-dependent diabetes mellitus	60
Tyrosinase	Albino mice	Tyrosinase negative albinism	Albino	61,62
β-Glucuronidase	Cone-head mouse	Sly syndrome	Lysosomal storage disease	63,64
X-Linked hypophosphatemic rickets	Hyp mice	HPDR	Hypophosphatemia	65,66
Pax-6	Small-eye mouse	Aniridia	Iris hypoplasia	67
APC	MIN (multiple intestinal neoplasia) mouse	Adenomatous polyposis coli	Colon cancer	68

Note: APC = adenomatous polyposis coli; CFTR = cystic fibrosis transmembrane receptor; HPDR = hypophosphatemic-dependent rickets; IDDM = insulin-dependent diabetes mellitus; Pax-6 = paired-like homeobox-containing.

QTLs identified in mice for human studies is to identify a human locus which is homologous to the mouse QTL and then to test for associations of the trait with the locus in humans. This method has been illustrated for diabetes. A locus on mouse chromosome 9 was identified in nonobese diabetic (NOD) mice as containing a gene for susceptibility to diabetes.[21] The homologous human chromosome, 11q, was then tested for linkage to diabetes in diabetic pedigrees; in this case, however, no linkage was found.

IX. CONCLUSION

Animal models are likely to be important in endeavors to understand the genetics of obesity. At present, the mapping of loci contributing to complex traits in animal models appears to be the most powerful general method for identifying new genetic factors contributing to obesity and its associated diseases. The approach is clearly feasible and, in fact, has already been applied to several diseases related to obesity in animal models.

REFERENCES

1. **Bray, G. and York, D. A.,** Genetically transmitted obesity in rodents, *Physiol. Rev.,* 51, 598, 1971.
2. **Bray, G. A. and York, D. A.,** Hypothalamic and genetic obesity in experimental animals: an autocrine and endocrine hypothesis, *Physiol. Rev.,* 59, 719, 1979.

3. **Festing, M. F. W.,** The inheritance of obesity in animal models of obesity, in *Animal Models of Obesity,* Festing, M. F. W., Ed., Oxford University Press, New York, 1979, 15.
4. **Price, R. A.,** Genetics of human obesity, *Ann. Behav. Med.,* 9, 9, 1987.
5. **Stunkard, A. J., Foch, T. T., and Hrubec, Z.,** A twin study of human obesity, *JAMA,* 256, 51, 1986.
6. **Bouchard, C.,** Variation in human body fat: the contribution of the genotype, in *Obesity: Towards a Molecular Approach,* Spiegelman, B. M. and Ricquier, E., Eds., Alan R. Liss, New York, 1990, 17.
7. **Bouchard, C., Tremblay, A., and Després, J.-P.,** The response to long-term overfeeding in identical twins, *N. Engl. J. Med.,* 322, 1477, 1990.
8. **Goldstein, J. L. and Brown, M. S.,** Familial hypercholesterolemia, in *The Metabolic Basis of Inherited Disease,* Stanbury, J. B., Wyngaarden, J. B., Fredrickson, D. S., Goldstein, J. L., and Brown, M. S., Eds., McGraw-Hill, New York, 1983, 672.
9. **Bouchard, C., Després, J.-P., and Tremblay, A.,** Genetics of obesity and human energy metabolism, *Proc. Nutr. Soc.,* 50, 139, 1991.
10. **Bouchard, C.,** Heredity and the path to overweight and obesity, *Med. Sci. Sports Exercise,* 23, 285, 1991.
11. **Bouchard, C.,** Genetic factors in obesity, *Med. Clin. North Am.,* 73, 67, 1989.
12. **Bray, G. A.,** Weight homeostasis, *Annu. Rev. Med.,* 42, 205, 1991.
13. **Breslow, J. L.,** Lipoprotein transport gene abnormalities underlying coronary heart disease susceptibility, *Annu. Rev. Med.,* 42, 357, 1991.
14. **Lusis, A. J.,** Genetic factors affecting blood lipoproteins: the candidate gene approach, *J. Lipid Res.,* 29, 397, 1988.
15. **Breslow, J. L.,** The genetic basis of lipoprotein disorders. Introduction and overview, *J. Intern. Med.,* 231, 627, 1992.
16. **Groden, J., Thilveris, A., Samowitz, W., Carlson, M., Gelbert, L., Albertson, H., Joslyn, G., Stevens, J., Spiro, L., Robertson, M., Sargeant, L., Krapcho, K., Wolff, E., Burt, R., Hughes, J. P., Warrington, J., McPherson, J., Wasmuth, J., LePaslier, D., Abderrahim, H., Cohen, D., Leppert, M., and White, R.,** Identification and characterization of the familial adenomatous polyposis coli gene, *Cell,* 66, 589, 1991.
17. **Kinzler, K. W., Nilbert, M. C., Su, L.-K., Vogelstein, B., Bryan, T. M., Levy, D. B., Smith, K. J., Preisinger, A. C., Hedge, P., McKechnie, D., Finniear, R., Markham, A., Groffen, J., Boguski, M. S., Altschui, S. F., Horii, A., Ando, H., Miyoshi, Y., Miki, Y., Nishisho, I., and Nakamura, Y.,** Identification of FAP locus genes from chromosome 5q21, *Science,* 253, 661, 1991.
18. **Rommens, J. M., Ianuzzi, M. C., Kerem, B.-S., Drumm, M. L., Melmer, G., Dean, M., Rozmahel, R., Cole, J. L., Kennedy, D., Hidaka, N., Zsiga, M., Buchwald, M., Riordan, J. R., Tsui, L.-C., and Collins, F. S.,** Identification of the cystic fibrosis gene: chromosome walking and jumping, *Science,* 245, 1059, 1989.
19. **Riordan, J. R., Rommens, J. M., Kerem, B.-S., Alon, N., Rozmahel, R., Grzelczak, Z., Zielenski, J., Lok, S., Plavsic, N., Chou, J.-L., Drumm, M. L., Iannuzzi, M. C., Collins, F. S., and Tsui, L.-C.,** Identification of the cystic fibrosis gene: cloning and characterization of complementary DNA, *Science,* 245, 1066, 1989.
20. **Kerem, B.-S., Rommens, J. M., Buchanan, J.A., Markiewicz, D., Cox, T. K., Chakravarti, A., Buchwald, M., and Tsui, L.-C.,** Identification of the cystic fibrosis gene: genetic analysis, *Science,* 245, 1073, 1989.
21. **Hyer, R. N., Julier, C., Buckley, J. D., Trucco, M., Rotter, J., Spielman, R., Barnett, A., Bain, S., Boitard, C., Deschamps, I., Todd, J. A., Bell, J. I., and Lathrop, G. M.,** High-resolution linkage mapping for susceptibility genes in human polygenic disease: insulin-dependent diabetes mellitus and chromosome 11q, *Am. J. Hum. Genet.,* 48, 243, 1991.

22. **Lander, E. S. and Botstein, D.,** Mapping Mendelian factors underlying quantitative traits using RFLP linkage maps, *Genetics,* 121, 185, 1989.
23. **Jacob, H. J., Lindpaintner, K., Lincoln, S. E., Kusumi, K., Bunker, R. K., Mao, Y. P., Ganten, D., Dzau, V. J., and Lander, E. S.,** Genetic mapping of a gene causing hypertension in the stroke-prone spontaneously hypertensive rat, *Cell,* 67, 213, 1991.
24. **Paterson, A. H., Lander, E. S., Hewitt, J. D., Peterson, S., Lincoln, S. E., and Tanksley, S. D.,** Resolution of quantitative traits into Mendelian factors by using a complete linkage map of restriction fragment length polymorphisms, *Nature,* 335, 721, 1988.
25. **Warden, C. H., Fisler, J. S., Pace, M. J., Svenson, K. L., and Lusis, A. J.,** Coincidence of genetic loci for plasma cholesterol levels and obesity in a multifactorial mouse model, *J. Clin. Invest.,* 92, 773, 1993.
26. **Hilbert, P., Lindpaintner, K., Beckmann, J. S., Serikawa, T., Soubrier, F., Dubay, C., Cartwright, P., De Gouyon, B., Julier, C., Takahasi, S., Vincent, M., Ganten, D., Georges, M., and Lathrop, G. M.,** Chromosomal mapping of two genetic loci associated with blood-pressure regulation in hereditary hypertensive rats, *Nature,* 353, 521, 1991.
27. **Montagutelli, X., Serikawa, T., and Guenet, J.-L.,** PCR-analyzed microsatellites: data concerning laboratory and wild-derived mouse inbred strains, *Mamm. Genome,* 1, 255, 1991.
28. **Dietrich, W., Katz, H., Lincoln, S. E., Shin, H.-S., Friedman, J., Dracopoli, N. C., and Lander, E. S.,** A genetic map of the mouse suitable for typing intraspecific crosses, *Genetics,* 131, 423, 1992.
29. **Lander, E. S., Green, P., Abrahamson, J., Barlow, A., Daly, M. J., Lincoln, S. E., and Newburg, L.,** MAPMAKER: an interactive computer package for constructing primary genetic linkage maps of experimental and natural populations, *Genomics,* 1, 174, 1987.
30. **Fisler, J. S., Warden, C. H., Pace, M. J., and Lusis, A. J.,** BSB: a new mouse model of multigenic obesity, *Obes. Res.,* 1, 271, 1993.
31. **Rapp, J. P., Wang, S.-M., and Dene, H. A.,** A genetic polymorphism in the renin gene of Dahl rats cosegregates with blood pressure, *Science,* 243, 542, 1989.
32. **Kurtz, J. W., Simonet, L., Potear, K. M., Wolfe, S., Chan, L., and Hjelle, P. I.,** Cosegregation of the renin allele of the spontaneously hypertensive rat with an increase in blood pressure, *J. Clin. Invest.,* 85, 1328, 1990.
33. **Mullins, J.J., Peters, J., and Ganten, D.,** Fulminant hypertension in transgenic rats harbouring the mouse Ren-2 gene, *Nature,* 344, 541, 1990.
34. **Ohkobo, H., Kawakami, H., Kakehi, Y., Arai, H., Yokota, Y., Iwai, M., Tanabe, Y., Masu, M., Hata, J., Iwao, H., Okamoto, H., Yokayama, M., Nomura, J., Katsuki, M., and Nakanishi, J.,** Generation of transgenic mice with elevated blood pressure by introduction of the rat renin gene and angiotensin genes, *Proc. Natl. Acad. Sci. U.S.A.,* 87, 5153, 1990.
35. **O'Brien, S. J., Womack, J. E., Lyons, L. A., Moore, K. J., Jenkins, N. A., and Copeland, N. G.,** Anchored reference loci for comparative genome mapping in mammals, *Nature Genet.,* 3, 103, 1993.
36. **Taketomi, S., Tsuda, M., Matsuo, J., Iwatska, H., and Suzuoki, Z.,** Alterations of hepatic enzyme activities in KK and yellow KK mice with various diabetic states, *Horm. Metab. Res.,* 5, 333, 1973.
37. **Fenton, P. F. and Carr, C. J.,** The nutrition of the mouse. XI. Response of four strains to diets differing in fat content, *J. Nutr.,* 45, 225, 1951.
38. **West, D. B., Boozer, C. N., Moody, D. L., and Atkinson, R. L.,** Dietary obesity in nine inbred mouse strains, *Am. J. Physiol. Regul. Integr. Comp. Physiol.,* 262, R1025, 1992.

39. **Bielschowsky, M. and Bielschowsky, F.,** A new strain of mice with hereditary obesity, *Proc. Otago Med. School,* 31, 29, 1953.
40. **Nakamura, M. and Yamada, K.,** A further study of the diabetic (KK) strain of the mouse. Fl and F2 offspring of the cross between KK and C57BL/6J mice, *Proc. Jpn. Acad.,* 39, 489, 1963.
41. **Butler, L. and Gerritsen, G.,** A comparison of the modes of inheritance of diabetes in the Chinese hamster and the KK mouse, *Diabetologia,* 6, 163, 1970.
42. **Crofford, O. B. and Davis, C. K.,** Growth characteristics, glucose tolerance and insulin sensitivity of New Zealand Obese mice, *Metabolism,* 14, 271, 1965.
43. **Veroni, M. C., Proietto, J., and Larkins, R. G.,** Evolution of insulin resistance in New Zealand Obese mice, *Diabetes,* 40, 1480, 1991.
44. **Herrberg, L., Doeppen, W., Major, E., and Gries, F. A.,** Dietary induced hypertrophic-hyperplastic obesity in mice, *J. Lipid Res.,* 6, 580, 1974.
45. **Festing, M. F. W.,** Inbred strains of mice, in *Genetic Variants and Strains of the Laboratory Mouse,* Lyon, M. F. and Searle, A. G., Eds., Oxford University Press, New York, 1989, 636.
46. **Nakamura, M. A.,** A diabetic strain of the mouse, *Proc. Jpn. Acad.,* 38, 348, 1962.
47. **Jones, E. E.,** Spontaneous hyperplasia of the pancreatic islets associated with glucosuria in hybrid mice, in *The Structure and Metabolism of the Pancreatic Islets,* Brolin, S. E., Hellman, B., and Knutson, H., Eds., Pergamon Press, Oxford, 1964, 189.
48. **Gleason, R. E., Lauris, V., and Soeldner, J. S.,** Studies on experimental diabetes in the Wellesley hybrid mouse, *Diabetologia,* 3, 175, 1967.
49. **Coleman, D. L.,** Obesity genes: beneficial effects in heterozygous mice, *Science,* 203, 663, 1979.
50. **Levan, G., Szpirer, J., Szpirer, C., Klinga, K., Hanson, C., and Islam, M. Q.,** The gene map of the Norway rat *(Rattus norvegicus)* and comparative mapping with mouse and man, *Genomics,* 10, 699, 1991.
51. **Serikawa, T., Kuramoto, T., Hilbert, P., Mori, M., Yamada, J., Dubay, C. J., Lindpaintner, K., Ganten, D., Guénet, J.-L., Lathrop, G. M., and Beckmann, J. S.,** Rat gene mapping using PCR-analyzed microsatellites, *Genetics,* 131, 701, 1992.
52. **Schemmel, R., Mickelson, O., and Gill, J. L.,** Dietary obesity in rats: body weight and body fat accretion in seven strains of rats, *J. Nutr.,* 100, 1041, 1970.
53. **Bray, G. A., York, D. A., and Fisler, J. S.,** Experimental obesity: a homeostatic failure due to defective nutrient stimulation of the sympathetic nervous system, *Vitam. Horm. N.Y.,* 45, 1, 1989.
54. **Bahary, N., Leibel, R. L., Joseph, L., and Friedman, J. M.,** Molecular mapping of the mouse db mutation, *Proc. Natl. Acad. Sci. U.S.A.,* 87, 8642, 1990.
55. **Bahary, N., Pachter, J. E., Felman, R., Leibel, R. L., Albright, K., Cram, S., and Friedman, J. M.,** Molecular mapping of mouse chromosomes 4 and 6: use of a flow-sorted Robertsonian chromosome, *Genomics,* 13, 761, 1992.
56. **Nadeau, J. H. and Taylor, B. A.,** Lengths of chromosomal segments conserved since divergence of man and mouse, *Proc. Natl. Acad. Sci. U.S.A.,* 81, 814, 1984.
57. **Snouwaert, J. N., Brigman, K. K., Latour, A. M., Malouf, N. N., Boucher, R. C., Smithies, O., and Koller, B. H.,** An animal model for cystic fibrosis made by gene targeting, *Science,* 257, 1083, 1992.
58. **Dorin, J. R., Dickinson, P., Alton, E. W. F. W., Smith, S. N., Geddes, D. M., Stevenson, B. J., Kimber, W. L., Fleming, S., Clarke, A. R., Hooper, M. L., Anderson, L., Beddington, R. S. P., and Porteous, D. J.,** Cystic fibrosis in the mouse by targeted insertional mutagenesis, *Nature,* 359, 211, 1992.
59. **Tybulewicz, V. L., Tremblay, M. L., LaMarca, M. E., Willemsen, R., Stubblefield, B. K., Winfield, S., Zablocka, B., Sidransky, E., Martin, B. M., and Huang, S. P.,**

Animal model of Gaucher's disease from targeted disruption of the mouse glucocerebrosidase gene, *Nature,* 357, 407, 1992.

60. **Prochazka, M., Leiter, E. H., Serreze, D. V., and Coleman, D. I.,** Three recessive loci required for insulin-dependent diabetes in nonobese diabetic mice, *Science,* 237, 286, 1987.
61. **Tomita, Y., Takeda, A., Okinaga, S., Tagami, H., and Shibahara, S.,** Human oculocutaneous albinism caused by single base insertion in the tyrosinase gene, *Biochem. Biophys. Res. Commun.,* 164, 990, 1989.
62. **Kwon, B. S., Haq, A. K., Wakulchik, M., Kestler, D., Barton, D. E., Francke, U., Lamoreux, M. L., Whitney, J. B., and Halaban, R.,** Isolation, chromosomal mapping, and expression of the mouse tyrosinase gene, *J. Invest. Dermatol.,* 93, 589, 1989.
63. **Kyle, J. W., Birkenmeier, E. H., Gwynn, B., Vogler, C., Hoppe, P. C., Hoffmann, J. W., and Sly, W. S.,** Correction of murine mucopolysaccharidosis VII by a human beta-glucuronidase transgene, *Proc. Natl. Acad. Sci. U.S.A.,* 87, 3914, 1990.
64. **Birkenmeier, E. H., Davisson, M. T., Beamer, W. G., Ganschow, R. E., Vogler, C. A., Gwynn, B., Lyford, K. A., Maltais, L. M., and Wawrzyniak, C. J.,** Murine mucopolysaccharidosis type VII. Characterization of a mouse with beta-glucuronidase deficiency, *J. Clin. Invest.,* 83, 1258, 1989.
65. **Kay, G., Thakker, R. V., and Rastan, S.,** Determination of a molecular map position for Hyp using a new interspecific backcross produced by in vitro fertilization, *Genomics,* 11, 651, 1991.
66. **Scriver, C. R. and Tenenhouse, H. S.,** Conserved loci on the X chromosome confer phosphate homeostasis in mice and humans, *Genet. Res.,* 56, 141, 1990.
67. **Jordan, T., Hanson, I., Zaletayev, D., Hodgson, S., Prosser, J., Seawright, A., Hastie, N., and Van Heyningen, V.,** The human PAX6 gene is mutated in two patients with aniridia, *Nature Genet.,* 1, 328, 1992.
68. **Su, L.-K., Kinzler, K. W., Vogelstein, B., Preisinger, A. C., Moser, A. R., Luongo, C., Gould, K. A., and Dove, W. F.,** A germline mutation of the murine homolog of the APC gene causes multiple intestinal neoplasia, *Science,* 256, 668, 1992.

Chapter 14

Genetics and Molecular Biology of Adipose Cell Characteristics

Gérard P. Ailhaud, Paul A. Grimaldi, and Raymond L. Négrel

TABLE OF CONTENTS

I. INTRODUCTION

During the last two decades, growth and development of white adipose tissue (WAT) and brown adipose tissue (BAT), at the cellular and molecular levels, have been studied extensively in various mammals and humans. *In vitro* approaches have provided data regarding similarities and differences between cells of preadipocyte clonal lines from rodents and adipose precursor cells from humans. Various molecular events associated with the recruitment and differentiation of adipose cells have been delineated. However, key information is lacking in regard to the origin of fat cells and is minimal in regard to adipose tissue development during embryogenesis and site-related differences in body fat distribution. Another important point with respect to the human embryo are the relationships between BAT and WAT since it is commonly accepted that BAT and WAT are present in newborns. This chapter examines the current understanding of the cellular and molecular mechanisms that ultimately determine the hyperplastic development of adipose tissue and discusses some of the controversial issues.

II. COMPARATIVE PROPERTIES OF ADIPOSE PRECURSOR CELLS FROM PREADIPOCYTE CLONAL LINES AND ADIPOSE TISSUES

The process of adipose cell differentiation has been investigated primarily in adipose precursor cells from established clonal lines, such as 3T3-L1, 3T3-F442A, Ob17, 1246, 3T3-T, and ST13, which are all aneuploid. Some investigators have turned to the study of adipose precursor cells derived from the stromal-vascular (SV) fraction of adipose tissues from various species, including humans; these cells are diploid, but have a limited life span. When transplanted into animals, cells from both sources develop into mature

0-8493-4880-3/94/$0.00+$.50

fat cells. It is worth pointing out that "differentiation" as applied to adipose precursor cells can have distinct meanings and that this can lead to confusion since, from a developmental perspective, all precursor cells (adipoblasts) are differentiated (or determined) because they are not progenitors of any other cell type. The process of determination (step1, Figure1) from multipotential stem cells to unipotential adipoblasts cannot be studied easily. However, a determination-like process can be induced by treatment of mouse 10T1/2 and 3T3 cells[1] and hamster CHEF-18 cells[2] with 5-azacytidine, whereas it is spontaneous in T984 cells isolated from a mouse teratocarcinoma.[3] In most cases, these cells are then able to differentiate into adipocytes, chondrocytes, and fibroblasts. Adipose precursor cells or adipoblasts have been cloned from this mixed population of cells.[4-6]

As shown in Figure 1, when dealing with preadipocyte clonal lines, differentiation is characterized by a sequence of events during which adipoblasts become committed and acquire early markers, but do not yet accumulate triacylglycerol (step2, Figure1). Terminal differentiation of early marker-expressing cells (preadipose cells) refers to late events, i.e., the acquisition of the protein machinery required for lipogenesis and triacylglycerol accumulation, which includes glycerol-3-phosphate dehydrogenase (GPDH; step3, Figure1). Very late events include the emergence of the α2-adrenoreceptor-mediated antilipolytic response (step4, Figure1). Overall, adipose cell differentiation corresponds to the following phenotypic changes: adipoblast $\rightarrow$ preadipose cell (usually termed preadipocyte) $\rightarrow$ immature adipose cell $\rightarrow$ mature adipose cell (adipocyte). The differentiation process in a primary culture of adipose precursor cells isolated from fat tissue (i.e., from the SV fraction) primarily corresponds to the sequence preadipose cell (preadipocyte) $\rightarrow$ immature adipose cell $\rightarrow$ mature adipose cell, although the presence of adipoblasts cannot be excluded. This tentative conclusion is based on the fact that rat, mouse, and human SV cells contain the bulk of A2COL6/pOb24 mRNA and express lipoprotein lipase (LPL) and insulin-like growth factor-I (IGF-I) mRNAs. In other words, these cells have already undergone commitment (step2, Figure1) and express early markers of differentiation. However, there is evidence that SV cells are present at different stages of differentiation. As an example, at least two populations of rat adipose precursor cells respond differently to insulin for terminal differentiation.[7] Once differentiated, rodent adipose cells from clonal lines or primary cultures show biochemical properties similar to those reported for mature adipocytes isolated from adipose tissue. Similar extensive studies remain to be performed in human adipose precursor cells once differentiated, despite the difficulties in obtaining a sufficient number of cells from biopsies or surgical samples.

The availability of preadipocyte clonal lines and the ability to grow and differentiate SV cells from various animal species, under serum-free chemically defined conditions, have allowed comparative studies. Mouse cells established from BAT appear five- to tenfold more sensitive to β-adrenergics than cells established from WAT. Since the same differences are observed between adipose precursor cells in primary culture from WAT and BAT of C57/BL6J mice, it appears that some intrinsic differences between these cells observed *ex vivo* remain present in preadipocyte clonal lines after cell immortalization, selection, and differentiation *in vitro*.[8,9] Altogether, this would suggest the existence of distinct precursor cells for brown and white adipocytes, but does not exclude the possibility of a transformation of brown precursor cells into white precursor cells, as shown by the rapid extinction of the uncoupling protein (UCP) gene expression observed in brown preadipocytes from lamb.[10] In contrast, no intrinsic differences were found between cells of clonal lines established from epididymal fat pads of genetically obese (Ob17 cell line) and genetically nonobese (HGFu cell line) mice.[11] In both cases, the adipsin gene is expressed *in vitro* at similar levels despite the fact that its expression *in vivo* is severely diminished in adult *ob/ob* mice compared to the lean animals.[12] This observation suggests that extracellular factors

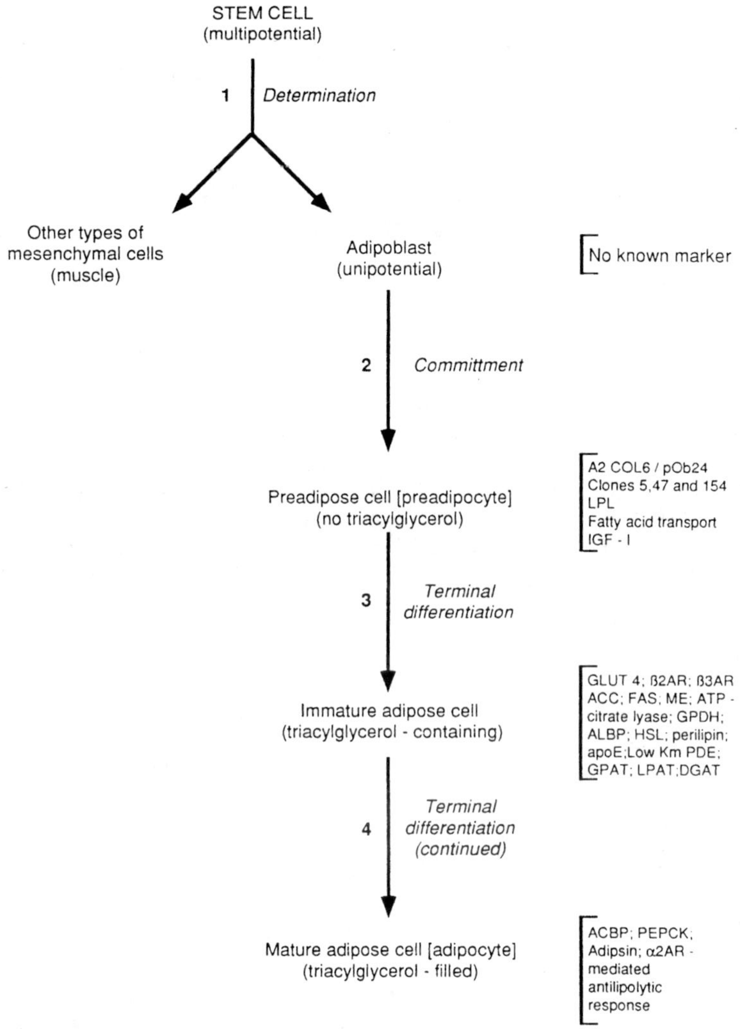

Figure 1. Multiple stages of adipose cell differentiation *in utero* and postnatally. This tentative scheme is based on data obtained with precursor cells from preadipocyte clonal lines. The abbreviations are: LPL, lipoprotein lipase; FA transport, fatty acid transport; A2COL6/pOb24, α2-chain of collagen VI; IGF-I, insulin-like growth factor-I; GLUT4, insulin-sensitive glucose transporter 4; ME, malic enzyme; ACC, acetyl-CoA carboxylase; FAS, fatty acid synthetase; GPDH, glycerol-3-phosphate dehydrogenase; ALBP, adipocyte lipid-binding protein (aP2); HSL, hormone-sensitive lipase; apoE, apolipoprotein E; low-Km PDE, low-Km phosphodiesterase; GPAT, glycerophosphate acyltransferase; LPAT, lysophosphatidate acyltransferase; DGAT, diglyceride acyltransferase; ACBP, acyl CoA binding protein; PEPCK, phosphoenolpyruvate carboxykinase; β2AR, β2-adrenoreceptor; β3AR, β3-adrenoreceptor; α2AR, α2-adrenoreceptor.

such as hyperinsulinemia and hypercorticosteronemia,[13] which are observed in genetically obese animals, may be responsible for this difference since insulin down-regulates the expression of the adipsin gene *in vitro.*[14] However, these results do not exclude the possibility that intrinsic differences yet to be characterized exist between adipose cells from lean and genetically obese mice.

III. ADIPOSE PRECURSOR CELLS DURING POSTNATAL AND LATE DEVELOPMENT

Methods of determining fat cell number and size have been used for a few decades to study the postnatal development of WAT, particularly in rodents. Unfortunately, these techniques are not sufficiently accurate to detect modest changes in cell number and, in any event, they only count triacylglycerol-filled cells. In other words, preadipocytes (Figure1), i.e., cells that have expressed early phenotypes but do not yet contain triacylglycerol droplets, are not counted. This technique excludes *a priori* a true estimate of the developmental potential of the various adipose depots. In preadipocytes, the transient expression of early markers, i.e., A2COL6/pOb24 mRNA,[15] the fat-tissue-specific expression of clone 5 (AP27 protein; see Reference 16), clone 47 (FSP27 protein; see Reference 17) and clone 154 (ADR protein, see Reference 18), and the expression of S-100 proteins[19] could help to better estimate the adipose tissue cellularity when using *in situ* hybridization and immunochemical techniques. Despite these limitations, the ability of adult mammals to increase their number of adipocytes, depending on the localization of the adipose depot, the nature of the diet, and the environmental conditions to which they have been exposed, has been long known.[20]

When triacylglycerol-devoid cells of the SV fraction are separated from triacylglycerol-filled cells of the adipocyte fraction after collagenase treatment of the adipose tissues from adult mice and centrifugation, the bulk of A2COL6/pOb24 mRNA is confined to the SV fraction and that of adipsin mRNA to the adipocyte fraction. Unexpectedly, adipose tissue from various sites of very old mice has been shown to contain high amounts of A2COL6/pOb24 mRNA, demonstrating that dormant preadipocytes are indeed present even at a very late age.[6] A similar situation applies to man: although the number of adipose precursor cells from subcutaneous adipose tissue diminishes with age, it is evident that preadipocytes remain present as dormant cells in elderly men and women since they can be revealed *in vitro* after differentiation under chemically defined conditions.[21] In other words, the potential to acquire new fat cells appears to remain throughout life.

Although sex- and site-related differences in body fat distribution are well known in humans and various animal species, the reasons for this differential development remain unclear. It is assumed that the differences in growth and differentiation between depots, or between individuals for a given depot, are due to (1) differences in the number of remaining adipose precursor cells able to respond to a given set of stimuli which are identical on a qualitative and quantitative basis, (2) differences in the nature or concentration of some stimuli (locally produced) triggering (or inhibiting) growth and/or differentiation of adipose precursor cells, and (3) a combination of both events. Regarding point 1, in Cushing's syndrome, hypercortisolism, which leads to centrally localized adipose tissue as in abdominal obesity, is likely to be accompanied by cell hyperplasia. A higher density of glucocorticoid receptors is found in abdominal fat tissue than in other fat depots, and investigators have proposed that glucocorticoids may regulate this differential development.[22] Differences in this depot between individuals with respect to the number of glucocorticoid-responsive adipose precursor cells remain to be seen. Clearly, however, differences in ability to differentiate into adipose cells *in vitro* are observed between SV cells from the abdominal and femoral adipose tissue of obese women,[23] but differences at the molecular level also remain to be seen. Regarding point 2, a way to look at differences in the nature or concentration of locally produced, low-molecular-weight stimuli is clearly a difficult goal to achieve; nevertheless, it can be approached *in vivo* using the microdialysis technique.[24]

One of the most critical questions on the development of adipose tissue remains the relationship between BAT and WAT. The existence of distinct precursor cells is based on important observations:[25-27] SV cells isolated from the interscapular BAT of young mice are able to express UCP mRNA and UCP protein and to differentiate into lipid-filled cells, and the stimulation of UCP gene expression is primarily regulated via β-adrenoreceptors. Under the same conditions, SV cells isolated from WAT express neither UCP mRNA nor UCP protein. The transformation of BAT precursors into WAT precursors appears to take place in ovine after birth:[10] the expression of UCP mRNA takes place in precursor cells from perirenal BAT of newborn lambs, and glucocorticoids promote a stimulating effect on this expression. However, UCP mRNA is not expressed and a glucocorticoid effect is not observed with precursor cells from 3-week-old lambs. Therefore, the extinction of the UCP gene appears to be a rapid process *in vivo.* The degree of completeness and irreversibility of this phenomenon have become important issues since it has been shown recently that, in rats, UCP mRNA is detected in tissues considered as typical WAT (epididymal, inguinal, mesenteric, retroperitoneal, and, particularly, periovarian). Upon exposure of the animals to cold or after β_3-agonist treatment, UCP expression is increased in the periovarian adipose tissue as it occurs in typical BAT.[28] Upon exposure to a β_3-agonist that has thermogenic and antiobesity properties in adult dog, a potent increase of the UCP content is also observed in extracts of perirenal, peribladder, and pericardiac adipose tissue.[29] Clearly, adipocytes expressing UCP are present in adipose depots considered as white fat, suggesting that the proportion of brown and white adipocytes can vary greatly between various sites and possibly could be modulated pharmacologically, at least in rat and dog and perhaps in humans. The latter possibility is suggested by the fact that, in humans, UCP is still observed in the perirenal, peristernal, and retroperitoneal adipose depots of young infants, but also in *adult* patients suffering from pheochromocytoma and primary aldosteronism.[30] Taken together, these observations do not exclude in normal subjects a possible "reactivation" of UCP expression in tissues formerly considered as white adipose depots and, therefore, do not exclude a means to increase thermogenesis.

IV. EXTRACELLULAR SIGNALS AND SIGNALING PATHWAYS INVOLVED IN THE TERMINAL DIFFERENTIATION OF ADIPOSE PRECURSOR CELLS

The observation that dormant preadipocytes are present in old animals as well as in elderly people has led to the identification of a panoply of adipogenic signals which are required *in vitro* for the terminal differentiation of preadipocytes. The role played by various hormones and factors in *differentiating* cells should not be confused with the role of the same hormones and factors in *differentiated* cells. In addition, because of uncertainty about the developmental stage of precursor cells from various sources at the time of inoculation, the characterization of cellular factors (adipogenic and antiadipogenic factors) has been and remains controversial. To add further complication, the (fetal) bovine serum used in most experiments contains positive and negative effectors, the proportions of which cannot be controlled. This makes comparisons difficult and has led investigators to use serum-free, chemically defined culture media.

A. CIRCULATING HORMONES

In both serum-supplemented and serum-free medium, growth hormone (GH) stimulates the terminal differentiation of 3T3-F442A and Ob17 cells. In the presence of GH, which acts as a protein kinase C (PKC) activator by means of diacylglycerol production from phosphatidylcholine, a potent increase in the adipogenic activity of the culture medium is observed. In the presence of IGF-I, the adipogenic activity of GH is mimicked by other PKC activators. Triiodothyronine also appears to be involved in the terminal differentiation of Ob17 cells and 3T3-L1 cells.[4] The role of insulin as a positive modulator of terminal differentiation has been clearly shown: it up-regulates the activity of glucose transporters GLUT1 and GLUT4 and increases the steady-state levels of lipogenic enzymes and triacylglycerol stores. Taken together, the various data suggest that, besides GH and T_3, there is a subtle interplay between insulin, IGF-I, and their own receptors to modulate the maximal expression of terminal differentiation. Glucocorticoids or the glucocorticoid analogue dexamethasone have been reported to stimulate terminal differentiation of preadipocytes from various clonal lines as well as that of adipose precursor cells from rat, rabbit, and human: in Ob17 cells, glucocorticoids appear to stimulate specifically the production of prostacyclin, a local paracrine/autocrine factor active in the differentiation of preadipose cells to adipose cells (see below).

B. PARACRINE/AUTOCRINE FACTORS

Using serum-free, chemically defined culture conditions, arachidonic acid has been characterized as being the main adipogenic factor leading to terminal differentiation of Ob17 cells.[31] Arachidonic acid increases in a rapid and dramatic manner the production of cyclic AMP (cAMP) and, in parallel, the late expression of GPDH activity and triacylglycerol accumulation; it is also able to amplify the terminal differentiation promoted by other cAMP-elevating agents and to induce polyphosphoinositide breakdown. Since these effects of arachidonic acid are prevented by indomethacin or aspirin, it has been postulated that one or more of the various prostaglandins produced by Ob17 cells, i.e., PGE_2, PGI_2 and $PGF_2\alpha$, actually could be involved. Prostacyclin and $PGF_2\alpha$ are indeed involved, and a combination of signals — each present above a threshold level — is required for terminal differentiation of cells having expressed early markers. This combination involves prostacyclin[32,33] (acting via the cAMP pathway) and IGF-I playing a cardinal role and $PGF_2\alpha$ and insulin playing a modulating role. According to this model, it has been predicted (and actually shown) that (1) antibodies able to neutralize PGI_2 and $PGF_2\alpha$ are able to block the terminal differentiation induced by arachidonic acid; (2) any hormone active on the release of arachidonic acid and/or on the production of prostaglandins should behave as an adipogenic stimulus (this is indeed the case with glucocorticoids, which are able to trigger terminal differentiation of Ob1771 cells by means of an increased production of PGI_2[34]); and (3) a critical "window" of hormone action should be expected (this is the case since prostacyclin becomes unable to stimulate cAMP production once the cells become differentiated, a phenomenon likely due to the disappearance of the prostacyclin receptor). The critical role of prostacyclin in promoting the terminal differentiation of preadipocytes has been extended to rat and human adipose precursor cells.[33] Recent results have shown that adenosine could also play a *positive* role in this respect, in addition to the fact that adenosine is already known to behave as an antilipolytic effector by means of a negative modulation of adenylate cyclase mediated by the A_1 receptor. By contrast, the A_2 receptor subtype, which is positively coupled to adenylate cyclase, is expressed in preadipocytes and, thus, potentiates the positive effect of PGI_2.[35]

Recently, striking results have been obtained in regard to the action of sex steroids, if one recalls that adipocytes can synthesize androgens and estrogens from adrenal steroid precursors[36] and that different sex steroid receptors (androgen, estrogen, and progesterone receptors) exist in these cells: in male and female hamsters, androgens are able to up-regulate the expression of $\alpha 2$-adrenoreceptors by means of an increase in the $\alpha 2$-adrenoreceptor mRNA level with no change in adenylate cyclase activity and coupling efficiency to G_i proteins.[37] A similar phenomenon takes place *in vitro* using primary cultures of hamster adipose precursor cells[68] in which α2-adrenoreceptor-mediated antilipolytic response is the latest event of terminal differentiation so far reported.[38] Taken together, the results obtained in preadipose cells from clonal lines lead to a prediction in regard to precursor cells isolated from fat tissue: since the latter cells have already expressed early markers and possibly have been "primed" by various hormones *in vivo,* their hormonal requirements for terminal differentiation *ex vivo* should be rather limited. This is indeed the case for mouse,[69] rabbit,[39] and human preadipocytes,[21] which require only IGF-I, insulin, and glucocorticoids. Last, but not least, since these stimuli must be present *ex vivo* at the same time above threshold levels, it is assumed that these hormonal signals must be in phase with each other *in vivo.* Since dormant preadipocytes are present *in vivo,* it can be postulated that frequent ill-timed hormone secretion, induced by diet or other means, increases the probability of an "in-phase" event taking place and, therefore, may lead to hyperplasia of adipose tissue.

C. FATTY ACIDS

In addition to circulating hormones and paracrine/autocrine factors, recent observations have shown that long-chain fatty acids are able to regulate at the transcriptional level the expression of adipocyte lipid-binding protein (ALBP) and acyl CoA synthetase (ACS) genes.[40,41] Nonmetabolized long-chain fatty acids are more potent in this process, demonstrating that fatty acids per se are active.[42] It is hypothesized that fatty acids, like all-*trans* and 9-*cis* retinoic acids, which are also nonmetabolized fatty acids, are able to stimulate gene transcription by means of nuclear receptors. In any event, these observations may provide a link between high-fat diets and the regulation of the expression of lipid-related genes and raise some intriguing questions relative to insulin resistance and dyslipoproteinemia.

D. ANTIADIPOGENIC FACTORS

Altogether, the above results underline the importance of characterizing various factors that inhibit or abolish differentiation of adipose precursor cells (see Reference 4 for review). In contrast to platelet-derived growth factor (PDGF), the inhibitory effect of transforming growth factor-β (TGF-β) appears to be independent of its mitogenic property. Epidermal growth factor (EGF) is required for terminal differentiation of 3T3-L1 cells, whereas it is inhibitory for that of adipose precursor cells from rat fat tissue. The latter observation is consistent with a recent report showing that subcutaneous administration of EGF to newborn rats results in a large decrease in the weight of inguinal fat pads. The effects of tumor necrosis factor α (TNF-α) have been studied extensively, since it can alter the energy balance *in vivo* by a selective action on adipose tissue. In differentiated cells from several clonal lines, TNF-α inhibits the expression of several differentiation-specific genes such as LPL, GPDH, adipsin, and ALBP mRNAs in a dose-dependent manner. Moreover, it stimulates lipolysis and induces a phenotypic "dedifferentiation" on a long-term basis.

Retinoids are also able to modulate terminal differentiation. In the case of 3T3-F442A cells, their inhibitory action is reversible and takes place after expression of LPL, but before expression of GPDH and accumulation of triacylglycerol.[43] Adipose tissue is a target for retinoid action; the nuclear retinoid acid receptors RAR α and γ are detected in Ob17 cells,[70] whereas RAR α, β, and γ are detected in rat adipose tissue.[44] Moreover, the expression of cellular retinol binding protein is high in preadipocytes only, whereas that of the secreted and circulating retinol binding protein is strong in adipocytes.[45] It would be of interest to gain some insights in the near future into the regulation of the expression of the genes coding for the various retinoic acid receptors and the retinol binding proteins in adipose cells from lean and genetically obese rodents.

V. MOLECULAR REGULATION OF ADIPOSE-RELATED GENES

The intracellular events that direct the complete differentiation of adipoblasts to mature adipose cells involve large changes in gene expression. Adipocyte-lipid binding protein does not appear to be an exclusive marker of adipose cells, but nevertheless remains the most characteristic phenotype since (1) limited information on the specific expression of clones 5,47 and 154[16-18] in adipose tissue has been reported; and (2) A2COL6/pOb24 mRNA, a marker of the preadipose state both *in vitro* and in adult animal,[6] is also present during embryogenesis as a marker of muscle differentiation.[46] Although the mechanisms which control gene expression can be numerous, the rate of transcription appears to be the major control point. This has been shown for early-expressing genes such as LPL and A2COL6/pOb24 as well as for various late markers such as ALBP, GPDH, and adipsin. In the past few years a large number of transcription regulatory factors have been described in adipose cells. This list includes proto-oncogenes (c-raf-1, c-*fos,* c-*jun*),[47-49] the glucocorticoid receptor,[50] NF-1-like factor,[51] CHOP10,[52] and C/EBP α, β, and γ.[53] From these studies it appears that C/EBP α plays the major role in terminal differentiation events since it appears to be both necessary and sufficient.[54-56] However, none of these factors are fat tissue specific, and in the case of the ALBP gene the C/EBPα response element is neither necessary nor sufficient.[57] A 518-base-pair enhancer region, upstream of the C/EBPα and AP-1 *(jun/fos)* binding sites, is sufficient for fat-tissue-specific expression in transgenic mice. Among the four cis response elements of the ALBP promoter, two are bound and regulated by an ARF2 factor (ARE2, ARE4) and the remaining two bind another nuclear factor, ARF6 (ARE6, ARE7).[58] It is of interest that ARE6 binds nuclear extracts from adipocytes only and that this sequence is not found in other genes expressed in adipocytes, in agreement with the fact that ALBP appears to be the most specific marker of adipose cells. It is also of interest to note that an overtranscription of the fatty acid synthetase (FAS) gene has been reported in genetically obese rats,[59] providing a basis for future investigation on the transcription regulatory factor(s) of the FAS gene, which may play a critical role in the development of genetic obesity. At present, little is known about the intracellular machinery and the mechanisms by which the multiple signaling pathways operate in the process of terminal differentiation. Recent observations indicate that Ras proteins are involved in the transduction signals initiated by insulin and IGF-I in differentiating 3T3-L1 cells.[60] The c-Myc protein, the expression of which is abolished at the time of early marker emergence, prevents the same cells from entering terminal differentiation,[61] and a reciprocal regulation of differentiation by c-Myc and C/EBP is observed.[62] Growth hormone, which in Ob17 cells activates a PKC-dependent pathway, induces the expression of c-*fos* gene and c-Fos protein which in turn regulates the expression of the LPL gene.[63]

VI. EXCESS OF ADIPOSE TISSUE MASS AND ADIPOSE CELLS AS SECRETORY CELLS

The excess of adipose tissue mass, particularly in the abdominal region, is correlated with hypertension, non-insulin-dependent diabetes, and dyslipoproteinemia. It is assumed that such an excess leads indirectly to these various and major metabolic disturbances. However, a more direct effect of adipose tissue on these disturbances can be postulated as the concept of adipocytes being secretory cells has emerged (Figure 2). In addition to secreting LPL, adipocytes are another important extrahepatic source of cholesterol ester transfer protein[64] and possibly of apolipoprotein E,[65] suggesting a link between excess adipose tissue mass and dyslipoproteinemia. Moreover, adipocytes are the most important extrahepatic source of angiotensinogen; although its role after conversion to angiotensin II is supposed to be the regulation of blood flow in adipose tissue,[66] the question of a

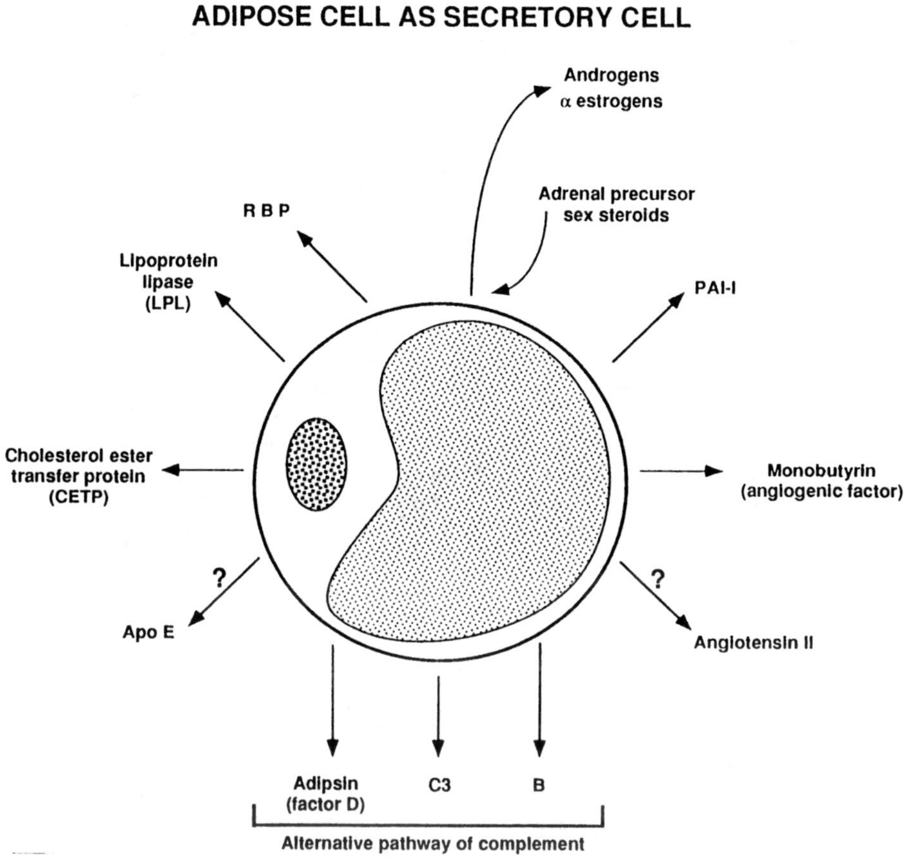

Figure 2. Adipose cells as secretory cells. ApoE, apolipoprotein E; RBP, retinol binding protein, PAI-I, plasminogen-activator inhibitor-I.

possible link between excess adipose tissue mass and hypertension remains open. Adipocytes are also able to secrete three major proteins of the alternative system of complement — i.e., factor D or adipsin, factor C_3, and factor B — and a role for adipsin in energy balance has been proposed.[67] Adipocytes synthesize the cellular-retinol binding protein and also synthesize and secrete the retinol binding protein, favoring the participation of adipose tissue in retinoid storage and metabolism in addition to storage and mobilization of triacylglycerol and unesterified cholesterol.[45] Last, but not least, the ability of adipocytes to synthesize significant amount of sex steroids is now recognized.[36] Together these observations emphasize that adipocytes secrete peptide and nonpeptide factors which can be active in cells from other organs. Thus, the importance of excess adipose tissue mass in the development of physiopathological situations may be more direct than postulated at the present time. Future research in that direction will be necessary to support this hypothesis.

ACKNOWLEDGMENTS

G. Ailhaud and R. Négrel are Professors of Biochemistry and P. Grimaldi is an established investigator from Institut National de la Santé et de la Recherche Médicale

(INSERM). This research has been supported by funds from Centre National de la Recherche Scientifique (CNRS) and grants from INSERM, Institut National de la Recherche Agronomique (INRA), and Association de Recherche Contre le Cancer (ARC). We thank C. Dani, C. Forest, D. Gaillard, and C. Vannier for their valuable contributions over the years. The important contributions of a large number of other investigators are also gratefully acknowledged. Special thanks are due to Mrs. G. Oillaux for expert secretarial assistance.

ABBREVIATIONS

WAT, white adipose tissue; BAT, brown adipose tissue; SV, stromal-vascular cells; GPDH, glycerol-3-phosphate dehydrogenase; LPL, lipoprotein lipase; IGF-I, insulin-like growth factor-I; GH, growth hormone; PKC, protein kinase C; cAMP, cyclic AMP; ALBP, adipocyte lipid-binding protein; ACS, acyl CoA synthetase; PDGF, platelet-derived growth factor; TGF-β, transforming growth factor-β; TNF-α, tumor necrosis factor-α; FAS, fatty acid synthetase; UCP, uncoupling protein; C/EBP, CCAAT/enhancer-binding protein; CHOP-10, C/EBP-homologous protein 10; NF-1, nuclear factor-1; ARF, adipocyte regulatory factor; ARE, adipocyte regulatory element.

REFERENCES

1. **Taylor, S. M. and Jones, P. A.,** Multiple new phenotypes induced in 10T1/2 and 3T3 cells treated with 5-azacytidine, *Cell,* 17, 771, 1979.
2. **Sager, R. and Kovac, P.,** Pre-adipocyte determination either by insulin or by 5-azacytidine, *Proc. Natl. Acad. Sci. U.S.A.,* 79, 480, 1982.
3. **Darmon, M., Serrero, G., Rizzino, A., and Sato, G.,** Isolation of myoblastic, fibroadipogenic, and fibroblastic clonal cell lines from a common precursor and study of their requirements for growth and differentiation, *Exp. Cell Res.,* 132, 313, 1981.
4. **Ailhaud, G.,** Extracellular factors, signalling pathways and differentiation of adipose precursor cells, *Curr. Opin. Cell Biol.,* 2, 1043, 1990.
5. **Ailhaud, G., Amri, E., Bertrand, B., Barcellini-Couget, S., Bardon, S., Catalioto, R.-M., Dani, C., Deslex, S., Djian, P., Doglio, A., Pradines-Figuères, A., Forest, C., Gaillard, D., Grimaldi, P., and Vannier, C.,** Cellular and molecular aspects of adipose tissue growth, in *Obesity: Towards a Molecular Approach,* Bray, G., Ricquier, D., and Spiegelman,B., Eds., Alan R. Liss, New York, 1990, 133.
6. **Ailhaud, G., Grimaldi, P., and Négrel, R.,** Cellular and molecular aspects of adipose tissue development, *Annu. Rev. Nutr.,* 12, 207, 1992.
7. **Swierczewski, E., Pello, J.-Y., Arapinis, C., Aron, Y., and Krishnamoorthly, R.,** Characterization of rat preadipocytes from normal rat adipose tissue by their effector response, *Biochem. J.,* 248, 383, 1987.
8. **Forest, C., Doglio, A., Ricquier, D., and Ailhaud, G.,** A preadipocyte clonal line from mouse brown adipose tissue. Short- and long-term responses to insulin and β-adrenergics, *Exp. Cell Res.,* 168, 218, 1987.
9. **Ailhaud, G., Amri, E., Barbaras, R., Casteilla, L., Catalioto, R.-M., Dani, C., Deslex, S., Doglio, A., Forest, C., Gaillard, D., Grimaldi, P., Négrel, R., Ricquier, D., and Vannier, C.,** Adipose cell differentiation: differential expression of specific mRNAs and protein markers in cells from white and brown adipose tissues, in *Recent Advances in Obesity Research,* Vol. 5, Berry, E. M., Blondheim, S. H., Eliahou, H. E., and Shafrir, E., Eds., John Libbey, London, 1987, 174.
10. **Casteilla, L., Nouguès, J., Reyne, Y., and Ricquier, D.,** Differentiation of ovine brown adipocyte precursor cells in a chemically defined serum-free medium. Importance of glucocorticoids and age of animals, *Eur. J. Biochem.,* 198, 195, 1991.

11. **Forest, C., Czerucka, D., Grimaldi, P., Vannier, C., Négrel, R., and Ailhaud, G.,** Metabolic characteristics of murine adipocyte precursor clones, in *The Adipocyte and Obesity: Cellular and Molecular Mechanisms,* Angel, A., Hollenberg, C. H., and Roncari, D. A. K., Eds., Raven Press, New York, 1983, 53.
12. **Flier, J. S., Cook, K. S., Usher, P., and Spiegelman, B. M.,** Severely impaired adipsin expression in genetic and acquired obesity, *Science,* 37, 405, 1987.
13. **Spiegelman, B. M., Lowell, B., Napolitano, A., Dubic, P., Barton, D., Francke, U., Groves, D. L., Cook, K. S., and Flier, J. S.,** Adrenal glucocorticoids regulate adipsin gene expression in genetically obese mice, *J. Biol. Chem.,* 264, 1811, 1989.
14. **Dani, C., Bertrand, B., Bardon, S., Doglio, A., Amri, E., and Grimaldi, P.,** Regulation of gene expression by insulin in adipose cells: opposite effects on adipsin and glycerophosphate dehydrogenase genes, *Mol. Cell. Endocrinol.,* 63, 199, 1989.
15. **Dani, C., Doglio, A., Amri, E., Bardon, S., Fort, P., Bertrand, B., Grimaldi,P., and Ailhaud, G.,** Cloning and regulation of a mRNA specifically expressed in the preadipose state, *J. Biol. Chem.,* 264, 10119, 1989.
16. **Wenz, H.-M., Hinck, L., Cannon, P., Navre, M., and Ringold, G. M.,** Reduced expression of AP27 protein, the product of a growth factor-repressible gene, is associated with diminished adipocyte differentiation, *Proc. Natl. Acad. Sci. U.S.A.,* 89, 1065, 1992.
17. **Danesch, U., Hoeck, W., and Ringold, G. M.,** Cloning and transcriptional regulation of a novel adipocyte-specific gene, FSP27. CAAT-enhancer-binding-protein (C/EBP) and C/EBP-like proteins interact with sequences required for differentiation-dependent expression, *J. Biol. Chem.,* 267, 7185, 1992.
18. **Jiang, H.-P. and Serrero, G.,** Isolation and characterization of a full-length cDNA coding for an adipose differentiation-related protein, *Proc. Natl. Acad. Sci. U.S.A.,* 89, 7856, 1992.
19. **Cinti, S., Cigolini, M., Morroni, M., and Zingaretti, M. C.,** S-100 protein in white preadipocytes: an immunoelectronmicroscopy study, *Anat. Rec.,* 224, 466, 1989.
20. **Faust, I. M. and Miller, W. H., Jr.,** Hyperplastic growth of adipose tissue in obesity, in *The Adipocyte and Obesity: Cellular and Molecular Mechanisms,* Angel,A., Hollenberg, C. H., and Roncari, D. A. K., Eds., Raven Press, New York, 1983, 41.
21. **Hauner, H., Entenmann, G., Wabitsch, M., Gaillard, D., Ailhaud, G., Négrel,R., and Pfeiffer, E.,** Promoting effect of glucocorticoids on the differentiation of human adipocyte precursor cells cultured in chemically defined serum, *J. Clin. Invest.,* 84, 1663, 1989.
22. **Rebuffé-Scrive, M., Krotkiewski, M., Elfverson, J., and Björntorp, P.,** Muscle and adipose tissue morphology and metabolism in Cushing's syndrome, *J. Clin. Endocrinol. Metab.,* 67, 1122, 1988.
23. **Hauner, H. and Entenmann, G.,** Regional variation of adipose differentiation in cultured stromal-vascular cells from the abdominal and femoral adipose tissue of obese women, *Int. J. Obes.,* 15, 121, 1991.
24. **Lönroth, P., Jansson, P. A., and Smith, U.,** A microdialysis method allowing characterization of intercellular water space in humans, *Am. J. Physiol.,* 253, E228, 1987.
25. **Rehnmark, S., Kopecky, J., Jacobsson, A., Néchad, M., Herron, D., Nelson, B., Obregon, M. J., Nedergaard, J., and Cannon, B.,** Brown adipocytes differentiated in vitro can express the gene for the uncoupling protein thermogenin: effects of hypothyroidism and norepinephrine, *Exp. Cell Res.,* 182, 75, 1989.
26. **Rehnmark, S., Néchad, M., Herron, D., Cannon, B., and Nedergaard, J.,** α- And β-adrenergic induction of the expression of the uncoupling protein thermogenin in brown adipocytes differentiated in culture, *J.Biol. Chem.,* 265, 16464, 1990.
27. **Kopecky, J., Baudysova, M., Zanotti, F., Janikova, D., Pavelka, S., and Houstek, J.,** Synthesis of mitochondrial uncoupling protein in brown adipocytes differentiated cell culture, *J. Biol. Chem.,* 265, 22204, 1990.

28. **Cousin, B., Cinti, S., Morroni, M., Raimbault, S., Ricquier, D., Pénicaud, L., and Casteilla, L.,** Occurrence of brown adipocytes in rat white adipose tissue: molecular and morphological characterization, *J. Cell Sci.,* 103, 931, 1992.
29. **Champigny, O., Ricquier, D., Blondel, O., Mayers, R. M., Briscoe, M. G., and Holloway, B. R.,** β3-Adrenergic receptor stimulation restores message and expression of brown-fat mitochondrial uncoupling protein in adult dogs, *Proc. Natl. Acad. Sci. U.S.A.,* 88, 10774, 1991.
30. **Garruti, G. and Ricquier, D.,** Analysis of uncoupling protein and its mRNA in adipose tissue deposits of adult humans, *Int. J. Obes.,* 16, 383, 1992.
31. **Gaillard, D., Négrel, R., Lagarde, M., and Ailhaud, G.,** Requirement and role of arachidonic acid in the differentiation of pre-adipose cells, *Biochem. J.,* 257, 389, 1989.
32. **Négrel, R., Gaillard, D., and Ailhaud, G.,** Prostacyclin as potent effector of adipose cell differentiation, *Biochem. J.,* 257, 399, 1989.
33. **Vassaux, G., Gaillard, D., Ailhaud, G., and Négrel, R.,** Prostacyclin is a specific effector of adipose cell differentiation: its dual role as a cAMP- Ca^{2+}-elevating agent, *J. Biol. Chem.,* 267, 11092, 1992.
34. **Gaillard, D., Wabitsch, M., Pipy, B., and Négrel, R.,** Control of terminal differentiation of adipose precursor cells by glucocorticoids, *J. Lipid Res.,* 32, 569, 1991.
35. **Vassaux, G., Gaillard, D., Mari, B., Ailhaud, G., and Négrel, R.,** Differential expression of adenosine A_1 and A_2 receptors in preadipocytes and adipocytes, *Biochem. Biophys. Res. Commun.,* 193, 1123, 1993.
36. **Labrie, F., Simard, J., Luu-The, V., Trudel, C., Martel, C., Labrie, C., Zhao, H.F., Rhéaume, E., Couet, J., and Breton, N.,** Expression of 3β-hydroxysteroid dehydrogenase/Δ5-Δ4 isomerase (3β-HSD) and 17β-hydroxysteroid dehydrogenase (17β-HSD) in adipose tissue, *Int. J. Obes.,* 15, 91, 1991.
37. **Saulnier-Blache, J.-S., Bouloumie, A., Valet, P., Devedjian, J.-C., and Lafontan, M.,** Androgenic regulation of adipocyte α2-adrenoreceptor expression in male and female Syrian hamsters: proposed transcriptional mechanism, *Endocrinology,* 130, 316, 1992.
38. **Saulnier-Blache, J.-S., Dauzats, M., Daviaud, D., Gaillard, D., Ailhaud, G., Négrel, R., and Lafontan, M.,** The α2-adrenoreceptor is a very late marker of adipose conversion in cultured hamster preadipocytes, *J. Lipid Res.,* 32, 1489, 1991.
39. **Reyne, Y., Nougès, J., and Dulor, J. P.,** Differentiation of rabbit adipocyte precursor cells in a serum-free medium, *In Vitro Cell. Dev. Biol.,* 25, 747, 1989.
40. **Amri, E., Bertrand, B., Ailhaud, G., and Grimaldi, P.,** Regulation of adipose cell differentiation. I. Fatty acids are inducers of the aP2 gene expression, *J. Lipid Res.,* 32, 1449, 1991.
41. **Amri, E., Ailhaud, G., and Grimaldi, P.,** Regulation of adipose cell differentiation. II. Kinetics of induction of the aP2 gene by fatty acids and modulation by dexamethasone, *J. Lipid Res.,* 32, 1457, 1991.
42. **Grimaldi, P., Knobel, S. M., Whitesell, R. R., and Abumrad, N. A.,** Induction of the aP2 gene by nonmetabolized long chain fatty acids, *Proc. Natl. Acad. Sci. U.S.A.,* 89, 10930, 1992.
43. **Pairault, J., Quignard-Boulangé, A., Dugail, I., and Lasnier, F.,** Differential effects of retinoic acid upon early and late events in adipose conversion of 3T3 preadipocytes, *Exp. Cell Res.,* 177, 27, 1988.
44. **Zovich, D. C., Orologa, A., Okuno, M., Wong Yen Kong, L., Talmage, D. A., Piantedosi, R., Goodman, D. W. S., and Blaner, W. S.,** Differentiation-dependent expression of retinoid-binding proteins in BFC-1β adipocytes, *J. Biol. Chem.,* 267, 13884, 1992.

45. **Tsutsumi, C., Okuno, M., Tannous, L., Piantedosi, R., Allan, M., Goodman, D. W. S., and Blaner, W. S.,** Retinoids and retinoid-binding protein expression in rat adipocytes, *J. Biol. Chem.,* 267, 1805, 1992.
46. **Ibrahimi, A., Bertrand, B., Bardon, S., Amri, E.-Z., Grimaldi, P., Ailhaud, G., and Dani, C.,** Cloning of α2 chain of type VII collagen and expression during mouse development, *Biochem. J.,* 289, 141, 1993.
47. **Zmuidzinas, A., Gould, G., and Yager, J.,** Expression of c-raf-1 and A-raf-1 during differentiation of 3T3-L1 preadipocyte fibroblasts into adipocytes, *Biochem. Biophys. Res. Commun.,* 162, 1180, 1989.
48. **Gurland, G., Ashcom, G., Cochran, B., and Schwartz, J.,** Rapid events in growth hormone action. Induction of c-*fos* and c-*jun* transcription in 3T2-F442A preadipocytes, *Endocrinology,* 127, 3187, 1990.
49. **Gaskins, H. R., Kim, J.-W., and Hausman, G. J.,** A decrease in local hormone biosynthesis and c-Fos gene expression accompany differentiation of porcine preadipocytes, *In Vitro Cell Dev. Biol.,* 26, 1049, 1990.
50. **Cook, J., Lucas, J., Sibley, E., Bolanswski, M., Christy, R., Kelly, T., and Lane, M.,** Expression of the differentiation-induced gene for fatty acid binding protein is activated by glucocorticoid and cyclic AMP, *Proc. Natl. Acad. Sci. U.S.A.,* 85, 2949, 1988.
51. **Graves, R. A., Tontonoz, P., Ross, S. R., and Spiegelman, B.,** Identification of a potent adipocyte-binding enhancer: involvement of an NF-1 like factor, *Genes Dev.,* 5, 428, 1991.
52. **Ron, D. and Habener, J.,** CHOP, a novel developmentally regulated nuclear protein that dimerizes with transcription factors C/EBP and LAP and functions as a dominant-negative inhibitor of gene transcription, *Genes Dev.,* 6, 439, 1992.
53. **Cao, Z., Umek, R. M., and McKnight, S. L.,** Regulated expression of three C/EBP isoforms during adipose conversion of 3T3-L1 cells, *Genes Dev.,* 5, 1538, 1991.
54. **Umek, R., Friedman, A., and McKnight, S.,** CCAAT/enhancer binding protein: a component of a differentiation switch, *Science,* 251, 288, 1991.
55. **Samuelsson, L., Stromberg, K., Vilman, K., Bjursell, G., and Enerback, S.,** The CCAAT/enhancer binding protein and its role in adipocyte differentiation: evidence for direct involvement in terminal adipocyte development, *Embo J.,* 10, 3787, 1991.
56. **Lin, F. and Lane, M. D.,** Antisense CCAAT/enhancer-binding protein RNA suppresses coordinate gene expression and triglyceride accumulation during differentiation of 3T3-L1 preadipocytes, *Genes Dev.,* 6, 533, 1992.
57. **Ross, S., Graves, R., Greenstein, A., Platt, K., Shyu, H., Mellovitz, B., and Spiegelman, B.,** A fat-specific enhancer is the primary determinant of gene expression for adipocyte P2 *in vivo, Proc. Natl. Acad. Sci. U.S.A.,* 87, 9590, 1990.
58. **Graves, R. A., Tontonoz, P., Ross, S. R., and Spiegelman, B.,** Analysis of a tissue-specific enhancer: ARF6 regulates adipogenic gene expression, *Mol. Cell Biol.,* 12, 1202, 1992.
59. **Guichard, C., Dugail, I., Le Liepvre, X., and Lavau, M.,** Genetic regulation of fatty acid synthetase expression in adipose tissue: overtranscription of the gene in genetically obese rats, *J. Lipid Res.,* 33, 679, 1992.
60. **Benito, M., Porras, A., Nebreda, R., and Santos, E.,** Differentiation of 3T3-L1 fibroblasts to adipocytes induced by transfection of *ras* oncogenes, *Science,* 253, 565, 1991.
61. **Freytag, S. O.,** Enforced expression of the c-*myc* oncogene inhibits cell differentiation by precluding entry into a distinct preadifferentiation state in G_0/G_1, *Mol. Cell Biol.,* 8, 1614, 1988.
62. **Freytag, S. and Geddes, T.,** Reciprocal regulation of adipogenesis by *myc* and C/EBP, *Science,* 256, 379, 1992.

63. **Barcellini-Couget, S., Pradines-Figuères, A., Roux, P., Dani, C., and Ailhaud, G.,** The regulation by growth hormone of lipoprotein lipase gene expression is mediated by *c-fos* proto-oncogene, *Endocrinology,* 132, 53, 1993.
64. **Jiang, X. C., Moulin, P., Quinet, E., Goldberg, I. J., Yacoub, L. K., Agellon, L. B., Compton, D., Schnitzer-Polokoff, R., and Tall, A. R.,** Mammalian adipose tissue and muscle are major sources of lipid transfer protein mRNA, *J. Biol. Chem.,* 266, 4631, 1991.
65. **Zechner, R., Moser, R., Newman, T. C., Fried, S. K., and Breslow, J. L.,** Apolipoprotein E gene expression in mouse 3T3-L1 adipocytes and human adipose tissue and its regulation by differentiation and lipid content, *J. Biol. Chem.,* 266, 10583, 1991.
66. **Frederich, R. C., Jr., Kahn, B. B., Peach, M. J., and Flier, J. S.,** Tissue-specific nutritional regulation of angiotensinogen in adipose tissue, *Hypertension,* 19, 339, 1992.
67. **Choy, L. N., Rosen, B. S., and Spiegelman, B. M.,** Adipsin and an endogenous pathway of complement from adipose cells, *J. Biol. Chem.,* 267, 12736, 1992.
68. **Lafontan, M.,** personal communication.
69. **Gaillard, G.,** unpublished results.
70. **Grimaldi, P.,** unpublished results.

Chapter 15

Molecular Genetic Approaches to Obesity

Streamson C. Chua, Jr. and Rudolph L. Leibel

TABLE OF CONTENTS

I. INTRODUCTION

A major role for genotype in the development of obesity is supported by data from twin,[1] adoption,[2,3] and population studies.[4] However, environmental and developmental factors also play an important role in this phenotype. Obesity cannot occur in an environment which does not permit the individual to ingest calories in excess of those needed for basal metabolism and physical activity. This situation is in contrast to other genetic diseases, e.g., sickle cell anemia or cystic fibrosis, which will be manifest in virtually all environmental circumstances. For these reasons, obesity-related genes are best regarded as conferring *susceptibility* to obesity, rather than producing the phenotype per se. Age, environmental dependence for the development of obesity, the likelihood of genetic heterogeneity, and the undoubted existence of phenocopies (nongenetic obesity) in the population severely complicate efforts to identify and quantify the genetic contributions to this disorder. Genetic analysis of obesity is paradigmatic of the difficulties in the genetic dissection of a quantitative trait. Such traits show continuous variation within a population and result from the interactions of multiple genes with environmental factors.

This chapter discusses the conceptual framework for genetic analysis of this complex phenotype and describes some of the newer molecular techniques and reagents available for such studies.

II. ASSESSING THE GENETIC CONTRIBUTION TO OBESITY IN MAN

Since it is likely that obesity is polygenic in man — or at least that different genes are responsible in different families — segregation analysis of families from diverse genetic backgrounds is unlikely to be fruitful. The ultimate goal of such analyses is to indicate the likely mode of inheritance of those genes with major influence on the risk of development of obesity. Such information may be used, in turn, to direct linkage analyses designed to identify specific genes or regions of the genome which confer such risk. The high likelihood of genetic heterogeneity, and of epistatic interaction of relevant genes, favors the initial use of linkage methods which are not dependent on prior knowledge of

0-8493-4880-3/94/$0.00+$.50

the mode(s) of inheritance. Affected sib pair analysis — in which affected siblings are examined for the inheritance of alleles linked to the phenotype of interest — is an example of such a model-free method.[5] A fully informative locus unlinked to the disease should be coinherited in Mendelian ratios of 1:2:1 for two, one, or zero alleles, respectively. If the marker allele is linked to the gene responsible for the phenotype, the likelihood of sib pair identity by descent (IBD) for two alleles is increased while the likelihood of IBD for zero alleles is reduced. IBD for a locus refers to the inheritance by sibs of identical alleles from a common ancestor.

In circumstances in which there is no prior knowledge of candidate genes or genomic regions for the phenotype being investigated and in which any relevant gene may not account for the major portion of the phenotype, the number of genetic markers which would have to be scored to insure a reasonable likelihood of demonstrating linkage is daunting. Spanning the human genome at 5 centiMorgan (cM) intervals would, for example, require 3200 cM per genome/5 cM = 640 markers. Under such circumstances, the likelihood of a type I error (erroneous acceptance of linkage) is increased because the search is performed without a hypothesis as to either the location or the nature (specific sequence) of the gene(s). A recent analysis of this problem by Terwilliger et al.[6] indicated that, even with the availability of extremely polymorphic molecular markers which increase the likelihood of interindividual difference and, hence, the informativeness of available meiotic events, the most efficient means of increasing the likelihood of demonstrating linkage is to increase the number of informative subjects/families in the analysis.

For complex phenotypes such as obesity, in which it seems highly likely that the same phenotype can be caused by different genes or gene combinations, the identification of individuals/families likely to have identical molecular etiologies is of critical importance. Amongst adults in the Pima Indian population, for example, the prevalence rates for obesity and type II diabetes exceed 35%. It has been suggested that a drought/famine imposed by the drying up of the Gila River in the late 19th century resulted in a restriction bottleneck which selected (by virtue of their enhanced survival) individuals enriched for energy-conserving "thrifty" genes.[7] Thus, obese individuals in the present population — by virtue of this earlier selective pressure and maintenance of a high degree of intermarriage on the reservation — are likely to have a common genetic contribution to their susceptibility to obesity and non-insulin-dependent diabetes mellitus (NIDDM).[8]

Even when such a relatively homogeneous population is available, there is still a need to identify an optimal set of molecular markers which can be used to implicate specific genes or regions of the genome in the development of the phenotype. Several autosomal recessive and dominant mutations resulting in obesity have been described in both humans and rodents. Whether alleles of the genes which produce obesity in rodents are operative in either the rare Mendelian forms of obesity in man (e.g., Alstrom, Bardet-Biedl, Cohen syndromes) or the much more frequent non-Mendelian forms is not known.

As noted, the application of regularly spaced molecular markers which span the genome to individuals in families segregating for an obese phenotype is fraught with logistic difficulties and a variety of potential statistical artifacts. However, with the rapidly increasing density of microsatellite maps and the development of techniques for rapid assay and detection of these polymorphisms, this approach undoubtedly will become more common, particularly for phenotypes with no outstanding candidate genes. For obesity and diabetes, the initial search can be based on genes which play a role in these phenotypes in animals.

III. USE OF RODENT MODELS TO IDENTIFY CANDIDATE GENES FOR HUMAN OBESITY

Several autosomal mutations producing obesity have been mapped genetically in the mouse and rat: Yellow *(A^y)*, mouse chromosome 2; diabetes *(db)*, chromosome 4; obese *(ob)*, chromosome 6; tubby *(tub)*, chromosome 7; fat *(fat)*, chromosome 8; Adipose *(Ad)*, chromosome 7; fatty *(fa)*, rat chromosome 5.[9-13] While A^y and *Ad* are dominant, the others are recessive. All of these rodent mutations are in regions of the mouse genome with high homology to regions of the human genome. The A^y mutation in the agouti (*a*) locus which produces obesity was recently cloned. The *agouti* gene codes for a protein which apparently has paracrine activity and which has a sequence with no significant homology to known proteins. The A^y mutation is in the regulatory sequence for this gene, causing it to be expressed in tissues in which it is not usually expressed.[14] The molecular basis for the obesity in these animals remains unknown. In no other instance of rodent obesity has the culpable gene been identified.

Important aspects of phenotype are common amongst these obese animals: all show hyperphagia, increases in body fat, enhanced metabolic efficiency (e.g., weight gain per kilocalorie fed), varying degrees of hyperinsulinemia and insulin resistance, and evidence of autonomic dysfunction (e.g., defective thermogenesis when subjected to cold stress or reduced thermic effect of feeding).[15] These rodent mutations themselves define different subgroups of mouse obesity that conceivably could have analogues in man. For example, the degree of hyperinsulinemia is greater in *ob* and *db* than in *tub* or A^y. The distribution of body fat also varies amongst these mutations. A^y, *fat*, and *tub* show diffuse increases in body fat, while *ob* and *db* tend to deposit fat axially and in the inguinal region ("pear shape").[10]

Comparative gene mapping between mammals has revealed a striking degree of homology in both chromosomal cytology and gene organization. The most extensive comparisons have been made between man and mouse. In man, over 2300 genes have been mapped and over 10,000 loci defined by DNA markers.[16,17] Over 3000 loci (genes, DNA markers) have been mapped in the mouse,[18] and more than 600 loci homologous between mouse and man have been identified.[19] The mouse is particularly useful in the molecular genetic analysis of single and polygene phenotypes because of the availability of inbred strains, extensive classical genetic resources (phenotype analysis, linkage maps, recombinant inbred strains), and the ability to manipulate the genome using transgenic techniques. The extent of homology between mouse and human genomes ranges from single-locus gene identities to conservations of groups of genes within a region in which gene order may or may not be conserved.

Homologous genes have been located on all mouse (19) and human (22) autosomes, as well as the X and Y chromosomes. A total of 65 conserved autosomal segments have been identified between mouse and man.[19] The average length of conserved autosomal linkages is 10.1 cM (±2.2 cM) in the mouse; the range is from 5.5 cM for mouse chromosome 2 and human chromosome 15 to 32.5 cM for mouse chromosome 2 and human chromosome 20.[20] Nadeau[21] estimated that ~37% of the 1500 cM autosomal genome of the mouse is located within segments in which both synteny and gene order have been conserved and that only 138 (±32 SD) linkage disruptions have occurred since mouse and man diverged (~1 disruption per million years). Once all of the conserved segments between mouse (or rat) and man have been identified, it will be possible to predict the likely position of any gene in one species from its location in the other.

Molecular genetic linkage maps around two mouse obesity mutations, *ob* and *db*, indicate the existence of extensive regions of conserved synteny between the mouse and human genomes in these regions. Around the mouse *obese* mutation there appears to be a region of at least 20 cM which shows conservation of gene order and distance between proximal mouse chromosome 6 and human chromosome 7q. Two markers, collagen type IV and the skeletal muscle chloride channel (Clc-1), appear to define the extent of the syntenic region. For the mouse *diabetes* mutation there is a smaller 15-cM region of mouse mid-chromosome 4 with synteny to human chromosome 1p. Two other mouse obesity mutations, *tub* and *fat,* are located on mouse chromosomes 7 and 8, respectively.[10] Since molecular maps around *tub* and *fat* are less developed, the exact regions of homology in the human genome are not definitely known. The identification of molecular markers (genes) from a specific human chromosome which flank each of these mouse mutations will pinpoint the region of synteny to the human genome. Molecular maps of such syntenic regions can be used to predict the respective locations of homologous genes between species.[22] Such a relationship was exploited recently to demonstrate the likely correspondence of the mouse *db* to the rat *fa* mutation.[13]

IV. MOLECULAR MAPPING TOOLS

The application of the polymerase chain reaction (PCR) to segments of DNA which are highly polymorphic within populations has allowed the rapid construction of complete maps of the human,[23] mouse,[24] and rat genomes.[25] The rapid development of the genomic maps which have permitted such interspecies comparison has been made possible by the observation that simple sequences of mono-, di-, tri-, and tetranucleotide repeats are highly polymorphic within a given species.[26,27] Since these simple sequence repeats (SSRs) are flanked by unique sequences, the SSRs can be amplified readily from genomic DNA by the PCR. Different sized alleles are resolved by appropriate gel electrophoretic systems. SSRs are estimated to occur once every 6 kilobase pairs (kbp) in the human genome. The most frequently used microsatellite, $(AC)_n$, occurs approximately once every 30 kbp in man and every 18 or 21 kbp in mice and rats, respectively.[28] The length of these SSRs determines their utility, with those having greater than 20 repeats being the most polymorphic. Rodent SSRs are larger in average length than those in man: for example, 43% of rat and 12% of human SSRs are >40 base pairs (bp). The power of SSRs in the generation of molecular maps is reflected in the recent publication of SSR maps for mouse (317 loci),[24] rat (125 loci),[25] and man (813 loci).[23] These maps were prepared by systematically searching data base sequences and genomic clones for such microsatellites, synthesizing flanking oligonucleotides, and then mapping the SSR relative to previously mapped genes and other SSRs in genetic crosses between polymorphic rodent strains or in three-generation human families. These SSRs have been used to scan the mouse and rat genomes rapidly for molecular markers linked to a variety of complex phenotypes. Such scanning led to the implication of the renin genes and angiotensin-converting enzyme (ACE) in rat models of hypertension in the salt-sensitive rat,[29] to the identification of several additional loci conferring diabetes susceptibility in the mouse[30] and rat,[31] and to specification of epilepsy-associated loci in mice.[32]

V. DO HOMOLOGS OF MOUSE OBESITY GENES CONTRIBUTE TO HUMAN OBESITY?

The autosomal recessive mutations which result in obesity in mice and rats reflect loss of function in genes which must act normally to suppress the body weight by effects on both food intake and energy expenditure. In virtually all of these single gene mutations, extensive studies of the metabolic/behavioral phenotypes of affected animals suggest that components of a central integrator for body fat are dysfunctional. This integrator probably exerts its actions through mediators of body fat content which are present in the central nervous system. This concept is supported by the fact that mechanical, chemical, or electrolytic lesions of specific brain regions (e.g., ventromedial hypothalamus, medial forebrain bundle) can produce a phenotype (hyperphagia, hypometabolism, hyperinsulinemia) very similar to that seen in the genetic obesities. There are data in normal rodents[33] and humans[34] which suggest that body weight is regulated physiologically by integrated effects on both food intake and energy expenditure. It seems likely that comparable control mechanisms are operant in man and animals and that the genes which encode the components of this system would be highly conserved in evolution. Thus, allelic variants of these rodent weight-regulating genes may be segregating in the human population. As mentioned, the positions of the rodent mutations in their respective genomes are well known, and in most instances the regions of homology in man are known as well. Such information can be used to identify those specific regions of the human genome which should be investigated for genetic linkage to an obese phenotype. Since the rodent genes (with the exception of A^y) have not yet been cloned, polymorphic molecular markers in the region of these genes must be used to detect the presence of probable allelic variants in affected human individuals by some type of linkage analysis. Such markers can be selected from the rapidly growing number of highly polymorphic microsatellites being mapped in the human genome.[23,35]

VI. POSITIONAL CLONING

Detailed molecular genetic maps of the regions containing mouse obesity mutations can be exploited in several ways. As described, areas of linkage conservation can be used to identify molecular markers for linkage analyses in human pedigrees segregating for an obese phenotype. The same maps provide the basis for "positional cloning" of the mutations. Positional cloning refers to the isolation of a gene based on its placement in the genome without prior knowledge of the nature of the gene product or even its primary organ(s) of expression. This approach has, for example, been used to clone the genes for chronic granulomatous disease,[36] Duchenne's muscular dystrophy,[37] cystic fibrosis,[38] neurofibromatosis,[11] and Huntington's disease.[39] The gene products or regulatory sequences encoded by the rodent obesity mutations are unknown. The secondary metabolic derangements which accompany the development of the obese/diabetic phenotype have confounded efforts to identify the primary biochemical lesion produced by these mutations. Hence, there have been recent efforts to clone these genes by positional genetics.[40]

In positional cloning one starts by identifying genes or DNA markers which flank the mutation. All of the DNA between the two closest flanking markers is then cloned by a chromosome "walk". Such a walk entails using a cloned segment of DNA containing a marker known by conventional genetic analysis to be near the mutation to identify another genomic clone containing a shared sequence. This process is repeated sequentially until a clone is obtained which contains a sequence known by conventional genetics to be on the other side of (i.e., to flank) the mutation. The enormous amount of labor which was initially required to clone loci by positional information has been reduced to more manageable levels by the cloning of large segments of DNA (0.3 to 1.0 million bp) with yeast artificial chromosome (YAC)[41] and P1[42] cloning systems.

YACs are generated by the ligation of large fragments (0.3 to 2 Mb) of genomic DNA to two vector arms which contain elements needed for DNA replication in yeast cells. These elements include a centromere, two telomeres, and a sequence equivalent to an origin of replication. Also included in the vector arms are genes (URA3, TRP1 [auxotrophic mutations which confer necessity of uracil and tryptophan, respectively, for growth]) for selection in transformed yeast and an ampicillin resistance cassette for selection in *Escherichia coli.* Yeast spheroplasts are transformed with these YACs, and the URA3 and TRP1 genes are used to enrich the resulting yeast pool for transformants by growth in appropriate media. The YAC replicates in synchrony with the normal chromosomes of *Saccharomyces cerevisiae* so that one copy is made per yeast cell.

In practice, an effort is made to generate a YAC library containing three to five genome equivalents. Obviously, the larger the insert size, the fewer the number of clones required. Various strategies are used to array such libraries in a manner which facilitates their screening for specific clones. By pooling individual YAC clones in sequentially larger pools and screening from larger to smaller pools by PCR with an STS (sequence tagged site) for a particular locus, individual YACs can be rapidly identified and recovered from libraries with over 20,000 YAC clones.[43]

YACs generally display low transformation efficiency, which decreases with increasing insert size. In addition, copy number is low, making it difficult to obtain large amounts of insert DNA from transformed cells. A bacteriophage P1 cloning system has been described recently which accepts DNA fragments up to 100 kb, has high transformation efficiency, and can be amplified readily within an *E. coli* host.[44] The recent publication of YAC physical maps (contigs) spanning entire chromosomes[45,46] suggests that chromosome walks may be superseded by extremely dense genetic linkage maps.

These vector systems, combined with contigs of the genome, can be used to access large segments of genomic DNA which span a region demonstrated by classical genetic studies (linkage or deletion analysis) to contain a gene of interest. The next step is usually the most difficult: the identification of expressed genes from the large stretch of genomic DNA obtained with the chromosome walk. There is no method currently available which will reliably identify all of the genes in a given stretch of genomic DNA. Each mutation must be identified by a mutation-specific strategy. If no prior information exists about the nature of the mutant gene, the identification of the gene may be extremely difficult. The gene may be located in a gene-rich region, with a density of one gene in every 10,000 bp. Positional information, which is derived from translocations or meiotic recombinations, generally has a resolution of 100,000 to 1 million bp. Thus, up to 100 genes may be candidates for the mutation, and each gene must be tested. However, if it is known that the mutation is expressed in a given tissue (e.g., pancreas), the search can be limited to those genes which are expressed in that organ. All other genes which are not expressed in the pancreas can be ignored. An additional consideration is the stage of development at which the mutated gene is expressed in a specific tissue. One might miss an expressed gene if the mRNA used is isolated from the right organ at an inappropriate stage of organogenesis.

If the entire sequence of a clone containing such a gene is known, a search can be made for CpG islands, which are methylation sites frequently found upstream of genes with expressed genes being frequently unmethylated in CpG sequences. Intron-exon boundaries can be detected by searching for consensus splice sequences, but such sequences are not invariant. Likewise, searches for open reading frames (ORFs) are frequently confounded by the fact that stop codons (3/64 codons) occur more frequently than the start codon, making it difficult to determine which ORFs are actual genes.

Recent strategies devised to identify coding regions without access to the genomic sequence within a clone include exon amplification[47] and hybridization of cDNAs to cosmids[48] or YACs.[49,50] These techniques hold promise not only for efficient cloning of genes from a specific genomic region, but also for use in generating organ-specific cDNA maps of genomic regions of interest and, eventually, the entire genome.

Confirmation that the gene of interest has been found is provided by the identification of the mutated sequence in the gene of an affected individual. Further confirmation can be obtained by correcting the phenotype of affected individuals with a functional gene or gene product and by replicating the mutant phenotype by replacing the wild-type gene with the mutated sequence through homologous recombination in embryonal stem cells.

The arguments described above which favor the brain (and specific regions within) as an organ in which genes critical to energy balance are expressed suggest another strategy for the identification and mapping of genes relevant to human obesity. cDNA libraries can be prepared from mRNA isolated from human and/or rodent brain (or specific regions). If desired, such libraries can be enriched for brain-specific clones by "substraction" of clones which are also expressed in other organs (e.g., liver). Using hybrid cell lines, irradiation-reduced hybrids, chromosomes-specific libraries, and YACs, cDNAs can be selected which map to regions of the mouse or human genome known by classical genetic studies to contain genes which affect energy balance. Large genetic crosses segregating for specific obesity-related mutations (e.g., *ob* or *db*) can be used to map such candidate genes relative to the desired mutation. Any clone which is nonrecombinant with the mutation in a sufficiently large number of meioses is potentially the gene itself. This approach is useful in efforts to clone mutations in unknown genes by positional techniques, but also generates an increasingly high-resolution map of organ-specific expressed sequences in a particular region of the genome. Such transcriptional maps of the genome will be extremely useful in facilitating the application of molecular genetic information to the study of integrated physiology.[51]

VII. GENETIC SUSCEPTIBILITY TO OBESITY-RELATED DISEASES

The major causes of excess morbidity in association with obesity are NIDDM, atherosclerosis, and hypertension. The reasons for the association between obesity and NIDDM is not known, but not all individuals with NIDDM are obese and not all obese subjects develop NIDDM.[52] Among patients with NIDDM there is great variability in the frequency with which overt diabetes mellitus develops. The magnitude and mechanism of the genetic contribution to this variability are not known. The susceptibility to pancreatic β-cell failure in rodents segregating for the *ob, db,* and *fa* mutations is highly dependent on the strain in which the mutation is segregating.[53,54] By segregating these mutations in genetic crosses between diabetes susceptible and resistant strains and haplotyping offspring for SSRs which span the genome, it should be possible to identify genes conferring susceptibility or resistance to the diabetogenic effects of these obesity mutations. Map positions of such genes in the mouse (and regions of linkage conservation in humans) can then be used to identify candidate genes and for positional cloning efforts.

The genetic analysis of susceptibility genes is more tractable when animal models are used. The major advantage to this strategy is that the same set of alleles can be tested repetitively in crosses designed to limit (usually to two, one for each parental strain) the number of possible alleles at any locus. Thus, genetic heterogeneity has been limited.

The rapidity and ease with which disease susceptibility loci can be identified in animal models can be appreciated by an analysis of the literature for Type I diabetes mellitus, hypertension, and seizure susceptibility. As described earlier, the use of a large number of polymorphic markers which span the genome has led to the identification of chromosomal regions which account for a substantial fraction of genetic susceptibility to these phenotypes. Strategies used to identify single gene mutations can be used to isolate the genes which influence susceptibility. Thus, diseases which are the result of multiple, interacting genes can be dissected genetically.

REFERENCES

1. **Borjeson, A. M.,** The aetiology of obesity in children, *Acta Paediat. Scand.,* 65, 279, 1976.
2. **Sørensen, T. I. A., Price, R. A., Stunkard, A. J., and Schulsinger, F.,** Genetics of obesity in adult adoptees and their biological siblings, *Br. Med. J.,* 298, 87, 1989.
3. **Stunkard, A. J., Harris, J. R., Pedersen, N. L., and McClearn, G. E.,** The body-mass index of twins who have been reared apart, *N. Eng. J. Med.,* 322, 1483, 1990.

4. **Moll, P. P., Burns, T. L., and Lauer, R. M.,** The genetic and environmental sources of body mass index variability: the Muscatine ponderosity family study, *Am. J. Hum. Genet.,* 49, 1243, 1991.
5. **Haseman, J. K. and Elston, R. C.,** The investigation of linkage between a quantitative trait and a marker locus, *Behav. Genet.,* 2, 3, 1972.
6. **Terwilliger, J. D., Ding, Y., and Ott, J.,** On the relative importance of marker heterozygosity and intermarker distance in gene mapping, *Genomics,* 13, 951, 1992.
7. **Neel, J.V.,** Diabetes mellitus: a "thrifty" genotype rendered detrimental by "progress"?, *Am. J. Hum. Genet.,* 14, 353, 1962.
8. **Knowler, W. C., Pettitt, D. J., Saad, M. F., and Bennett, P. H.,** Diabetes mellitus in the Pima Indians: incidence, risk factors and pathogenesis, *Diabetes Metab. Rev.,* 6, 1, 1990.
9. **Coleman, D. L.,** Diabetes-obesity syndromes in mice, *Diabetes,* 31, 1, 1982.
10. **Coleman, D. L. and Eicher, E. M.,** Fat *(fat)* and tubby *(tub):* two autosomal recessive mutations causing obesity syndromes in the mouse, *J. Hered.,* 81, 424, 1990.
11. **Wallace, M., Marchuk, D., Andersen, L., Letcher, R., Odeh, H., Saulino, A., Fountain, J., Brereton, A., Nicholson, J., Mitchell, A., Brownstein, B., and Collins, F.,** Type 1 neurofibromatosis gene: identification of a large transcript disrupted in three NF1 patients, *Science,* 249, 181, 1990.
12. **Wolff, G. L., Roberts, D. W., and Galbraith, D. B.,** Prenatal determination of obesity, tumor susceptibility and coat color in viable Yellow (Avy/a) mice, *J Hered.,* 77, 151, 1986.
13. **Truett, G. E., Bahary, N., Friedman, J. M., and Leibel, R. L.,** Rat obesity gene fatty (fa) maps to chromosome 5: evidence for homology with the mouse gene diabetes (db), *Proc. Natl. Acad. Sci.,* 88, 7806, 1991.
14. **Bultman, S. J., Michaud, E. J., and Woychik, R. P.,** Molecular characterization of the mouse agouti locus, *Cell,* 71, 1195, 1992.
15. **Bray, G. A. and York, D. A.,** Genetic and hypothalamic mechanisms for obesity — finding the needle in the haystack, *Am. J. Clin. Nutr.,* 50, 891, 1979.
16. **McAlpine, P. J., Shaws, T. B., Huenber, M., and Anderson, W. A.,** The 1991 catalog of mapped genes and report of the nomenclature committee, *Cytogenet. Cell Genet.,* 58, 5, 1991.
17. **Group, N. C. M.,** A comprehensive genetic linkage map of the human genome, *Science,* 258, 67, 1992.
18. **Silver, L. M.,** Bouncing off microsatellites, *Nature Genet.,* 2, 8, 1992.
19. **Davisson, M. T., Lalley, P. A., Peters, J., Doolittle, D. P., Hillyard, A. L., and Searle, A. G.,** Report of the comparative committee for human, mouse and other rodents, *Cytogenet. Cell Genet.,* 58, 1152, 1991.
20. **Copeland, N. G. and Jenkins, N. A.,** Development and applications of a molecular genetic linkage map of the mouse genome, *Trends Genet.,* 7, 113, 1991.
21. **Nadeau, J. H.,** Maps of linkage and synteny homologues between man and mouse, *Trends Genet.,* 5, 82, 1989.
22. **Lyon, M. F. and Kinby, M. C.,** Mouse Chromosome Atlas, in *Mouse Genome,* Peters, J., Ed., 1993, 91, 40.
23. **Weissenbach, J., Gyapay, G., Dib, C., Vignal, A., Morissette, J., Millasseau, P., Vaysseix, G., and Lathrop, M.,** A second-generation linkage map of the human genome, *Nature,* 359, 794, 1992.
24. **Dietrich, W., Katz, H., Lincoln, S. E., Shin, H. S., Friedman, J., Dracopoli, N. C., and Lander, E. S.,** A genetic map of the mouse suitable for typing intraspecific crosses, *Genetics,* 131, 423, 1992.
25. **Serikawa, T., Kuramoto, T., Hilbert, P., Mori, M., Yamada, J., Dubay, C. J., Lindpainter, K., Ganten, D., Guenet, J. L., Lathrop, G. M., and Beckmann,**

J. S., Rat gene mapping using PCR-analyzed microsatellites, *Genetics,* 131, 701, 1992.

26. **Hamada, H., Petrino, M. G., and Kakunaga, T.**, A novel repeated element with Z-DNA-forming potential is widely found in evolutionarily diverse eukaryotic genomes, *Proc. Natl. Acad. Sci. U.S.A.,* 79, 6465, 1982.
27. **Weber, J. L. and May, P. E.**, Abundant class of human DNA polymorphisms which can be typed using the polymerase chain reaction, *Am. J. Hum. Genet.,* 44, 388, 1989.
28. **Beckmann, J. S. and Weber, J. L.**, Survey of human and rat microsatellites, *Genomics,* 12, 627, 1992.
29. **Jacob, H. J., Petterson, A., Wilson, D., Mao, Y., Lernmark, A., and Lander, E. S.**, Genetic dissection of autoimmune type I diabetes in the BB rat, *Nature Genet.,* 2, 56, 1992.
30. **Todd, J. A., Aitman, T. J., Cornall, R. J., Ghosh, S., Hall, J. R. S., Hearne, C. M., Knight, A. M., Love, J. M., McAleer, M. A., Prins, J. B., Rodrigues, N., Lathrop, M., Pressey, A., DeLarato, N. H., Peterson, L. B., and Wicker, L. S.**, Genetic analysis of autoimmune type I diabetes mellitus in mice, *Nature,* 351, 542, 1991.
31. **Jacob, H. J., Lindpaintner, K., Lincoln, S. E., Kusumi, K., Bunker, R. K., Mao, Y., Ganten, D., Dzau, V. J., and Lander, E. S.**, Genetic mapping of a gene causing hypertension in the stroke-prone spontaneously hypertensive rat, *Cell,* 67, 213, 1991.
32. **Rise, M. L., Frankel, W. N., Coffin, J. M., and Seyfried, T. N.**, Genes for epilepsy mapped in the mouse, *Science,* 253, 669, 1991.
33. **Keesey, R. E.**, A set point analysis of the regulation of body weight, in *Obesity,* Stunkard, A.J., Ed., W.B. Saunders, New York, 1986, 144.
34. **Leibel, R. L.**, Is obesity due to a heritable differences in "set point" for adiposity?, *West. J. Med.,* 153, 429, 1990.
35. **Hearne, C. M., Ghosh, S., and Todd, J. A.**, Microsatellite linkage analysis of genetic traits, *Trends Genet.,* 8, 288, 1992.
36. **Royer-Pokora, B., Kunkel, L. M., Monaco, A. P., Goff, S. C., Newburger, P. E., Baehner, R. L., Cole, F. S., Curnutte, J. T., and Orkin, S. H.**, Cloning the gene for an inherited human disorder-chronic granulomatous disease-on the basis of its chromosomal location, *Nature,* 322, 32, 1986.
37. **Koenig, M., Hoffman, E. P., Bertelson, C. J., Monaco, A. P., Feener, C., and Kunkel, L. M.**, Complete cloning of the Duchenne muscular dystrophy (DMD) gene and preliminary genomic organization of the DMD gene in normal and affected individuals, *Cell,* 50, 509, 1987.
38. **Riordan, J. R., Rommens, J. M., Kerem, B., Alon, N., Rozmahel, R., Grzelczak, Z., Zielenski, J., Lok, S., Plavsic, N., Chou, J. L., Drumm, M. L., Iannuzzi, M. C., Collins, F. S., and Tsui, L. C.**, Identification of the cystic fibrosis gene; cloning and characterization of complementary DNA, *Science,* 245, 1066, 1989.
39. **The Huntington's Disease Collaborative Research Group,** A novel gene containing a trinucleotide repeat that is expanded and unstable on Huntington's disease chromosomes, *Cell,* 72, 971, 1993.
40. **Friedman, J. and Leibel, R. L.**, Tackling a weighty problem, *Cell,* 69, 217, 1992.
41. **Burke, D. R., Carle, G. F., and Olson, M. V.**, Cloning of large segments of DNA into yeast by means of artificial chromosome vectors, *Science,* 236, 806, 1987.
42. **Sternberg, N.,** Bacteriophage P1 cloning system for this isolation, amplification, and recovering of DNA fragments as large as 100 kilobase pairs, *Proc. Natl. Acad. Sci.,* 87, 103, 1990.
43. **Green, E. D. and Olson, M. V.**, Systematic screening of yeast artificial-chromosomes libraries by use of the polymerase chain reaction, *Proc. Natl. Acad. Sci. U.S.A.,* 87, 1213, 1990.

44. **Pierce, J. C., Sternberg, N., and Sauer, B.,** A mouse genomic library in the bacteriophage P1 cloning system: organization and characterization, *Mamm. Genome,* 3, 550, 1992.
45. **Foote, S., Vollrath, D., Hilton, A., and Page, D. C.,** The human y chromosome: overlapping DNA clones spanning the euchromatic region, *Science,* 258, 60, 1992.
46. **Chumakov, I., Rigault, P., Guillou, S., Ougen, P., Billaut, A., Guasconi, G., Gervy, P., LeGall, I., Soularue, P., Grinas, L., Bougueleret, L., Ballane-Chantelot, C., Lacroix, B., Barillot, E., Gesnouin, P., Pook, S., Vaysseix, G., Frelat, G., Schmitz, A., Sambucy, J. L., Bosch, A., Estivill, X., Weissenbach, J., Vignal, A., and Riethman, H.,** Continuum of overlapping clones spanning the entire human chromosome 21q, *Nature,* 359, 380, 1992.
47. **Buckler, A. J., Chang, D. D., Graw, S. L., Brook, D., Haber, D. A., Sharp, P. A., and Housman, D. E.,** Exon amplification: a strategy to isolate mammalian genes based on RNA splicing, *Proc. Natl. Acad. Sci. U.S.A.,* 88, 4005, 1991.
48. **Korn, B., Sedlacek, Z., Manca, A., Kioschis, P., Konecki, D., Lahrach, H., and Poustka, A.,** A strategy for the selection of transcribed sequences in the Xq28, *Hum. Mol. Genet.,* 1, 235, 1992.
49. **Parimco, S., Patanjali, S. R., Shukla, H., Chaplin, D. D., and Weissman, S. M.,** cDNA selection: efficient PCR approach for the selection of cDNAs encoded in large chromosomal DNA fragments, *Proc. Natl. Acad. Sci. U.S.A.,* 88, 9623, 1991.
50. **Lovett, M., Kere, J., and Hinton, L. M.,** Direct selection: a method for the isolation of cDNAs encoded by large genomic regions, *Proc. Natl. Acad. Sci. U.S.A.,* 88, 9628, 1991.
51. **Hochgeschwender, U.,** Toward a transcriptional map of the human genome, *Trends Genet.,* 8, 41, 1992.
52. **DeFronzo, R. A., Bonadonna, R. C., and Ferrannini, E.,** Pathogenesis of NIDDM: a balanced overview, *Diabetes Care,* 15, 317, 1992.
53. **Leiter, E. H.,** The genetics of diabetes susceptibility in mice, *FASEB J.,* 3, 2231, 1989.
54. **Ikeda, H., Shino, A., Matsuo, T., Iwatsuka, H., and Suzuoki, Z.,** A new genetically obese-hyperglycemic rat (Wistar fatty), *Diabetes,* 30, 1045, 1981.

Chapter 16

Genetics of Obesity: Overview and Research Directions

Claude Bouchard

TABLE OF CONTENTS

I. INTRODUCTION

Obesity is a highly prevalent chronic disease that carries enormous human and economical costs in Western nations. As revealed by the content of this book, we have barely begun to define the genetic basis of human obesities. The complexity and the diversity of the paths leading to an overweight or an obesity status require that scientists interested in the genetics of human obesities be imaginative and avoid simplistic schemes and pronouncements. The same view applies to the broad topic of the role played by genetic differences in the metabolic and clinical consequences of the various obese states. Nothing is simple in obesity as a disease entity: etiology, causes, associated morbidity, treatment, economic burden of the disease, cost/benefit ratio of weight loss, genetic basis, prevention, and other aspects are all highly complex and intimately associated with other diseases whose prevalence is augmented by our present way of life.

This chapter will provide a brief overview of the current status of knowledge concerning the genetic basis of human obesities based on the content of the book and on recent publications that could not be reviewed at the time most chapters were written. Finally, a brief discussion of useful concepts and of strategies to improve the odds of defining the genetic and molecular basis of human obesities is presented.

II. A PERSONAL VIEW OF THE CURRENT STATUS

The early chapters of the book revealed that the prevalence of overweight and obesity was already quite high in Western societies and on the rise in developing countries of the world. Moreover, the prevalence of overweight and obesity continues to increase in the most affluent countries.[1] On the other hand, the chapter by Hill and collaborators[2] has emphasized the notion that large variation in body mass and body composition can occur under the influence of behavioral factors, indicating that the prevalence of overweight and obesity cannot be explained only by genetic inheritance. As a matter of fact, it would not be surprising if behavioral differences would turn out to be more important than genetic differences in the etiology of overweight and obesity in technologically advanced societies.

0-8493-4880-3/94/$0.00+$.50

A. GENETIC EPIDEMIOLOGY DATA

The genetic epidemiology features of body fat content and overweight or obesity phenotypes were reviewed in Chapters 4 to 8. The results were generally quite heterogeneous. Trends in the data, as perceived by this author, are summarized in Tables 1 and 2. Table 1 describes these trends in terms of the various designs used to generate the data. Thus, the heritability level is highest with twin studies, intermediate with nuclear family data, and lowest when derived from adoption data. When several types of relatives are used jointly in the same design, the heritability estimates typically cluster around 25 to 40% of the age- and gender-adjusted phenotype variance. There is no clear evidence for a specific maternal or paternal effect, and the common familial environmental effect is marginal. The presence of a nonadditive genetic effect is often suggested from this research.

Table 2 summarizes the trends in the complex segregation analysis results obtained on body mass index (BMI), weight adjusted for height, or percent body fat in various studies. All studies are unanimous in reporting evidence for a multifactorial component and a major effect. However, in two reports the major effect was non-Mendelian. In a third paper the major effect became Mendelian only when age- and sex-related variations in the major effect were considered. In five of the seven studies, the estimated gene frequence of the putative recessive gene ranged from about 0.2 to 0.3.

Table 1. **Overview of the genetic epidemiology of human body fat/obesity**

	Heritability/ transmission	Maternal/ paternal	Familial environment
Nuclear families	30 to 50	No	Minor
Adoption studies	10 to 30	Mixed results	Minor
Twin studies	50 to 80	No	No
Combined strategies	25 to 40	No	Minor

Table 2. **Overview of segregation analysis results for body mass index/obesity**

Multifactorial transmission (%)	Major effect	Major gene	Gene frequency	Ref.
41	Yes, 20%	Yes	0.25	27
34	Yes	Yes	0.21	28
42	Yes, 35%	Yes	0.25	29
39	Yes	No	Non-Mendelian	30[a]
42	Yes, 20%	No	Non-Mendelian	31
Yes	Yes	Age and sex related	0.22	32
25	Yes, 45%	Yes	0.30	33[b]

[a] Weight adjusted for height; [b] Percent body fat.

B. MOLECULAR MARKERS

The investigation of the association between DNA sequence variation at specific genes and obesity phenotypes has just begun. Table 3 summarizes the results of the studies reported at the time this chapter was written. Thus far, no association has been found with molecular markers of GLUT1, GLUT4, insulin, insulin receptor, glucocorticoid receptor, and uncoupling protein genes. On the other hand, statistically significant associations have been found with red blood cell acid phosphatase, low-density lipoprotein (LDL) receptor, apoprotein (apo) B, apo D, and Na/K ATPase genes and the D-loop of mitochondrial DNA. It is obvious that these findings are generally based on small sample sizes and, thus, there may well be false positive as well as false negative results. However, it is also clear that the pace of molecular studies is accelerating and that a large number of genes are likely to be investigated in the next few years.

The data on linkage between obesity phenotypes and candidate genes or other molecular markers are even less abundant. The currently available results are summarized in Table 4. Significant linkage has been found with markers at the adenosine deaminase, Kell, esterase D, and α-2 and β-loci of the Na/K ATPase and 3-β-hydroxysteroid dehydrogenase genes. Lack of linkage has been reported for GLUT1 and the α-1 locus of the Na/K ATPase. Conflicting results have been obtained for adenylate kinase-1.

C. OTHER TYPES OF EVIDENCE

The limited molecular marker studies published so far suggest that there will likely be several genes associated and/or linked with human obesity. The number of genes may increase even more when studies on regional fat distribution phenotypes become available. In addition, other lines of evidence indicate that other important loci also may be involved. For instance, five mouse mutations causing obesity are encoded on five different mouse chromosomes. These mouse obesity genes are in coding regions that have homologous equivalents in humans. These human homologous regions are also located on five different human chromosomes.[3,4] Interestingly, the mouse *db* gene may be homologous to the rat *fa* obesity gene,[5] and they both appear to have a human homologous coding region on human chromosome 1p31.[3]

Using the quantitative trait locus (QTL) mapping approach, a new mouse gene for obesity may have been identified recently. Fisler et al.[6] obtained a backcross between the

Table 3. **Studies of body mass index/obesity association with candidate genes**

Gene	Number of Cases	Association	Ref.
Apo B	232	Yes	34
RBC-AcP	75	Yes	35
GLUT1	52	No	36
GLUT4	48	No	37
Insulin	35	No	37
Insulin receptor	35	No	37
Glucocorticoid receptor	55	No	38
LDL receptor	84	Yes	39
Apo D	114	Yes	40
Uncoupling protein	100	No	41
Mitochondrial DNA, D-loop	42	Yes	42
Na/K ATPase	113	Yes	43

Note: Apo B (D), apoprotein B (D); RBC-AcP, red blood cell acid phosphatase; LDL, low-density lipoprotein.

Table 4. **Overview of sib-pair linkage analysis — results for body mass index/obesity phenotypes**

Number of Pairs	Gene/ marker	Linkage	Ref.
~500	AK-1	Yes	44
402	ADA	Yes	45
	AK-1	No	
	Kell	Yes	
	ESD	Yes	
55 families	GLUT-1	No	46
110	Na/K ATPase		42
	α-1	No	
	α-2 (haplotype)	Yes	
	β (haplotype)	Yes	
140	3-β-HSD	Yes	47

Note: AK-1, adenylate kinase-1; ADA, adenosine deaminase; ESD, esterase D; 3-β-HSD, 3-β-hydroxysteroid dehydrogenase.

strains *Mus spretus* and C57BL/6J which they called the BSB mouse. BSB exhibits a wide range of carcass lipid, from 1 to 50%. Based on the QTL approach with a large number of markers, Warden et al.[7] reported that a locus on BSB chromosome 7 determines the lipid content of the carcass (log-of-the-odds [LOD] score of 3.8). Mouse chromosome 7 is also known to encode the tubby and Adipose genes. Although the BSB locus seems to be different from these two other genes, further characterization is needed before a definitive conclusion can be reached. It is interesting to note that the percent carcass lipid locus on chromosome 7 also contributes to an elevated plasma cholesterol level (LOD score of 5.8).[7]

Results from transgenic mouse models also reveal that dysfunction in certain genes can cause obesity. For example, a transgenic mouse with impaired corticosteroid receptor function was created by a partial knockout of the type II glucocorticoid receptor with an antisense RNA transgene.[8] The transgenic animals had increased fat deposition with a body mass twice as high as controls by 6 months of age. This was observed despite the fact that the transgenic animals ate about 15% less than normal mice. More recently, it has been reported that a transgenic mouse that expresses GLUT4 constitutively in the adipose tissue becomes quite fat with only a moderate elevation in body mass.[9]

A good number of genes, therefore, would seem to have the capacity to cause obesity or increase the likelihood of becoming obese when they are altered or dysfunctional in mammalian organisms. To the growing list one must also add the loci associated with the Mendelian disorders that have obesity as one of their features. For instance, the paternally imprinted Prader-Willi syndrome, imputed to a locus encoded on chromosome 15q11–13, is one of these cases.[10] Table 5 provides a listing of the genes or loci that are exhibiting associations or linkages with body mass for height or body fat content in animal models or in humans. The table includes only the genes, loci, or human homologous regions that are identified in the present chapter, plus the lipoprotein lipase (LPL) gene, for which there is now unpublished evidence of association with body fat content, its changes over time in a prospective study, and its response to long-term overfeeding. Even though it is obvious that the investigation of the molecular markers of obesity has barely begun, Table 5 indicates that already at least 20 genes, loci, or chromosomal regions have been identified that may be of importance in determining the human obesity phenotypes. They are located on about a dozen different chromosomes. We believe that many additional

Table 5. **Summary of loci associated with body mass index/obesity in animal models and human studies (May 1993)**

Gene	Chromosomal assignment	Gene	Chromosomal assignment
3-β-HSD	1p11–13	LPL	8p22
Na/K ATPase		AK-1	9q34
β	1q	Mouse BSB	(10, 11, 16)
α-2	1cen-q32	Mouse tub	(11p15.1)
Rat fa	(1p31)	ESD	13q14
Mouse db	(1p31-ter)	Prader-Willi	15q11–13
GLUT-1	1p31–35	Mouse fat	(16q22–24)
RBC-AcP	2p25	GLUT-4	17p13
HGR	5q31–32	Mouse A^y	(20q13)
Mouse ob	(7q31)	ADA	20q13
Kell	7q33	Mitochondrial D-loop	Mitochondrial DNA

Note: Parentheses denote human homologous regions of the rodent genome equivalent. 3-β-HSD, 3-β-hydroxysteroid dehydrogenase; LPL, lipoprotein lipase; AK-1, adenylate kinase-1; ESD, esterase D; RBC-AcP, red blood cell acid phosphatase; ADA, adenosine deaminase; HGR, human glucocorticoid receptor.

genes will be identified in the future, such that the panel of the human obesity genes, based on association, linkage, or animal models, will grow and become quite large. This may be a reflection of how often human obesity cases come about and perhaps not a consequence of false positive results, as discussed below.

III. A KEY CONCEPT: SUSCEPTIBILITY GENES

We are convinced that most cases of human obesities cannot be readily reduced to simple Mendelian phenotypes. They are complex multifactorial traits evolving under the interactive influences of dozens of affectors from the social, behavioral, physiological, metabolic, cellular, and molecular domains. Segregation of the genes is not easily detected in familial or pedigree studies, and whatever the influence of the genotype on the etiology it is generally attenuated or exacerbated by nongenetic factors.[11]

Efforts to understand the genetic causes of human obesities can be successful only if they are based on an appropriate conceptual framework, adequate phenotype and intermediate phenotype measurements, proper samples of unrelated persons and nuclear families or extended pedigrees, and extensive candidate gene typing and other molecular markers. In this context, the distinction between "necessary" genes and "susceptibility" genes proposed recently by Greenberg[12] seems particularly relevant to obesity phenotypes. Although there are several examples of necessary loci resulting in excess body mass or body fat for height — i.e., carriers of one or two copies of the deficient alleles have the disease — they represent only a small fraction of the obese population.[13] An example of a necessary locus for human obesity is the paternally imprinted locus on chromosome 15q11–13 causing the Prader-Willi syndrome.[10] There are also several rodent models of obesity that can be explained by a necessary gene (see above and Chapters 12, 13, and 15 in this book).

Of particular importance for the human obesity phenotypes is the susceptibility gene concept. A susceptibility gene is defined as one that increases susceptibility or risk for the disease, but is not necessary for disease expression.[12] An allele at a susceptibility gene may increase the likelihood of the carrier becoming obese, but the presence of that allele is not sufficient by itself to explain the occurrence of the disease. It merely lowers the threshold for a person to develop the disease.[12] The concept implies that the true causes of obesity may be nongenetic (nongenetic determinants of energy balance in the presence of genetic susceptibility at one locus) or genetic, including genetic variation at gene(s) other than the susceptibility gene or additive or interactive effects at several susceptibility loci. As proposed by Greenberg,[12] if susceptibility genes are neither necessary nor sufficient for disease expression, linkage analysis is likely to yield little more information than is obtained from association studies. This is particularly true when the deficient allele at the locus under consideration carries less than about ten times the risk for the disease in comparison with the normal allele.

Figure 1 illustrates these concepts in a schematic manner. The figure allows for the contributions of necessary and susceptibility genes not only as causal factors for variation in body fat content and fat topography, but also for the metabolic and health consequences associated with the presence of obesity in some of its forms.

IV. CURRENT RESEARCH TRENDS

A. METHODOLOGICAL ADVANCES

Recent progress in animal genetics, transfection systems, transgenic animal models, recombinant DNA technologies applied to positional cloning, and methods to identify loci contributing to quantitative traits have provided a new impetus to this field. The stage is now set for major advances to occur in the understanding of the genetic and molecular basis of complex diseases such as human obesities. Table 6 provides an overview of some of the methods that now can be harnessed to bear upon the task of uncovering the genes and molecular mechanisms pertaining to the causes of human obesities and of the genetic susceptibility to the metabolic complications of obesity.

As evidenced by the various chapters of this book, most of the data accumulated so far have been generated by genetic epidemiologists. However, a small body of knowledge

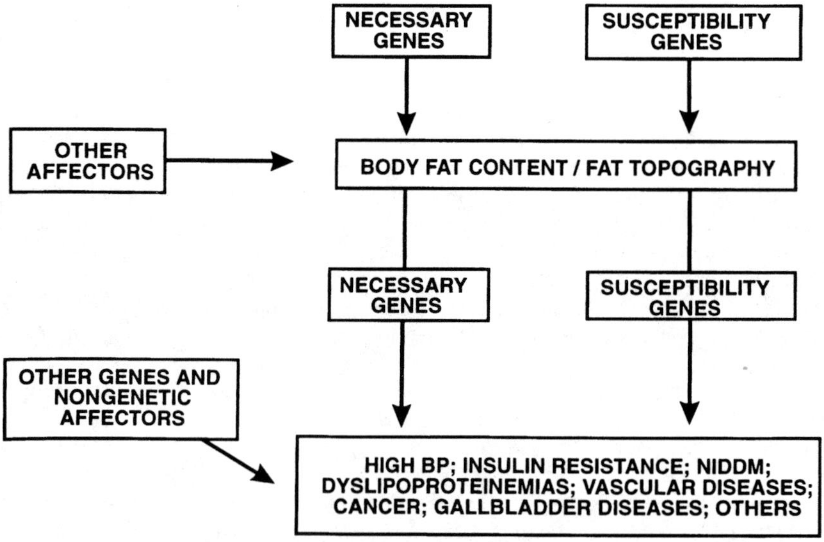

Figure 1. The concept of necessary genes vs. susceptibility genes[12] applied to the topic of human obesity and genetic susceptibility to obesity in terms of complications commonly observed in the metabolic syndrome. BP, blood pressure; NIDDM, non-insulin-dependent diabetes mellitus.

Table 6. **Families of research strategies to define the genetic basis of a multifactorial phenotype**

1. Genetic epidemiology (top down): heritability, segregation pattern, etc.
2. Association studies with candidate genes
3. Linkage studies with candidate genes and other markers
4. Quantitative trait loci (QTL) approach
5. Positional cloning
6. Transgenic models
7. DNA sequencing

derived from association and linkage research is emerging. It is fair to conclude that no major advances have been made thus far from these areas of research, but a better understanding of the genetic epidemiology characteristics of the obesity phenotypes and of the complexity of human obesities has been achieved.

Association and linkage studies are now reported more frequently. Based on the current understanding of the pathophysiology of human obesity, including upper body fat obesity and abdominal visceral obesity, we expect that the candidate gene approach will yield useful association and linkage results. Moreover, with the advent of a comprehensive human genetic linkage map,[14] linkage studies with a large number of markers covering most of the chromosomal length of the human genome are likely to be helpful in the identification of putative obesity genes or chromosomal regions. However, these approaches also have their limitations, particularly when confronted with a complex multifactorial phenotype.

An important methodological advance in this area has been the development of the QTL approach.[15] The method allows the identification of the loci linked with a phenotype, such as obesity, and the isolation of the loci by genetic crosses so that the genes eventually can be defined by positional cloning.[16,17] We anticipate that major progress will be made by a combination of the QTL and positional cloning technologies, particularly as progress is being made in the definition of the mouse and rat genetic linkage maps.

Another area that undoubtedly will contribute in a major way to our understanding of the genetic and molecular basis of human obesity is that involving transgenic models.[18-20] Several studies are currently in progress with a variety of transgenes, and the preliminary data reported at meetings in the past year or so suggest that much will be learned about gene expression and dysfunction as a common feature of obesity by this approach. Indeed, it is progressively becoming apparent that dysregulation in the expression of an otherwise normal gene product even in pathways that appear to be totally unrelated to the disease has the potential to cause obesity. A recent intriguing example is the report about dysregulation in the expression of the gene potentially responsible for obesity in the Yellow mouse.[21] One of the lessons from the latter paper, and from the findings of transgenic animals, is in our view that the genes that play a role in the etiology of human obesities may turn out to be markedly different from those that are listed in the panel of best candidate genes by the geneticists interested in this common disease.

B. A CHALLENGING PROBLEM AREA

An important contemporary issue is whether there are genotype-environment effects and/or gene-gene effects which influence the events leading to the various obesity phenotypes or to some of their outcomes. They remain very difficult to investigate even with present-day technology. Using the unmeasured genotype approach, we recently proposed[22] that one way to test for the presence of a genotype-environment (diet or exercise) effect in humans was to challenge several genotypes in a similar manner by submitting both members of monozygotic (MZ) twin pairs to a standardized treatment and comparing the within- and the between-pair variances of the response to the treatment. The finding of a significantly higher variance in the response between pairs than within pairs suggests that the changes induced by the treatment are more heterogeneous in genetically dissimilar individuals. In a series of experiments conducted on MZ twins over the last 10 years in our laboratory, we used either exercise training (with or without negative energy balance) or chronic overfeeding as a means to investigate these effects. In general, these studies have revealed that genotype-environment interaction effects seem to be ubiquitous in human variation.[22,23]

The study of the genotype-environment effect in humans can be extended to a measured genotype approach. An important advantage of the measured genotype approach over the unmeasured genotype approach is that it eventually makes possible the identification of the responsible genes, thereby providing a means of detecting individuals at a higher risk, say for a disease, because of differences in susceptibility to risk factors. Thus, molecular markers can be used in the MZ twin intervention design defined above to delineate both the quantitative importance of the genotype-treatment interaction effect and its molecular basis. This approach can be extended to several genes or molecular markers in order to look for evidence of gene-gene interaction effects on quantitative phenotypes or common multifactorial diseases such as obesity.

In the search for genes associated with genotype-environment effects, one could also use the method proposed by Berg.[24,25] The method is clearly less demanding from an experimental point of view since it can be carried out on cross-sectional observations made in pairs of MZ twins of the same sex. However, a relatively large number of MZ pairs is required for the findings to be robust and conclusive. Briefly, since MZ brothers or sisters have the same genes, any difference between two members of a given pair in a multifactorial phenotype is caused by nongenetic factors. One can then compare the mean within-pair difference in the phenotype between MZ pairs who have a given allele at a locus with those who have other alleles of the same gene. Berg has argued that if an allele has a permissive effect the within-pair variance would be greater in those pairs with the allele than in those lacking the particular allele. The opposite would be true for an allele with a restrictive effect. This essentially amounts to a method allowing one to test for genotype-environment interaction effect considering one gene at a time. Berg[26] has applied this approach to plasma lipids and lipoproteins in a series of studies and has reported several cases of apolipoprotein genes having significant effects on within-MZ-pair phenotype variability. The method has not been used yet to any extent in the investigation of the genetic determinants of obesity.

Among the issues that have not been considered at all so far, gene-gene interaction effects must be mentioned. It seems to us that the whole field of the genetic basis of human obesities and of the genetic susceptibility to metabolic derangements in the presence of an obese state is one in which gene-gene interactions are ubiquitous. There is no doubt that the topic will attract a lot of attention over the next decade. It will likely be a complicated area of research, however, in the sense that large sample sizes will be needed if several genes are to be considered in the same analysis, new and innovative experimental designs will have to be developed, and the panel of the most important genes to investigate will probably emerge only when strong data become available from association, linkage, QTL, positional cloning, or transgenic studies.

REFERENCES

1. **Bray, G. A.,** Etiology and prevalence of obesity, in *Genetics of Obesity,* Bouchard, C., Ed., CRC Press, Boca Raton, FL, 1994, chap. 2.
2. **Hill, J. O., Pagliassotti, M. J., and Peters, J. C.,** Nongenetic determinants of obesity and body fat topography, in *Genetics of Obesity,* Bouchard, C., Ed., CRC Press, Boca Raton, FL, 1994, chap. 3.

3. **Friedman, J. M., Leibel, R. L., and Bahary, N.,** Molecular mapping of obesity genes, *Mamm. Genome,* 1, 130, 1991.
4. **Chua, S. C. and Leibel, R. L.,** Molecular genetic approaches to obesity, in *Genetics of Obesity,* Bouchard, C., Ed., CRC Press, Boca Raton, FL, 1994, chap. 15.
5. **Truett, G. E., Bahary, N., Friedman, J. M., and Leibel, R. L.,** Rat obesity gene fatty (fa) maps to chromosome 5: evidence for homology with the mouse gene diabetes (db), *Proc. Natl. Acad. Sci. U.S.A.,* 88, 7806, 1991.
6. **Fisler, J. S., Warden, C. H., Pace, M. J., and Lusis A. J.,** BSB: a new mouse model of multigenic obesity, *Obes. Res.,* 1, 271, 1993.
7. **Warden, C. H., Fisler, J. S., Pace, M. J., Svenson, K. L., and Lusis, A. J.,** Coincidence of genetic loci for plasma cholesterol levels and obesity in a multifactorial mouse model, *J. Clin. Invest.,* 92, 773, 1993.
8. **Pépin, M. C., Pothier, F., and Barden, N.,** Impaired type II glucocorticoid-receptor function in mice bearing antisense RNA transgene, *Nature,* 235, 725, 1992.
9. **Shepherd, P. R., Gnudi, L., Tozzo, E., Yand, H., and Kahn, B. B.,** Enhanced glucose disposal and obesity in transgenic mice overexpressing Glut4 selectively in fat, *Diabetes (Abstract Book),* 53rd Annual Meeting of American Diabetes Association, Las Vegas, 42(1), No. 239, 1993.
10. **McKusick, V. A.,** Catalogs of Autosomal Dominant, Autosomal Recessive, X-Linked, Y-Linked, and Mitochondrial Phenotypes, OMIM (Online Mendelian Inheritance in Man), The Johns Hopkins University, Baltimore, MD, 1993.
11. **Bouchard, C.,** Current understanding of the etiology of obesity: genetic and nongenetic factors, *Am. J. Clin. Nutr.,* 53, 1561S, 1991.
12. **Greenberg, D. A.,** Linkage analysis of "necessary" disease loci versus "susceptibility" loci, *Am. J. Hum. Genet.,* 52, 135, 1993.
13. **Bouchard, C. and Pérusse, L.,** Heredity and body fat, *Annu. Rev. Nutr.,* 8, 259, 1988.
14. **NIH/CEPH Collaborative Mapping Group,** A comprehensive genetic linkage map of the human genome, *Science,* 258, 67, 1992.
15. **Lander, E. S. and Botstein, D.,** Mapping Mendelian factors underlying quantitative traits using RFLP linkage maps, *Genetics,* 121, 185, 1989.
16. **Warden, C. H. and Fisler, J. S.,** Identification of genes underlying polygenic obesity in animal models, in *Genetics of Obesity,* Bouchard, C., Ed., CRC Press, Boca Raton, FL, 1994, chap. 13.
17. **Warden, C. H., Daluiski, A., and Lusis, A. J.,** Identification of new genes contributing to atherosclerosis: the mapping of genes contributing to complex disorders in animal models, in *Molecular Genetics of Coronary Artery Disease. Candidate Genes and Processes in Atherosclerosis,* Lusis, A. J., Rotter, J. I., and Sparkes, R. S., Eds., S. Karger, Basel, 1992, 419.
18. **Jaenisch, R.,** Transgenic animals, *Science,* 240, 1468, 1988.
19. **Merlino, G. T.,** Transgenic animals in biomedical research, *FASEB J.,* 5, 2996, 1991.
20. **Metsäranta, M. and Vuorio, E.,** Transgenic mice as models for heritable diseases, *Ann. Med.,* 24, 117, 1992.
21. **Bultman, S. J., Michaud, E. J., and Woychik, R. P.,** Molecular characterization of the mouse Agouti locus, *Cell,* 71, 1195, 1992.
22. **Bouchard, C., Tremblay, A., Després, J. P., Nadeau, A., Lupien, P. J., Thériault, G., Dussault, J., Moorjani, S., Pineault, S., and Fournier, G.,** The response to long-term overfeeding in identical twins, *N. Engl. J. Med.,* 322, 1477, 1990.
23. **Bouchard, C., Dionne, F. T., Simoneau, J. A., and Boulay, M. R.,** Genetics of aerobic and anaerobic performances, *Exercise Sport Sci. Rev.,* 20, 27, 1992.
24. **Berg, K.,** Twin research in coronary heart disease, in *Twin Research,* Vol. 3, Part C, Epidemiological and Clinical Studies, Gedda, L., Parisi, P., and Nance, W. E., Eds., Alan R. Liss, New York, 1981, 117.

25. **Berg, K.,** Molecular genetics and nutrition, in *Genetic Variation and Nutrition,* Simopoulos, A. P. and Childs, B., Eds., S. Karger, Basel, 1990, 49.
26. **Berg, K.,** Variability gene effect on cholesterol at the Kidd blood group locus, *Clin. Genet.,* 33, 102, 1988.
27. **Province, M. A., Amqvist, P., Keller, J., Higgins, M., and Rao, D. C.,** Strong evidence for a major gene for obesity in the large, unselected, total Community Health Study of Tecumseh, *Am. J. Hum. Genet.,* 47(Suppl.), A143, 1990.
28. **Price, R. A., Ness, R., and Laskarzewski, P.,** Common major gene inheritance of extreme overweight, *Hum. Biol.,* 62, 747, 1990.
29. **Moll, P. P., Burns, T. L., and Lauer, R. M.,** The genetic and environmental sources of body mass index variability: the Muscatine Ponderosity Family Study, *Am. J. Hum. Genet.,* 49, 1243, 1991.
30. **Tiret, L., André, J. L., Ducimetière, P., Herbeth, B., Rakotovao, R., Guegen, R., Spyckerelle, Y., and Cambien, F.,** Segregation analysis of height-adjusted weight with generation- and age-dependent effects: the Nancy Family Study, *Genet. Epidemiol.,* 9, 389, 1992.
31. **Rice, T., Borecki, I. B., Bouchard, C., and Rao, D. C.,** Segregation analysis of body mass index in an unselected French-Canadian sample: the Québec Family Study, *Obes. Res.,* 1, 288, 1993.
32. **Borecki, I. B., Bonney, G. E., Rice, T., Bouchard, C., and Rao, D. C.,** Influence of genotype-dependent effects of covariates on the outcome of segregation analysis of the body mass index, *Am. J. Hum. Genet.,* 53, 676, 1993.
33. **Rice, T., Borecki, I. B., Bouchard, C., and Rao, D. C.,** Segregation analysis of fat mass and other body composition measures derived from underwater weighing, *Am. J. Hum. Genet.,* 52, 967, 1993.
34. **Rajput-Williams, J., Wallis, S. C., Yarnell, J., Bell, G. I., Knott, T. J., Sweetnam, P., Cox, N., Miller, N. E., and Scott, J.,** Variation of apolipoprotein-B gene is associated with obesity, high blood cholesterol levels, and increased risk of coronary heart disease, *Lancet,* 2, 1442, 1988.
35. **Lucarini, N., Finocchi, G., Gloria-Bottini, F., Macioce, M., Borgiani, P., Amante, A., and Bottini, E.,** A possible genetic component of obesity in childhood. Observations on acid phosphatase polymorphism, *Experientia,* 46, 90, 1990.
36. **Weaver, J. U., Kopelman, P. G., and Hitman, G. A.,** Glucose transporter (Glut 1) as a possible candidate gene for obesity, in *Obesity in Europe 91. Proc. 3rd Eur. Cong. Obesity,* Ailhaud, G., Guy-Grand, B., Lafontan, M., and Ricquier, C., Eds., John Libbey, Paris, 1992, 89.
37. **Weaver, J. U., Kopelman, P. G., and Hitman, G. A.,** Central obesity and hyperinsulinaemia in women are associated with polymorphism in the 5′ flanking region of the human insulin gene, *Eur. J. Clin. Invest,* 22, 265, 1992.
38. **Weaver, J. U., Hitman, G. A., and Kopelman, P. G.,** An association between a BclI restriction fragment length polymorphism of the glucocorticoid receptor locus and hyperinsulinaemia in obese women, *J. Mol. Endocrinol.,* 9, 295, 1992.
39. **Zee, R. Y. L., Griffiths, L. R., and Morris, B. J.,** Marked association of a RFLP for the low density lipoprotein receptor gene with obesity in essential hypertensives, *Biochem. Biophys. Res. Commun.,* 189(2), 965, 1992.
40. **Vijayaraghavan, S., Hitman, G. A., Weaver, J. U., and Kopelman, P. G.,** Apolipoprotein D polymorphism: a shared genetic determinant between obesity and NIDDM, *Int. J. Obes.,* 17(Suppl. 2), 107, 1993.
41. **Oppert, J. M., Vohl, M. C., Chagnon, M., Dionne, F. T., Cassard-Doulcier, A. M., Ricquier, D., and Bouchard, C.,** DNA variation of the UCP gene and human body fat (Abstract), *Int. J. Obes.,* 17(2), 29, 1993.

42. **Truchon, J.,** Le génome mitochondrial et son polymorphisme, Thèse de maîtrise, Université Laval, Québec, 1992.
43. **Dériaz, O.,** Aspects génétiques et environnementaux du métabolisme de repos, Thèse de doctorat, Université Laval, Québec, 1993.
44. **Wilson, A. F., Elston, R. C., Tran, L. D., and Siervogel, R. M.,** Use of the robust sib-pair method to screen for single-locus, multiple-locus, and pleiotropic effects: application to traits related to hypertension, *Am. J. Hum. Genet.,* 48, 862, 1991
45. **Borecki, I. B., Rice, T., Pérusse, L., Bouchard, C., and Rao, D. C.,** An exploratory investigation of genetic linkage with obesity phenotypes: the Québec Family Study, *Obes. Res.,* in press.
46. **Clément, K., Driouch, K., Lesage, S., Philippi, A., Velho, G., and Froguel, P.,** Linkage analysis of a candidate gene for familial obesity (Abstract), *Int. J. Obes.,* 17(2), 107, 1993.
47. **Pérusse, L., Vohl, M. C., Dionne, F., Dériaz, O., Chagnon, M., and Bouchard, C.,** Linkage between a gene involved in the synthesis of sex steroids and obesity in humans, *Am. J. Hum. Genet.,* 53, 842 (Abstr.), 1993.

INDEX

A

B

C

D

E

F

G

H

I

N

O

P

Q

R

S

T

U

V

W

X

Y

Z